Obesity and Weight Management

The Exercise Professional's Guide to Fitness Programming

Alexios Batrakoulis,
PhD, CSCS,*D, ACSM-EP, FACSM

International Obesity Exercise Training Institute

Editor

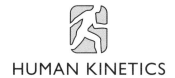

HUMAN KINETICS

Library of Congress Cataloging-in-Publication Data

Names: Batrakoulis, Alexios, 1975- editor
Title: Obesity and weight management : the exercise professional's guide to
  fitness programming / Alexios Batrakoulis, PhD, editor.
Other titles: Exercise professional's guide to fitness programming
Description: Champaign, IL : Human Kinetics, [2026] | Includes
  bibliographical references and index.
Identifiers: LCCN 2024061205 (print) | LCCN 2024061206 (ebook) | ISBN
  9781718230125 paperback | ISBN 9781718230132 epub | ISBN 9781718230149
  pdf
Subjects: LCSH: Reducing exercises | Weight loss | Health behavior
Classification: LCC RA781.6 .O24 2026 (print) | LCC RA781.6 (ebook) | DDC
  613.7071/171--dc23/eng/20250326
LC record available at https://lccn.loc.gov/2024061205
LC ebook record available at https://lccn.loc.gov/2024061206

ISBN: 978-1-7182-3012-5 (print)

The web addresses cited in this text were current as of November 2024, unless otherwise noted.

Senior Acquisitions Editor: Michelle Earle; **Developmental Editor:** Anne Hall; **Managing Editor:** Hannah Werner; **Copyeditor:** Jenny MacKay; **Proofreader:** Aliza Becker; **Indexer:** Ferreira Indexing; **Permissions Manager:** Laurel Mitchell; **Graphic Designer:** Dawn Sills; **Cover Designer:** Keri Evans; **Cover Design Specialist:** Susan Rothermel Allen; **Photograph (cover):** Jason Allen; © Human Kinetics; **Photographs (interior):** © Human Kinetics, unless otherwise noted; **Photo Asset Manager:** Laura Fitch; **Photo Production Specialist:** Amy M. Rose; **Photo Production Manager:** Jason Allen; **Senior Art Manager:** Kelly Hendren; **Printer:** Versa Press

We thank Crunch Fitness in Champaign, Illinois, for assistance in providing one of the locations for the photo shoot for this book.

Printed in the United States of America   10 9 8 7 6 5 4 3 2 1

The paper in this book is certified under a sustainable forestry program.

Human Kinetics	*United States and International*	*Canada*
1607 N. Market Street	Website: **US.HumanKinetics.com**	Website: **Canada.HumanKinetics.com**
Champaign, IL 61820	Email: info@hkusa.com	Email: info@hkcanada.com
USA	Phone: 1-800-747-4457	

Human Kinetics' authorized representative for product safety in the EU is Mare Nostrum Group B.V., Mauritskade 21D, 1091 GC Amsterdam, The Netherlands.
Email: gpsr@mare-nostrum.co.uk

E9539

Obesity and Weight Management

The Exercise Professional's Guide to Fitness Programming

Contents

PART III   The Application

PART IV   The Programming

Foreword

Obesity is the number one health crisis of our time. Once thought to afflict only the more affluent societies, it has now reached nearly all developed and developing countries, making this truly a global health struggle. The economic impact of obesity has been estimated to be in billions of U.S. dollars. When obesity is combined with chronic conditions such as heart disease, diabetes, and cerebrovascular disease, it almost certainly exacerbates the condition and exponentially increases health care costs. According to the World Health Organization (WHO) 2024 data, there were 2.5 billion adults over age 18 (43% of adults) who were considered overweight; among them, 890 million (16% of the world's population) were considered obese. And it's not just adults. The WHO estimated that 37 million children under the age of 5 were overweight, and 390 million children between the ages of 5 and 18 were overweight or obese, increasing from 8% of that age group in 1990 to 20% in the year 2022. The WHO estimated that 2% of the world's children were considered obese in 1990; that number was estimated to be 8% in 2022 (160 million children in the age group 5 to 19). This alarming trend has led some international organizations and governments to develop programs aimed at improving lifestyles and reducing overweight and obesity.

One attempt by the U.S. federal government was the development of Healthy People 2000, an effort by the U.S. Department of Health and Human Services to identify measurable objectives to focus on to reduce lifestyle-related diseases. These objectives were modified with Healthy People 2010; Healthy People 2020; and, most recently, Healthy People 2030 (which will no doubt be followed by Healthy People 2040). For nearly three decades, the U.S. government has been trying to make people healthier by identifying and tracking leading causes of death and making suggestions on how to become healthier. Unfortunately, many health and fitness professionals, including me, believe that these attempts have failed and that a new, more innovative approach needs to be developed. That is why this book, *Obesity and Weight Management: The Exercise Professional's Guide to Fitness Programming*, is so very important. This comprehensive, science-based professional resource focuses on the pivotal role of exercise in the fight against the greatest global public health challenge of the 21st century.

Dr. Alexios Batrakoulis has put together a team of worldwide experts to help the fitness professional develop effective exercise programs when working with anyone who has excess body weight or adiposity. The book is divided into four parts: part I, The Science; part II, The Assessment; part III, The Application; and part IV, The Programming. The text aims to translate evidence into practice that can be readily implemented in the real world. This unique textbook includes case studies that are presented by clients who have been to health clubs and have sought new ways to combat their condition. The case studies feature actual clients in real settings, not fictional examples as is common in other texts. The case studies are followed by detailed exercise programs designed for these clients, including effective warm-ups, continuous endurance training, high-intensity interval training, resistance training, balance and coordination, cool-downs, and stretching routines. This, combined with many other features, is why this book is so important. Fitness professionals can pull this book off their shelf and use it immediately for any obesity and weight management scenario. College and university professors from around the world should consider this book for classroom adoption, and it should be used in any setting fitness professionals are being trained.

Walter R. Thompson, PhD, FACSM, FAACVPR, FCEPA
Regents' Professor Emeritus of Kinesiology, Regents' Professor Emeritus of Public Health, Regents' Professor Emeritus of Nutrition, Regents' Professor Emeritus of Physical Therapy, and Retired Associate Dean for Graduate Studies and Research at Georgia State University
Former President of American College of Sports Medicine (2017-2018)

Preface

The aim of this all-new textbook is to be the most current and comprehensive obesity-related exercise resource to date, providing exercise professionals, fitness educators, and faculty members with science-based and practice-oriented strategies for empowering clients with overweight or obesity to participate in successful and engaging fitness experiences. This textbook is the first of its kind, blending science and application related to weight management and exercise to offer a complete guide of programming techniques and communication strategies for individuals with obesity. This approach presents theoretical concepts in a way that will enable exercise professionals to more easily apply theory to their practice.

The book empowers practitioners to help clients with excess weight achieve their health and fitness goals through pain-free, effective, and pleasant exercise programming solutions in various fitness settings. By providing wide-ranging information and tips for exercise professionals who serve individuals with excess weight of all fitness levels and ages, this resource is an evidence-based career tool for both current and aspiring professionals in the health and fitness industry.

How This Book Is Organized

Each chapter of this textbook ends with a summary, key points, multiple-choice recap questions (with answers provided in the appendix), and a short real-world case study with targeted essay or multiple-choice questions to help readers summarize and integrate the chapter's content. The book consists of 14 chapters, divided into four sections.

Part I, The Science (chapters 1 to 4), provides exercise professionals with a theoretical background for working with clients who have excess weight. These four chapters present in detail the current evidence regarding obesity and the role of exercise as a key behavioral strategy for preventing, managing, and treating this disease.

Chapter 1, Understanding Overweight and Obesity, provides current information regarding the epidemiology, definition, and classification of overweight and obesity. Readers will explore the pathophysiology of obesity, understand the mechanisms behind this disease, and learn how to translate research on exercise and obesity into practice in order to make informed exercise recommendations. This chapter provides a theoretical background of obesity to help exercise professionals apply the practical solutions provided in the rest of the chapters.

Chapter 2, The Role of an Exercise Professional, presents the rationale for positioning qualified exercise professionals at the forefront of the fight against the inactivity and obesity epidemics. This chapter identifies both the key role and the scope of practice of an exercise professional as a valuable member of a multidisciplinary team of allied health care practitioners helping clients manage obesity and overweight. Career development opportunities for exercise specialists in weight management and obesity within the medical fitness space are also presented. In addition, the rationale for accredited academic education in conjunction with recognized professional credentials and approved continuing education opportunities is explained.

Chapter 3, The Role of Exercise in Weight Management and Obesity, describes the vital role of physical activity and exercise in the prevention of bodyweight gain and increased adiposity and provides evidence that exercise interventions support bodyweight reduction and adiposity prevention efforts. This chapter explains the effects of physical activity and exercise on body composition and their role in bodyweight regulation. Readers will also explore factors that contribute to effective prevention and treatment of excess weight and adiposity.

Chapter 4, Coaching Lifestyle Modification and Behavior Change, identifies and explains key behavior-change theories related to lifestyle modifications that focus on physical activity and nutrition to improve weight loss outcomes. The chapter describes common, evidence-based strategies exercise professionals can use to facilitate behavior change, prevent relapses of unhealthy habits, and assist clients with achieving health and weight-based goals.

Part II, The Assessment, comprises chapters 5 and 6, providing the research-based information and actionable instructions exercise professionals should use when conducting field tests to evaluate various health-related physical fitness parameters among individuals with excess weight. In these two chapters, the health appraisal process is described in detail, aiming to equip exercise professionals with the latest research findings and adequate skills to administer the assessment procedures safely and efficiently.

Chapter 5, Exercise Preparticipation Interview and Health Screening, explores the interview and screening processes that should be conducted before clients participate in exercise and provides instructions on how to complete an analysis of cardiovascular disease risk factors with a client. This chapter will help exercise professionals determine a course of action once a client's medical risk has been established. In addition, methods to assess a client's stage of readiness for exercise-related change and to create a stage-matched intervention are presented.

Chapter 6, Health-Related Physical Fitness Assessments, teaches exercise professionals how to administer health-related physical fitness assessments and select appropriate field tests for clients with overweight or obesity, based on the client's functional abilities. In this chapter, readers will examine why conducting physical fitness assessments is valuable for program design and will learn how to explain physical fitness assessment results to their clients. The chapter will also teach readers how to supervise client-centered, multicomponent flexibility training programs and cool-down routines.

Part III, The Application, comprising chapters 7 through 11, presents practice-oriented information supported by evidence regarding various recommended exercise modes for clients with overweight or obesity. In these five chapters, cardiorespiratory and musculoskeletal fitness exercises, along with warm-up and cool-down activities, are analyzed in detail, providing readers with important practical skills to translate science into application in real-world fitness settings.

Chapter 7, Warm-Up Concepts, presents the rationale for and psychophysiological responses to a warm-up. A sample structure of a warm-up routine tailored for clients with overweight or obesity is also presented. This chapter provides readers with detailed instructions and tips for implementing engaging warm-up drills and feasible fitness games to provide positive exercise experiences in various settings.

Chapter 8, Muscular Fitness, explains psychophysiological adaptations to resistance training while exploring myths and misconceptions linked to muscle-strengthening activities. This chapter teaches exercise professionals how to implement exercises that use gym equipment, body weight, and partner-assisted manual resistance. Progressions and modifications of fundamental movement patterns are also presented, equipping practitioners with the knowledge and skills to conduct muscular fitness activities in various exercise settings.

Chapter 9, Neuromotor Fitness, describes physiological adaptations to neuromotor and functional training and clarifies the benefits of adapted agility, balance, and coordination training for people with excess weight. In this chapter, readers will learn how to use adjunct modalities for improving motor fitness and explore the role of mind–body fitness activities as a feasible neuromotor fitness modality.

Chapter 10, Cardiorespiratory Fitness, presents psychophysiological adaptations to aerobic training and explores the benefits and limitations of continuous endurance training and high-intensity interval training for individuals with excess weight. In this chapter, exercise professionals will learn the similarities and differences between traditional and hybrid-type interval training and explore the adjunct role of dance fitness activities as a feasible cardiorespiratory fitness modality.

Chapter 11, Flexibility Training and Cool-Down Techniques, presents the benefits of participating in an effective flexibility training program and describes the components of the cool-down phase. The chapter explains the value of cooling down following a workout and teaches exercise professionals how to design and supervise engaging cool-down routines and client-centered, multicomponent flexibility training programs for clients with overweight or obesity.

Part IV, The Programming, includes chapters 12 to 14, providing readers with wide-ranging, proven exercise solutions adapted for clients with excess weight. These three chapters include smart program-design strategies, applicable sample workouts, and case studies to translate theory into practice, helping exercise professionals work with clients who have overweight or obesity.

Chapter 12, Program Design, presents training principles for effective and safe exercise programming and explores the fundamental concepts of training and exercise prescription. In this chapter, readers will learn the components of a tailored exercise session and how to design client-centered, progressive cardiorespiratory and muscle-strengthening training programs in various fitness settings. Smart exercise-engagement strategies and feasible solutions for program design are also presented.

Chapter 13, Sample Workouts, provides 21 complete training plans for clients with overweight or obesity of various health statuses, fitness levels, and needs. This chapter familiarizes readers with comprehensive exercise solutions for individuals who have excess weight, with or without additional health complications. The chapter also provides several multicomponent workout programs using body weight and different types of stationary and portable equipment in settings such as commercial health clubs, boutique gyms, fitness studios, and home gyms.

Chapter 14, Case Study Scenarios, applies theory to practice through real-world cases, focusing on the needs and priorities of clients with excess weight and considering potential psychophysiological impairments. This chapter demonstrates how the scientific knowledge and practice-oriented information presented throughout the textbook are used by exercise professionals to manage specific considerations for individuals with excess weight and adiposity.

The appendix, Chapter Quiz and Case Study Answers, provides readers with insights into the practical applications of theoretical concepts, thus bridging the connection between theory and practice. The case studies aim to develop coaching skills that are applicable in the real world through the use of critical thinking, assessment, and active engagement with the chapter content.

Online Supplementary Content

The book's references and two sections of supplementary content can be accessed online at https://ancillaries.humankinetics.com/ObesityAndWeightManagement1E.

The first section available exclusively online is **Translating Overweight and Obesity Research Into Practice**, which helps exercise professionals understand how research findings can be incorporated into evidence-based practices in their own professions. Readers will also identify the most effective and safe exercise strategies for individuals with excess body weight and adiposity as well as the underlying mechanisms through which these conditions operate.

The second section of online content, **Business and Marketing Strategies**, presents basic business and marketing concepts exercise professionals should implement as an essential piece of the coaching puzzle when serving clients with overweight or obesity. Readers will also learn how to adapt their communication strategies for these clients in a real-world fitness setting.

The true goal of this textbook is to equip exercise professionals with better knowledge and understanding of how to work with clients who have overweight or obesity. These clients may have special concerns or health complications that must be managed during exercise in order for them to train safely, effectively, and enjoyably. Considering that a large majority of adults worldwide are overweight or have obesity, exercise professionals can greatly benefit from gaining more science-based knowledge about obesity and weight management, along with immediately actionable practical skills and effective communication strategies to work with these clients in real-world fitness settings.

This resource aims to serve as the exercise professional's authoritative guide to obesity and weight management, bridging the gap between research and practice and supporting the fight against the inactivity and obesity epidemics that are considered some of the greatest global public health challenges.

Acknowledgments

I would like to thank Human Kinetics for the amazing opportunity to provide exercise professionals around the globe with this definitive exercise training guide to obesity and weight management. It has been an honor to edit and heavily contribute to this exercise-related textbook dedicated to the masses fighting against the inactivity and obesity epidemics, as well as to the qualified exercise professionals working with these populations in the real world.

First and foremost, I would like to thank the authors who contributed their expertise to each of the respective chapters. This was true teamwork that involved the coordinated contributions of many experts, aiming to provide a science-based and practice-oriented resource on exercise and obesity. It was a privilege and great pleasure to work with such an outstanding group of academics, fitness educators, and leading practitioners. Their knowledge, experience, and professionalism were critically important to this major project, resulting in the most comprehensive and evidence-based exercise training guide to date for individuals with overweight or obesity.

Second, I sincerely thank the Human Kinetics staff for guiding and coordinating the publication process. In particular, I would like to acknowledge the efforts of Michelle Earle, who crucially assisted me through every stage of the process, ensuring that the project progressed smoothly and efficiently.

Third, I would also like to dedicate this work to my clients and students, past and present, who inspired me to learn, grow, and innovate and to be where I am today, seeking professional development and excellence in the professional and academic fields.

Lastly, and most of all, I am deeply grateful to my family—my wife, Ioanna, and my daughters, Emmanouela and Katerina—for supporting me throughout this challenging journey. Undertaking this project would have not been possible without their incredible encouragement, patience, and understanding.

PART I

THE SCIENCE

CHAPTER 1

Understanding Overweight and Obesity

Renee Rogers, PhD, and Sara Kovacs, PhD

After completing this chapter, you will be able to
- discuss the epidemiology of overweight and obesity,
- define and classify overweight and obesity,
- explain the pathophysiology of obesity,
- translate research into practice on exercise and obesity, and
- make informed exercise recommendations.

The latest global data on overweight and obesity indicate that 43% of adults aged 18 years or older were overweight and 16% were living with obesity. This suggests that more than one in two adults worldwide are affected by excess weight or adiposity (Phelps et al. 2024). In the Western world, almost two in three adults are overweight and more than one in four have obesity, while 31% of U.S. adults are overweight and approximately 43% are considered people with obesity. Importantly, 9% of those with obesity are classified as having class 3 or severe obesity in the United States (Bray et al. 2018; Hales et al. 2020; Jensen et al. 2014). Further, obesity prevalence in the U.S. is now similar in adult men and women at approximately 40%, with racial and ethnic minority groups disproportionately affected. It is estimated that Black, Native American, and Hispanic individuals have obesity rates of 50% or greater (Fryar et al. 2020). On a global scale, obesity rates are continuing to rise. Adult obesity rates are increasing very fast in Asia, especially in the Middle East (Phelps et al. 2024). In 2016, approximately two billion people worldwide were overweight or obese, with most of these individuals living in low- or middle-income countries. Since 1975, this prevalence has nearly tripled (WHO 2024). Of concern, the global increase in obesity prevalence in children and adolescents may further contribute to the percentage of adults with obesity in the future.

Overweight and obesity are associated with increased economic costs, both direct (medical costs, travel costs when seeking care) and indirect (productivity loss, absenteeism). The estimated cost by gross domestic product varies greatly due to the differing measurement methods but ranges from US$6 per capita in low-income countries to up to US$1,110 in high-income countries (Okunogbe et al. 2022). In the United States, adults with obesity experience annual medical costs that are 100% higher compared to their counterparts without obesity (Cawley et al. 2021). Obesity contributes to economic costs not only in the United States but worldwide, and the economic effects will increase if current trends continue (Okunogbe et al. 2022).

Definition and Classification of Overweight and Obesity

Public health recommendations for evaluating weight status commonly focus on the computed measure of body mass index (BMI), the ratio of an adult's height to weight. BMI can be calculated using either metric or imperial units. The metric units are weight (in kilograms) divided by height squared (in meters), and the resulting value is expressed as kg/m^2. The imperial units are weight (in pounds) divided by height squared (in inches), multiplied by 703, and the resulting value is expressed as $lb/in.^2$. An individual's BMI is a significant indicator of potential future health risks and has been extensively used as a criterion in the formulation of various public health policies (Nuttall 2015). BMI categories include normal (or healthy) weight categories and categories that indicate whether an individual's weight exceeds what is healthy for a given height (overweight or obesity). BMI categories for overweight and obesity are outlined in table 1.1. BMI is not used for children and adolescents; weight status categories for those age groups are determined using percentile ranges ("Clinical Guidelines" 1998; Purnell 2015).

Table 1.1   Overweight and Obesity BMI, Waist Circumference, and Risk Categories

BMI category	BMI (kg/m²)	Associated disease risk	Waist circumference*
Overweight	25.0-29.9 23.0-27.4 (Asians)	Increased	Women: 36 in. (91 cm) or greater Men: 39 in. (100 cm) or greater
Obesity class I	30.0-34.9 27.5-29.9 (Asians)	High	Women: 41 in. (140 cm) or greater Men: 43 in. (109 cm) or greater
Obesity class II	35.0-39.9 ≥30.0 (Asians)	Very high	Women: 45 in. (114 cm) or greater Men: 49 in. (124 cm) or greater
Obesity class III	≥40.0	Extremely high	Women: 45 in. (114 cm) or greater Men: 49 in. (124 cm) or greater

*Thresholds have been identified that indicate an increased health risk within each body mass index (BMI) category for white individuals. The aforementioned thresholds are 40 in. (102 cm) and 35 in. (89 cm), respectively, for African American men and women across all BMI categories. In various Asian populations (e.g., South Asian, Chinese, and Japanese), these thresholds are 36 in. (91 cm) and 32 in. (81 cm) across all BMI categories.

Adapted from Nuttall (2015) and WHO Expert Consultation (2004).

While BMI is the most common screening tool for determining weight status or category, there are limitations with this measure. BMI does not consider an individual's sex, ethnicity, body shape, or body composition. This distinction is important, because while the basic ratio of weight to height provides a quick screening assessment that can work well on a population level, it does not always predict health status on a personal level. Furthermore, focusing on BMI alone ignores potential adverse biases and stigma associated with this measure that can lead to health care avoidance (Alberga et al. 2019; Flegal 2023).

Alternative methods can be used to assess body composition and markers of weight and adiposity, such as waist and hip circumference (Ross et al. 2020) (see table 1.1); skinfold measurement; and body composition analyses using techniques such as bioelectrical impedance analysis (BIA), air displacement plethysmography, and dual-energy x-ray absorptiometry (DEXA) (Burridge et al. 2022). Currently, there is a push to evaluate obesity and the effects of obesity on health more broadly than just through BMI (AMA 2023) and to include additional body composition metrics and medical evaluations; however, this topic remains an area of continued debate and warrants further investigation.

Effects of Obesity on Health

As BMI increases, so does the risk of chronic health conditions. Epidemiological studies consistently reveal that obesity increases the risk for all-cause mortality and morbidity. Additionally, obesity increases the risk of developing cardiovascular diseases (coronary heart disease, ischemic stroke, and heart failure) and cardiovascular risk factors such as hypertension and dyslipidemia (Jin et al. 2023). The risks of type 2 diabetes, certain cancers, osteoarthritis, and liver disease are also associated with carrying excess body fat (Jin et al. 2023). Obesity is also linked with a reduction in health-related quality of life, reductions in physical function, and increases in stigma and discrimination (Jin et al. 2023).

Obesity as a Multifaceted and Complex Disease

Overweight and obesity develop as a result of energy imbalance; energy intake from caloric consumption exceeds the energy that is expended through the resting metabolic rate, the thermic effect of food, and movement (physical activity, exercise). When energy intake exceeds energy needs, the excess is stored and can lead to metabolic changes (Jin et al. 2023).

Given the sustained increase in prevalence, obesity is widely considered to be a major public health concern. The World Health Organization (WHO) (James 2008), European Commission (Burki 2021), and American Medical Association (AMA) (AMA 2013) all classify obesity as a disease. In its policy, the AMA explicitly states that the "multiple pathophysiological aspects (of obesity) require a range of interventions to advance obesity treatment and prevention." This policy includes lifestyle interventions that incorporate physical activity and exercise.

Obesity has been previously and simplistically characterized by having excessive accumulation and storage of fat in the body. The Obesity Medicine Association provides a more comprehensive definition of obesity as "a chronic, relapsing, multifactorial, neurobehavioral disease, wherein an increase in body fat promotes adipose tissue dysfunction and abnormal fat mass physical forces, resulting in adverse metabolic, biomechanical, and psychosocial health consequences" (Fitch and Bays 2022, p. 2).

While a disease classification for obesity is becoming more widely accepted, there is also some concern that the designation of obesity as a disease may inaccurately classify those living with obesity but without cooccurring metabolic conditions. This disparity further emphasizes the need to avoid making weight-related assumptions when working with an individual carrying excess body weight and to accurately evaluate health status before providing programming (Rubino et al. 2020).

Overweight and obesity are likely the result of a complex collision of biological, psychological, behavioral, and environmental factors (Schwartz et al. 2017). Figure 1.1 provides a theoretical model of some of the unique factors that may contribute to obesity.

The exercise professional must place importance on understanding the multitude of factors that may affect obesity disease status and the overlapping elements that add to the complexity of weight management treatment. Exercise professionals should also acknowledge that participants carrying excess body weight who engage in physical activity may choose to do so for reasons other than weight loss. This highlights the need for person-centered exercise prescription. For people carrying excess body weight, exercise can play a role in the prevention of weight gain and can assist with weight loss and long-term weight management. Exercise and physical activity also improve numerous health parameters independent of weight loss.

As with any complex disease, a collaborative, multidisciplinary team may be needed to address obesity, and this includes exercise professionals. As shown in figure 1.1, when participants present for weight loss assistance, many of the factors contributing to obesity may be outside the scope of practice for exercise professionals. It is important that exercise professionals not only understand the complexity of obesity but also have a strong referral network to provide holistic weight management treatment as appropriate. For individuals needing additional support related to weight loss, medical and mental health management (e.g., bariatric surgery, medication therapy, or behavioral therapy) in conjunction with changing lifestyle behaviors (modifying diet and increasing physical activity) can help improve weight-related outcomes. Exercise professionals should pay special attention to avoiding weight-related biases and stigmatizing behavior (Panza et al. 2018; Rubino et al. 2020). They should also be encouraged to focus on person-first language and participant-centered communication and to be aware of stereotypical exemplars that oversimplify a complex disease (Puhl et al. 2016; Rubino et al. 2020).

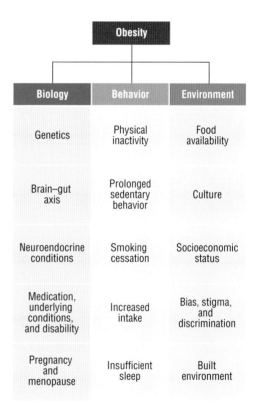

Figure 1.1   Biological, behavioral, and environmental factors that contribute to obesity.

Adapted from Schwartz et al. (2017).

CHAPTER SUMMARY

Obesity is a major public health concern. This multifaceted and complex disease affects more than two billion individuals worldwide and is associated with numerous adverse outcomes, including an increased risk of all-cause morbidity and mortality, a reduction in health-related quality of life, and increased economic costs. There are multiple biological, psychological, behavioral, and environmental factors that may affect obesity disease status. While many of these factors are outside the scope of practice for fitness professionals, it is important for exercise professionals to understand the complexity of this disease and have a strong referral network to provide holistic weight management treatment for participants with whom they work.

KEY POINTS

- Obesity rates continue to increase worldwide.
- Public health recommendations for evaluating weight status commonly focus on the measure of BMI.
- A BMI of 30 kg/m^2 or greater is classified as obesity and can be further broken down into class 1 obesity (BMI of 30.0 to <35.0 kg/m^2), class 2 obesity (BMI of 35.0 to <40.0 kg/m^2), and class 3 (severe) obesity (BMI of 40.0 kg/m^2 or greater).
- While BMI is the most common screening tool for determining weight status, it has limitations.
- As BMI increases, so does the risk of all-cause morbidity and mortality.
- In addition to chronic health conditions, obesity is also linked with an increase in stigma, discrimination, and economic costs as well as a reduction in health-related quality of life.
- While obesity is a complex and multifaceted disease, a major contributor to its development is energy imbalance.
- Biological, behavioral, and environmental factors can all affect obesity.
- A collaborative, multidisciplinary approach for weight management should include the exercise professional.

CHAPTER QUIZ

Quiz answers can be found in the appendix.

1. A BMI of 35.0 to less than 40.0 kg/m^2 is considered
   a. overweight
   b. class 1 obesity
   c. class 2 obesity
   d. class 3 obesity

2. BMI is calculated using an individual's body weight and
   a. waist circumference
   b. percentage of lean tissue mass
   c. percentage of body fat
   d. height

3. On a global scale, obesity rates are
   a. increasing
   b. decreasing
   c. remaining the same

4. Alternative methods for assessing body composition and markers of weight and adiposity include
   a. dual-energy x-ray absorptiometry (DEXA)
   b. skinfold measurement
   c. bioelectrical impedance analysis (BIA)
   d. all of the above

5. Obesity is associated with all of the following EXCEPT
   a. reduction in indirect costs
   b. reduction in health-related quality of life
   c. increased risk of all-cause mortality
   d. increases in stigma and discrimination

6. BMI categories consider an individual's sex, ethnicity, and body shape.
   a. true
   b. false

7. Behavioral factors that affect obesity include insufficient sleep, excessive calorie intake, and
   a. physical inactivity
   b. socioeconomic status
   c. bias and discrimination
   d. prenatal determinants

8. Exercise, independent of weight loss, can improve numerous health parameters.
   a. true
   b. false

9. Exercise professionals should understand the complexity of obesity, have a strong referral network, and take a _____ approach when prescribing exercise to participants who are overweight or obese.
   a. weight loss
   b. person-centered
   c. high-intensity

10. As BMI increases, the risk of chronic health conditions
    a. remains the same
    b. increases
    c. decreases

CASE STUDY

Case study answers can be found in the appendix.

You are working with a new client at your fitness facility. Before developing their exercise prescription, you screen the participant for exercise safety and use screening tools for determining weight status and BMI category.

1. You collect height and weight measurements and calculate that the participant's BMI is 32.3 kg/m^2. This BMI is considered
   a. overweight
   b. class 1 obesity
   c. class 2 obesity
   d. class 3 obesity

2. Based on the client's BMI, which of the following statements is true?
   a. At this BMI, the client has a high disease risk.
   b. At this BMI, the client has a very high disease risk.
   c. At this BMI, the client has an extremely high disease risk.

3. Identify two limitations of using BMI as the only measure of weight status when working with this participant.

4. Describe two behavioral factors that affect obesity and are within the scope of the exercise professional to discuss with the participant.

5. How can you take a person-centered approach to developing the exercise prescription and working with this participant?

CHAPTER 2

The Role of an Exercise Professional

Christie L. Ward-Ritacco, PhD, and Alison C. Berg, PhD

After completing this chapter, you will be able to

- explain why qualified exercise professionals should be at the forefront of the fight against the inactivity and obesity epidemics,
- identify the key role of an exercise professional as a valuable member of a multidisciplinary client health care team,
- describe the scope of practice for obesity and weight management exercise specialists working with allied health care practitioners,
- list career development opportunities available as an exercise specialist in weight management and obesity within the medical fitness space, and
- justify the rationale for accredited academic education in conjunction with recognized professional credentials and approved continuing education opportunities.

Worldwide rates of obesity in developed countries have continued to rise over the past two decades (World Health Organization 2022), with global obesity rates in 2025 predicted to grow to about 18% in men and about 21% in women (NCD Risk Factor Collaboration 2016). Relatedly, estimates show that almost 28% of the world's adult population does not meet current recommendations for physical activity (at least 150 minutes of moderate-intensity or 75 minutes of vigorous-intensity physical activity per week, or any equivalent combination) when the amount of physical activity accumulated via work, household activity, transport, and leisure time is evaluated (Guthold et al. 2018). Moreover, the prevalence of physical inactivity changes across the life span and by weight status. Young adults are more likely to be active compared to older adults (Johannsen et al. 2008), and individuals with obesity have been shown to have lower physical activity levels than individuals with a lower body mass index (Jackson et al. 2024). Additionally, because both aerobic and resistance training exercise is important for health-related outcomes, it is notable that when these types of exercise are analyzed separately, recent estimates show that only about 20% of adults meet the muscle strengthening and resistance training recommendations (Bennie et al. 2020).

Although many individuals with obesity are motivated to increase their physical activity levels and engage in regular programs of exercise for the purpose of managing their weight and improving their quality of life and physical fitness levels, they are often limited in their success, due to real and perceived barriers to becoming more active (Baillot et al. 2021). Commonly cited barriers to becoming more physically active include a perceived lack of self-discipline or motivation; fear of pain, injury, or physical discomfort with exercise; and a lack of time (Baillot et al. 2021; Hamer et al. 2021). Other barriers include fear of embarrassment, and a lack of professional guidance is also often cited by adults as a reason why they delay or avoid engaging in exercise programming. The culmination of these data show that exercise professionals have an important role to play in educating and assisting individuals ready to start a program of regular activity or enhancing their current exercise program. Because achieving the recommended levels of physical activity is associated with improved quality of life, better physical function, higher energy, and lower fatigue, all independent of weight loss (Physical Activity Guidelines Advisory Committee 2018), exercise professionals are at the forefront of helping to improve the health and wellness of adults with overweight or obesity.

Categories of Exercise Professionals

Exercise professional is a broad term used to describe individuals who provide instruction and education related to physical activity and exercise programming (U.S. Registry of Exercise Professionals 2023). This overarching term may be used to describe any of the following professionals: group exercise instructors, personal fitness trainers, exercise physiologists, clinical exercise physiologists, and strength and conditioning professionals.

Instructors and Trainers

Group exercise instructors are trained to lead groups of individuals through choreographed exercise programming, typically accompanied by music. Group exercise instruction can also use a variety of equipment in isolation or in combination, including but not limited to free weights, resistance bands and tubes, step benches, spin bicycles, treadmills, and rowing machines. Personal trainers are qualified to develop and deliver individualized exercise programming for individuals or small groups of participants. This programming differs from group exercise in that it is typically not choreographed.

Exercise Specialists

Exercise physiologists, clinical exercise physiologists, and strength and conditioning coaches are commonly distinguished from group exercise instructors and personal fitness trainers in that their advanced fitness credentials require a university degree in exercise science or an equivalent to be eligible to sit for the associated certification exam. Exercise physiologists receive formal education and training in the development and delivery of individualized exercise prescriptions and apply behavioral and motivational strategies when working with apparently healthy individuals and individuals with medically stable conditions (Overstreet et al. 2023). Strength and conditioning specialists apply the principles of individualized exercise prescription, typically with populations of athletes focused on improving sport and athletic performance (National Strength and Conditioning Association 2023). Clinical exercise physiologists are further distinguished from other fitness professionals due to additional clinical training in working with individuals with clinical conditions, which can include cardiovascular, pulmonary, metabolic, neuromuscular, immunological, and orthopedic disorders (Richardson 2022). Table 2.1 provides additional information on common titles for exercise professionals and their associated skills and workplaces.

Table 2.1   Common Exercise Profession Titles and Specialized Skills

Exercise professional	Education and expertise required	Specialized skills	Common workplaces
Group exercise instructor	High school diploma, minimum	Lead safe and effective choreographed exercise programs in diverse group settings	Worksite wellness, commercial, and community facilities
Personal trainer	High school diploma, minimum	Perform preparticipation screening and fitness assessments; develop exercise programs targeted at client goals	Worksite wellness, commercial, and community facilities
Strength and conditioning specialist	Bachelor's degree, minimum	Perform preparticipation screening and fitness assessments; develop customized strength and conditioning programs targeted at client goals, often aimed at improving athletic performance	Athletic facilities; commercial and community facilities
Exercise physiologist	Bachelor's degree, minimum	Perform comprehensive preparticipation screening and fitness assessments; develop customized exercise prescriptions; counsel on lifestyle modification and behavior change with the goal of improving health and wellness outcomes	Medical fitness facility; worksite wellness, commercial, and community facilities
Clinical exercise physiologist	Bachelor's or master's degree; clinical hours	Perform comprehensive preparticipation screening and fitness assessments; develop customized exercise prescriptions; counsel on lifestyle modification and behavior change specifically for individuals with chronic disease conditions, with the goal of improving health and wellness outcomes and enhancing chronic disease management	Medical fitness facility

Multidisciplinary Practitioners

Successful weight loss and maintenance are most often the result of a team of health care practitioners working together with a client to support them in their weight loss efforts. In addition to the exercise professional, members of this health care team can include medical doctors, physician assistants, licensed nurse practitioners, registered dietitian nutritionists (RDNs), licensed dietitian nutritionists (LDNs), certified diabetes educators, and mental health professionals, depending on the client and their health history (Soan et al. 2014). Each team member will play a unique role in developing a care plan for an individual with obesity, who may be working toward weight loss or the maintenance of lean mass through undergoing bariatric surgery, using weight loss medications, adopting a change in dietary intake, or simply beginning a program of regular physical activity. In the management of overweight and obesity, the growing use of bariatric surgery (Coen et al. 2018) and medications including glucagon-like peptide 1 (GLP-1) receptor agonists (Ghusn et al. 2022; Popoviciu et al. 2023) demonstrates the ever-increasing need for health care practitioners to work together to develop individualized care plans—including medical intervention (surgery or medication), dietary guidance, and exercise prescription—for optimal holistic health outcomes (Jakicic et al. 2024).

Integrating Exercise and Weight Management

Physical activity and exercise should be encouraged for individuals with obesity, independent of any effect on weight loss, due to the health benefits independently associated with exercise (Physical Activity Guidelines Advisory Committee 2018), especially because exercise alone has not been shown to result in substantial changes in weight or body composition (Bellicha et al. 2021). Additionally, there is strong evidence demonstrating that when dietary restriction is combined with regular exercise programming, the changes in body composition are more favorable, as individuals lose body fat while maintaining or increasing their lean body mass and bone mass (Cava et al. 2017). Therefore, it is important that exercise professionals become involved when an individual is engaging in physical activity and exercise as adjunctive therapy for weight loss, because they are uniquely qualified to assess physical fitness levels and create an exercise prescription that is targeted to meet a client's goals. However, significant changes in body weight in healthy adults require significant changes in total energy intake, and the resultant negative energy balance is needed for substantial weight loss to occur (Bellicha et al. 2021; Johns et al. 2014); therefore, it is important to understand the important role that trained nutrition professionals—RDNs and LDNs—play in the weight management process (Bleich et al. 2015). Nutrition assessment, development and monitoring of substantial changes in dietary intake, and delivery of nutrition counseling for persons with obesity should be directed by an RDN or LDN because their education, training, and credentialing position them as experts in nutrition and dietetic practice (Academy of Nutrition and Dietetics n.d.).

Licensed Dietitian Nutritionists

LDNs provide nutrition counseling and education to clients, but their scope of practice is more limited than that of RDNs. These health care professionals specialize in the study of nutrition, diet, and the relationship between food and health. LDNs provide nutrition coaching services, focusing on healthier food choices and eating habits. More specifically, they perform nutritional needs assessments, nutrition education and coaching, and client-centered evaluations of the relationship between diet and health. Importantly, LDNs collaborate with other allied health care professionals, such as physicians, nurses, behavior change specialists, physical therapists, and exercise professionals, to provide comprehensive care to clients with excess body weight or adiposity.

Registered Dietitian Nutritionists

To earn the RDN credential in the United States, individuals must complete a minimum of a graduate-level degree program at a regionally accredited university or college, with course work accredited by the Accreditation Council for Education in Nutrition and Dietetics of the Academy of Nutrition and Dietetics (Academy of Nutrition and Dietetics n.d.), in addition to an accredited supervised practice program. After completion of degrees, coursework, and supervised practice, individuals must pass a national examination, which is developed and administered by the Commission on Dietetic Registration (CDR), the credentialing arm of the Academy of Nutrition and Dietetics.

RDNs can also earn certifications in specialized areas of practice related to nutrition and dietetics, which are awarded via the CDR (Academy of Nutrition and Dietetics n.d.) and include specialization in adult weight management (Tewksbury et al. 2022). The Revised 2022 Standards of Practice and Standards of Professional Performance for Registered Dietitian Nutritionists (competent, proficient, and expert) in Adult Weight Management from the Academy of Nutrition and Dietetics (Tewksbury et al. 2022) further provide RDNs with guidance on how to support an individual with overweight or obesity who chooses weight loss to promote optimal physical and mental well-being during the person's weight management efforts. Thus, RDNs are uniquely qualified to develop and deliver nutrition care for persons with overweight or obesity who have a goal of weight loss and who may also have one or more other nutrition-related chronic diseases. RDNs should work alongside exercise professionals as part of the interdisciplinary care team.

Career Development for the Exercise Specialist

Exercise professionals should aim to enhance their knowledge and skill set as their career progresses. Passing an accredited certification examination is just the first step in one's career as an exercise professional. Credentialed exercise professionals should remain certified and continue building their knowledge base by engaging in professional development and continuing education programming offered by trusted certification or professional organizations, including the American Council on Exercise, the American College of Sports Medicine, the National Strength and Conditioning Association, the National Academy of Sports Medicine, the Clinical Exercise Physiology Association, the British Association of Sport and Exercise Sciences (BASES), the Canadian Society for Exercise Physiology, Exercise & Sports Science Australia (ESSA), and training providers recognized by national registers around the world that verify the qualifications of exercise professionals for distinct roles in health and fitness, such as the International Confederation of Registers of Exercise Professionals and the European Register of Exercise Professionals. Continuing educational offerings from accredited certification organizations can be completed via online synchronous or asynchronous

Scope of Practice for Obesity and Weight Management Specialists

The scope of practice for a health care professional outlines the activities that an individual licensed to practice in a health profession is permitted to perform (American Medical Association 2022). The scope of practice for both exercise and nutrition professionals is often determined at the state level in the United States and by the affiliated licensing entity for the profession. Exercise professionals are not currently licensed in the United States, except for clinical exercise physiologists in the state of Louisiana (Louisiana State Board of Medical Examiners 2023). Therefore, for most exercise professionals, minimal competency standards and related professional practice standards are set by accredited certification organizations, and exercise professionals are expected to obtain an accredited certification to establish their professional competency.

Some states require licensure for an RDN to legally provide nutrition-related care services in that state. The licensed dietitian nutritionist (LDN) credential distinguishes an RDN as someone who has met their state's education requirements to practice nutrition counseling in the state and who has been licensed to practice by that state, noting that not all states require a license to practice dietetics (Commission on Dietetic Registration n.d.). State licensure boards and the Commission on Dietetic Registration require continuing education to maintain certification and ensure nutrition professionals are staying current and competent.

Dietitians in Europe are recognized health care professionals, educated to at least the bachelor's degree level. The European Federation of the Associations of Dietitians (EFAD), which is open to national associations of dietitians from any European country and currently has 31 member associations representing over 30,000 dietitians in 25 European countries, defines a dietitian as a person with a qualification in nutrition and dietetics recognized by a national authority. According to the EFAD's position statement, dietitians play a key role in the management of obesity in adults and children at every level. They are uniquely qualified to translate the scientific evidence on energy intake and expenditure, nutrition, and behavior into practical dietary advice and the provision of healthy food to individuals with overweight or obesity (Fleurke et al. 2020).

trainings, webinars, and in-person or virtual conferences and workshops, and a certain amount of verified continuing education is typically required to renew one's professional certification, dependent on the requirements of the certifying organization.

Because the number of individuals undergoing bariatric surgery has risen steadily across the past several decades (Alalwan et al. 2021), and as the availability of prescription weight loss medications substantially increases, the need for well-trained exercise professionals with experience in working in the area of weight management will continue to grow. Recently, a group of experts reviewed patient-centric tasks that exercise professionals, most commonly exercise physiologists, performed in metabolic and bariatric surgery settings (Stults-Kolehmainen et al. 2024). In medical fitness facilities focused on weight management, exercise physiologists are most often engaged in conducting fitness testing, developing exercise prescriptions, and providing exercise supervision for program participants. Exercise professionals in these settings are highly qualified to conduct exercise-related health assessments, including body composition and cardiorespiratory and muscular fitness evaluations and assessments of physical activity levels and sedentary behavior; to educate participants on lifestyle change and on proper exercise technique and progression; and to provide social support (Stults-Kolehmainen et al. 2024). Individuals interested in working in positions related to weight management should focus on developing their skills in these areas to enhance their professional growth.

Finally, because clients with obesity often present with one to several other noncommunicable chronic disease conditions, including but not limited to cardiovascular disease, hypertension, and type 2 diabetes, it is essential that exercise professionals working with these individuals understand the complexities of managing conditions with multiple morbidities. As such, formal education in the exercise sciences in the form of undergraduate and graduate study is encouraged for exercise professionals. Furthermore, individuals interested in working as a degreed exercise professional should strongly consider studying at a university or college that has earned and maintained academic accreditation and should ensure that the curriculum covers the essential skills, knowledge, and abilities associated with competence in the exercise field (Ward-Ritacco and Magal 2020). In the United States, the Committee on Accreditation for the Exercise Sciences (Commission on Accreditation of Allied Health Education Programs 2023b) works under the umbrella of the Commission on Accreditation of Allied Health Education Programs (CAAHEP), an organization dedicated to the accreditation of education programs in the health sciences and health professions (Commission on Accreditation of Allied Health Education Programs 2023a). In Australia, ESSA establishes the accreditation standards for education programs (Exercise and Sports Science Australia 2023), while, in the United Kingdom, BASES offers an undergraduate endorsement scheme, which recognizes exercise science degree courses that provide undergraduate students with the knowledge and skills required by the profession (British Association of Sport and Exercise Sciences 2023). Enhancing the number of university programs in the exercise sciences that earn programmatic accreditation, ensuring that individuals educated as exercise professionals at the undergraduate and graduate level have similar knowledge, skills, and abilities and are competent to enter the workforce, will continue to enhance the employment opportunities available to exercise professionals across the world.

CHAPTER SUMMARY

Exercise professionals have an important role to play in helping to reverse the current trends in rates of overweight and obesity and physical inactivity. Physical activity behavior change is an important part of an individual weight loss program and can complement dietary changes by helping individuals to maintain or improve their body composition. Exercise professionals are important members of interdisciplinary health care teams and are uniquely qualified to support people with overweight or obesity by providing individualized exercise programming designed to support their weight loss efforts and promote overall health and wellness outcomes.

KEY POINTS

- The growing rates of obesity and physical inactivity among adults highlight the important role exercise professionals play in improving public health outcomes.
- *Exercise professional* is a broad term used to describe an individual who provides instruction and education related to physical activity and exercise programming.
- Exercise professionals include group exercise instructors, personal fitness trainers, exercise physiologists, clinical exercise physiologists, and strength and conditioning professionals.
- Multidisciplinary health care teams, including exercise professionals, are essential to helping individuals' weight loss efforts.
- Registered dietitian nutritionists play a vital role in weight loss programming.
- Exercise professionals should aim to maintain their certifications and training status and add to their skill set by regularly engaging in continuing education.

CHAPTER QUIZ

Quiz answers can be found in the appendix.

1. An exercise professional who typically leads group classes in a choreographed fashion is known as
   a. an exercise physiologist
   b. a group exercise instructor
   c. a personal trainer
   d. a clinical exercise physiologist

2. An exercise professional who performs comprehensive preparticipation screening and fitness assessments, develops customized exercise prescriptions, and counsels on lifestyle modification and behavior change specifically for individuals with chronic disease conditions, with the goal of improving health and wellness outcomes and enhancing chronic disease management, is best described as
   a. an exercise physiologist
   b. a group exercise instructor
   c. a personal trainer
   d. a clinical exercise physiologist

3. Global obesity rates in 2025 were predicted to grow to _____ in men and _____ in women.
   a. about 18%; about 21%
   b. about 20%; about 25%
   c. about 21%; about 18%
   d. about 50%; about 50%

4. Exercise professionals must pass a licensure examination to practice in their field.
   a. true
   b. false

5. A university or college degree is required to work as an exercise professional.
   a. true
   b. false

6. Because clients with obesity often present with one to several other noncommunicable chronic disease conditions, including but not limited to cardiovascular disease, hypertension, and type 2 diabetes, it is essential that exercise professionals working with these individuals understand the complexities of managing conditions with multiple morbidities.
   a. true
   b. false

7. Nutrition assessment, development, and monitoring of substantial changes in dietary intake and delivery of nutrition counseling for persons with obesity should be directed by _____, because their education, training, and credentialing position them as experts in nutrition and dietetic practice.
   a. exercise physiologists
   b. personal trainers
   c. clinical exercise physiologists
   d. registered dietitian nutritionists

8. In medical fitness facilities focused on weight management, exercise physiologists are most often engaged in which of the following activities?
   a. conducting fitness testing
   b. developing exercise prescriptions
   c. providing exercise supervision for program participants
   d. all of the above

9. All U.S. states require a license to practice dietetics.
   a. true
   b. false

10. Exercise alone, when done for the sole purpose of increasing energy expenditure, has typically been shown to result in substantial changes in weight or body composition.
    a. true
    b. false

CASE STUDY

Case study answers can be found in the appendix.

Martina is a 34-year-old woman with a body weight of 194 lb (88 kg) and a height of 5 ft 2 in. (158 cm). She has high blood pressure and type 2 diabetes. She lives in a busy New York City neighborhood with a park and a community center but no grocery store. She has three school-aged children (ages 6, 13, and 16 years) and works for the county government as an administrative professional; her work hours are 8:30 a.m. to 5:30 p.m. She takes the bus to work and walks 0.25 mi (0.40 km) from her bus stop to her office. Her workplace offers a discounted rate for employees on exercise classes at a recreation center on the same block as her office building. The exercise program offerings include yoga, cardio and dance programs, and strength training. Martina would like to lose weight and has tried to on several occasions but has fallen short of her goals. She does not feel confident about starting an exercise program; it makes her feel anxious because she does not feel like she knows what to do or how to get started. Additionally, Martina is unsure of how to change her diet to help her lose weight and manage her chronic conditions while also making meals that her children will eat and enjoy.

1. To which exercise professional would it be best to refer Martina if she is interested in using exercise as an adjunct therapy to manage her high blood pressure?
   a. exercise physiologist
   b. group exercise instructor
   c. personal trainer
   d. clinical exercise physiologist

2. A group exercise instructor is the preferred exercise professional to help Martina start a regular program of resistance training at the recreation center near her employer.
   a. true
   b. false

3. To which health care professional would it be best to refer Martina if she is interested in receiving nutrition counseling?
   a. exercise physiologist
   b. registered dietitian nutritionist
   c. personal trainer
   d. clinical exercise physiologist

4. What barriers to Martina's becoming more physically active can you identify from the information provided?

5. What are some of the challenges Martina may face when trying to change her dietary intake?

CHAPTER 3

The Role of Exercise in Weight Management and Obesity

John M. Jakicic, PhD, and Landon Deru, PhD

After completing this chapter, you will be able to

- describe the vital role of physical activity and exercise in the prevention of bodyweight gain and increased adiposity,
- implement effective exercise interventions to reduce body weight and boost adiposity prevention and treatment efforts,
- define the role of physical activity and exercise in bodyweight regulation and its effects on body composition, and
- name the factors that contribute to effective prevention and treatment of excess weight and adiposity.

Body weight is regulated by the balance between energy intake and energy expenditure. Simply expressed, when energy intake and energy expenditure are equal, body weight should theoretically remain stable. However, other factors that contribute to growth and development in the younger years of life and the aging that occurs in later years of life can affect body weight. Given this paradigm, it stands to reason that when energy intake and energy expenditure are not equal, body weight will be gained (when energy intake exceeds energy expenditure) or lost (when energy expenditure exceeds energy intake). This would also theoretically suggest that increasing physical activity, through either structured exercise or other nonexercise forms of physical activity, would result in an energy imbalance, leading to weight loss when just one component of physical activity is increased while other factors that contribute to energy expenditure remain stable and energy intake also remains stable. However, there is interindividual variability in response to the effects that physical activity has on bodyweight regulation, suggesting that energy balance is a dynamic process and that within the context of physical activity, other components of energy balance respond in a dynamic and variable manner. These considerations are briefly considered in the following sections.

Physical Activity and Energy Expenditure

Total energy expenditure includes several components, with one of these components being physical activity (Ravussin and Bogardus 1989). Physical activity can be further defined as energy expenditure from structured exercise and other, nonstructured forms of exercise (e.g., activities of daily living, transportation activity, and occupational activity). Physical activity is the most variable of the components that contribute to total daily energy expenditure (Ravussin and Bogardus 1989). Factors such as mode, intensity, and duration of physical activity contribute to energy expenditure, and phenotypic variables (e.g., body weight) contribute to individual variability in energy expenditure from physical activity. For a specific duration and intensity of physical activity, the energy expenditure may decrease with weight loss. This suggests the need to progressively increase components of physical activity within the context of weight loss to sustain the energy expenditure of the same activity prior to weight loss (Ravussin and Bogardus 1989).

Recovery from physical activity and structured exercise includes an elevation in energy expenditure during recovery from the activity, and this has been termed *excess postexercise* (or *postactivity*) *oxygen consumption* (EPOC) (Borsheim and Bahr 2003). However, the contribution of EPOC to bodyweight regulation is relatively minor (LaForgia et al. 2006).

Resting Energy Expenditure

The component that makes the greatest contribution to total daily energy expenditure is resting energy expenditure, which is also termed *resting metabolic rate*. This component of energy expenditure accounts for the energy needs of the body to sustain normal body functions. Factors that contribute to the magnitude of the resting energy expenditure include age, biological sex, body weight, lean body mass, muscle mass, and many physiological processes. The association between higher amounts of lean body mass or muscle mass and a higher resting energy expenditure may have implications for how physical activity and exercise influence resting energy expenditure (Aristizabal et al. 2015). Higher amounts of physical activity are associated with higher levels of lean body mass, and training studies have shown that some forms of physical activity and exercise can increase lean body mass and muscle mass (Lopez et al. 2022). However, after weight loss, there is typically a decrease in resting energy expenditure. Thus, a potential role of exercise within the context of weight loss may be to assist in the preservation of resting energy expenditure, although studies have demonstrated that even when weight loss is primarily achieved through an increase in physical activity, resting energy expenditure still decreases (Hopkins et al. 2014). This may be a result of weight loss adaptations to hormones and other physiological processes that are independent of the volume of lean body mass and muscle mass. This may also reflect findings supporting that the loss of adiposity, rather than lean body mass, is significantly associated with decreases in resting energy expenditure observed with weight loss (Martin et al. 2022).

Complementary Factors in Energy Expenditure

An additional consideration is how the various components of energy expenditure interact with each other to contribute to total energy expenditure. One perspective is that the components of energy expenditure are additive, suggesting that if any component of energy expenditure is increased, then the total energy expenditure is increased. This model is the basis for recommending physical activity and exercise to enhance total energy expenditure. However, an alternative to this additive energy-expenditure model is a constrained energy-expenditure model, which suggests that the body regulates overall energy expenditure within a narrow range (Pontzer 2015).

In this model, an increase in energy expenditure resulting from physical activity may trigger compensatory adjustments to other components of energy expenditure, such as energy expenditure from other types of physical or nonphysical activity, to maintain a stable level of energy balance. These proposed compensatory adaptations may partially explain interindividual variability in weight loss in response to physical activity (Donnelly and Smith 2005); however, some researchers have suggested that the variability in weight loss from a given dose of physical activity may be a result of compensation for factors that influence eating behaviors (Martin et al. 2019).

Effects of Physical Activity on Appetite

The converse of energy expenditure is energy intake. A potential pathway by which physical activity can regulate body weight is through its influence on mechanisms that affect appetite, hunger, and satiety. Selective factors that contribute to the regulation of energy intake are considered in this section.

Appetite is the desire to eat food and is largely influenced by both physiological hunger and hedonic hunger. Physiological hunger is the biological drive to consume food and is signaled through stomach contraction, low blood glucose, low body temperature, and hormones such as ghrelin. Hedonic hunger, in contrast, is the desire to consume food in the absence of physiological hunger for the purpose of pleasure and can override physiological hunger cues. **Satiety**, defined as the absence of hunger, is also influenced by several signals, such as stomach distension, increased blood glucose, and hormones such as leptin, glucagon-like peptide 1 (GLP-1), and insulin.

Appetite Suppression

Studies on the influence of physical activity on hunger and satiety provide an understanding of several mechanisms of appetite control. Acute bouts of exercise and short-term endurance training have been shown to temporarily suppress ghrelin, which is an orexigenic hormone that stimulates hunger (Broom et al. 2007; Deru et al. 2023). Additionally, exercise redirects blood away from digestive organs and to the muscles being used for the activity. This may decrease the rate of digestion and can increase signals of satiety that contribute to possible decreases in energy intake. Moreover, exercise has been shown to increase nutrient-stimulated hormones such as GLP-1 (Deru et al. 2023; Wu et al. 2022) and glucose-dependent insulinotropic polypeptide (GIP) (Kelly et al. 2009), which assist in cognitive signaling of satiety.

It is also well established that an acute response to exercise is an increase in lactate production, and there is a growing body of evidence to suggest that an exercise-induced elevation in lactate is associated with suppression of appetite (Chen et al. 2023). Collectively, these findings appear to support that physical activity and exercise may contribute to an acute increase in satiety and appetite suppression, which may contribute to bodyweight regulation. However, there is also variability in the magnitude of acute energy intake in response to a structured period of exercise, with some persons demonstrating an increase and some persons demonstrating a decrease in energy intake (Unick, Otto, et al. 2010). This variability in acute eating response may also provide a potential mechanism to explain the variability in weight change in response to physical activity and exercise.

Homeostatic Regulation

Energy expenditure resulting from higher amounts of physical activity may facilitate a physiological matching of energy intake to energy expenditure. While there is variation in the findings across different studies, the evidence indicates that engaging in physical activity proves to be successful in creating a temporary decrease in hunger and thus produces an energy deficit. Moreover, it is noteworthy that individuals typically do not offset the energy expended through exercise by adjusting their food consumption immediately after their workout (Schubert et al. 2013).

A greater daily energy expenditure resulting from a higher amount of physical activity may facilitate the homeostatic regulation of energy intake to match the caloric needs of energy expenditure (Blundell et al. 2015). At low levels of physical activity, dysregulation occurs that is not compensated for by the downregulation of energy intake, resulting in a positive energy balance that contributes to weight gain (Hill et al. 2012; Mayer et al. 1956). This lack of a homeostatic match between low energy expenditure from physical activity and energy intake that results in body weight not remaining stable has been termed the *nonregulated zone*. However, as physical activity increases and there is a corresponding increase in energy expenditure, there is compensatory regulation of satiety and hunger to match energy intake to energy expenditure. This proposed improved homeostatic match between higher energy expenditure from physical activity and energy intake to keep body weight stable has been termed the *regulated zone*. Thus, this model suggests that as physical activity increases and is maintained, there is a corresponding improvement in energy-intake regulation to facilitate energy balance.

Effects of Physical Activity on Body Weight

Within the context of the effects of physical activity on body weight, several scenarios warrant consideration. These include prevention of weight gain and treatments focused on weight loss. Considerations within each of these scenarios are addressed in this section.

Prevention of Weight Gain

It is important from public health and clinical perspectives to have interventions that effectively reduce body weight and maintain weight loss along with any associated health benefits. However, to effectively counter the deleterious effects of excess weight and adiposity, there is also a public health need for efforts focused on prevention of obesity and further weight gain. Physical activity is a key lifestyle approach to these prevention initiatives.

Evidence from prospective cohort studies shows that physical activity can contribute to preventing weight gain and obesity (Jakicic et al. 2019). However, there appears to be a threshold of dose and intensity needed to prevent weight gain. The current evidence suggests that to most effectively prevent weight gain, the physical activity should be at a moderate to vigorous intensity, and the dosage should accumulate to a threshold of at least 150 minutes per week (Jakicic et al. 2019). Despite the contemporary evidence supporting the possible health benefits of reducing sedentary behavior, the evidence does not support that a focus solely on reducing sedentary behavior, such as standing more and sitting less, will have a meaningful effect on prevention of weight gain (Katzmarzyk et al. 2019). This may be due to findings that the energy expenditure during standing is only moderately greater than the energy expenditure during periods of sitting (Creasy et al. 2016). Such findings suggest that any reduction in sedentary behavior needs to result in a sufficient increase in physical activity and energy expenditure to have an effect on prevention of weight gain. The evidence also supports that engagement in a sufficient dose of physical activity can prevent the transition to obesity in adults (Jakicic et al. 2019; Rosenberg et al. 2013; Su et al. 2017).

Weight Loss

Given the public health concerns over the association of excess weight and adiposity with numerous deleterious health outcomes, the focus for combating such outcomes is on implementing treatment approaches that result in weight loss. The following sections consider physical activity within the context of several obesity treatment approaches.

Physical Activity Without Energy Intake Restriction

One intervention approach is to solely target physical activity without a concurrent focus on modifying eating behaviors to reduce energy intake. Systematic reviews and meta-analyses have shown that an approach focused only on increasing physical activity results in average weight loss of 1 to 7 lb (0.5-3 kg) per person (Donnelly et al. 2009; Garrow and Summerbell 1995; O'Donoghue et al. 2021; Wing 1999). A meta-analysis also showed that resistance exercise was less effective than aerobic exercise for weight loss but that the combination of resistance and aerobic exercise was more effective for weight loss than either type of exercise alone (O'Donoghue et al. 2021).

Regardless of the type of exercise, its effect on weight loss remains modest compared to the weight loss that can be achieved with modest dietary restriction over the same duration of intervention. This outcome does not suggest that exercise should not be used as a method to induce weight loss but rather that the weight loss achieved by exercise alone may be modest compared to other treatment approaches. However, evidence also supports that the effect of physical activity and exercise on weight loss occurs in a dose-response manner (Donnelly et al. 2009; Jakicic et al. 2024) and that noticeable effects on weight loss are achieved with a dose of at least 150 minutes per week of physical activity at moderate to vigorous intensity, as previously mentioned (U.S. Department of Health and Human Services 2008). Moreover, the expected benefits of exercise extend beyond their effect on body weight to numerous other health benefits among persons with excess weight and adiposity (Piercy et al. 2018; Powell et al. 2019).

Physical Activity With Energy Intake Restriction

The combination of modest dietary restriction with physical activity is recommended in clinical guidelines as a foundational lifestyle approach for weight loss (Jensen et al. 2014). The evidence strongly supports this combined approach to maximize weight loss compared to using dietary restriction alone or physical activity alone (Donnelly et al. 2009). Of importance is that when an appropriate dose of physical activity is added to modest dietary restriction, the additional weight loss achieved is approximately 20% greater (4-7 lb [2-3 kg], on average) than what is achieved with dietary modification alone (Curioni and Lourenco 2005).

This finding has been observed in young and middle-aged adults and in adults across the spectrum of obesity classifications, including severe obesity (Goodpaster et al. 2010; Jakicic et al. 2015). An additional consideration is that physical activity is a key lifestyle behavior associated with enhanced long-term weight loss and prevention of weight gain recurrence following weight loss (Jakicic et al. 2003; Jakicic et al. 2008; Jakicic et al. 2014; Jakicic et al. 1999; Tate et al. 2007; Unick, Jakicic, et al. 2010; Wadden et al. 2009). These long-term effects on weight loss are typically observed with a dose of physical activity of approximately 200 to 300 minutes per week and at a moderate to vigorous intensity (Donnelly et al. 2009; Haskell et al. 2007; Jakicic et al. 2001; Saris et al. 2003).

Physical Activity With Metabolic and Bariatric Surgery

Metabolic and bariatric surgery (MBS) is an effective medical treatment for obesity, and more than 250,000 procedures are performed annually in the United States (American Society of Metabolic and Bariatric Surgery 2021). Physical activity is considered an important lifestyle behavior for patients undergoing MBS and is recommended in clinical practice guidelines (Mechanick et al. 2020; Oppert et al. 2021). Literature reviews and meta-analyses have concluded that, on average, the addition of physical activity to MBS contributes 4 to 6 lb (2-3 kg) more weight lost than what is achieved with MBS without physical activity (Oppert et al. 2021; Ren et al. 2018). This additional weight loss within the context of MBS is achieved with aerobic or resistance physical activity or a combination of these modes (Oppert et al. 2021). As with research on weight loss and exercise without the use of MBS, studies have concluded that the combination of aerobic and resistance modes of physical activity may be superior to either mode alone (Ren et al. 2018).

The effects of physical activity on this additional weight loss may not be observed in short-term periods following MBS (Coen, Tanner, et al. 2015) but may be more pronounced during periods of long-term follow-up (Ren et al. 2018). However, despite the possible benefits of physical activity to enhance long-term weight loss following MBS, the evidence currently does not support that physical activity will prevent weight recurrence following MBS (Bond et al. 2023).

Physical Activity With an Anti-Obesity Medication

Currently, there are highly effective pharmacotherapies for the treatment of obesity (Jastreboff et al. 2022; Wilding et al. 2021). These pharmacotherapies are commonly referred to as anti-obesity medications (AOMs). The current generation of AOMs is based on nutrient-stimulated hormones (NuSHs) that naturally occur in the human body and have been shown to assist in the regulation of eating behavior. The therapies target receptors of NuSHs, such as GIP and GLP-1. While NuSHs are the current targets of AOMs, additional obesity therapies also in development will need to be considered once approved for treatment (Jastreboff and Kushner 2023). These have been shown to be highly effective for weight loss (Jastreboff et al. 2022; Wilding et al. 2021) and for obesity treatment by inducing weight loss in persons with overweight or obesity, either with or without type 2 diabetes (Davies et al. 2021; Garvey et al. 2022; Garvey et al. 2023; Jastreboff et al. 2022; Kadowaki et al. 2022; Lin et al. 2023; Wadden, Chao, Machineni, et al. 2023; Wilding et al. 2021).

The studies that have examined the efficacy and effectiveness of these AOMs have reported that a lifestyle approach including physical activity was a component of the intervention that individuals received in addition to the AOMs (Jastreboff et al. 2022;

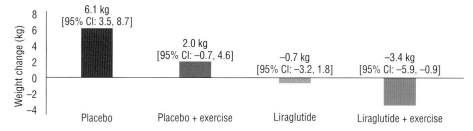

Figure 3.1 12-month change in body weight with liraglutide and exercise following an initial 8-week, lifestyle-based weight loss intervention.

Adapted from Lundgren et al. (2021).

Wilding et al. 2021). However, few studies have reported on the contribution of physical activity to the weight loss observed in response to these AOMs. One of the few currently available published studies examined the effect of an AOM (liraglutide), both combined and not combined with physical activity, on the 12-month change in body weight following an initial period of weight loss that did not include an AOM (Lundgren et al. 2021). As shown in figure 3.1, the addition of physical activity to the AOM resulted in significant weight loss, whereas the AOM alone did not result in significant further weight loss. The potential benefits of coupling physical activity with contemporary AOMs are described in a recent commentary and suggest that these benefits may reach beyond weight loss to outcomes related to enhancing holistic health and well-being (Jakicic et al. 2023).

Physical Activity and Body Composition

Bodyweight status, typically represented by the body mass index (BMI), is a common intervention target for the treatment of overweight and obesity. However, while the BMI is associated with several negative health outcomes, leading medical organizations now recommend that health status be evaluated with factors beyond BMI (American Medical Association 2023). An alternative to using BMI may be to consider effects on components of body composition within the context of treatment of overweight and obesity, with a particular consideration of how physical activity may contribute to changes in two main areas of body composition: adipose tissue and lean body mass.

Adipose Tissue

Adiposity, typically referred to as body fatness, is a major component of body composition that warrants consideration within the context of overweight and obesity. Body adiposity can be considered as the total volume of adipose tissue within the human body, and most measures of body composition quantify this component. Both total body fatness and the various components and distribution of adiposity are associated with several deleterious health outcomes. One area of interest is visceral adiposity, which accounts for the fat surrounding the vital organs within the abdominal cavity. A higher amount of visceral adiposity is associated with less favorable indicators of cardiometabolic health (Chartrand et al. 2022). There is also interest in fat that may be embedded in key organ tissues, and an organ of particular interest is the liver (Sarwar et al. 2018).

There are two primary types of adipose tissue—brown and white. Both types play key roles in body temperature regulation and hormone production. However, white adipose tissue is metabolically dormant and stores large fat droplets, which provide its characteristic white appearance, whereas brown adipose tissue contains smaller droplets of lipids and has many mitochondria that make it capable of metabolizing glucose and lipids (Dong et al. 2023). Brown adipose tissue is generally regarded as the healthier of the two because of its ability to aid in energy balance and glucose regulation (Dong et al. 2023). The distribution of white adipose tissue exhibits considerable variation among different animal species. Typically, white adipose tissue is located in two distinct regions of the body, namely subcutaneous adipose tissue and visceral (intra-abdominal) adipose tissue, where it is stored. Brown adipose tissue is located in the neck, kidneys, adrenal glands, heart (aorta), and chest (mediastinum). The quantity of brown fat is minimal in adults (Dong et al. 2023).

Physical Activity and Total Body Adiposity

Physical activity is inversely associated with total body adiposity (Bradbury et al. 2017; Lindsay et al. 2022). A study of data from the UK Biobank found that physical activity of 100 or more metabolic equivalent (MET)–hours per week was associated with a 2.8% lower body fat percentage in men and a 4.0% lower body fat percentage in women (Bradbury et al. 2017). Despite the strong evidence to support an association between lower body adiposity and higher levels of physical activity (Bellicha et al. 2021), some studies have found that as much as 7 hours of physical activity per week (60 minutes per day), performed at a moderate to vigorous intensity, may be needed to contribute to meaningful reductions in total body adipose mass (Saris et al. 2003; Weinsier et al. 2002). Studies of the mode of physical activity support that aerobic physical activity and high-intensity interval training result in significant reductions in total body adiposity (Bellicha et al. 2021).

Physical Activity and Adiposity Distribution

Physical activity reduces adiposity in the abdominal region of the human body. A systematic review and meta-analysis showed that aerobic exercise effectively lowered visceral adiposity, whereas resistance training did not have the same effect (Ismail et al. 2012). Moreover, the addition of resistance exercise training to aerobic modes of physical activity does not appear to further enhance reductions in total body adiposity (Willis et al. 2012). The studies that showed an effect of aerobic exercise on visceral adiposity in general included at least 150 minutes per week of moderate-intensity aerobic activity, and it is unclear whether there are effects at lower doses of physical activity. Moreover, a higher dose of physical activity may be associated with even greater effects on visceral adiposity (Ohkawara et al. 2007). However, when physical activity is coupled with dietary restriction to result in weight loss, the reduction in visceral adiposity may not be enhanced with additional physical activity, particularly in the presence of higher overall body adiposity (Goodpaster et al. 2010). This finding applies to any type of activity beyond the recommended 150 minutes per week.

Physical activity may also contribute to lowering the amount of adipose tissue located in the subcutaneous areas of the human body. A meta-analysis of over 40 studies and more than 3,500 participants found that aerobic exercise, resistance training, and a combination of the two led to significant decreases of subcutaneous adipose tissue, with aerobic exercise showing greater efficacy (Yarizadeh et al. 2021). It has been proposed that the effect of physical activity on subcutaneous adipose tissue may result from an increase in adrenaline, a decrease in insulin, and the release of natriuretic peptides during periods of physical activity (de Glisezinski et al. 2009). However, when physical activity is coupled with dietary restriction to result in weight loss, the reduction in subcutaneous adiposity may not be enhanced with the addition of more volume of physical activity, particularly in the presence of higher overall body adiposity (Goodpaster et al. 2010). Also similar to findings on visceral adiposity, this finding applies to any type of activity beyond the recommended 150 minutes per week.

Physical Activity and Type of Adipose Tissue

Physical activity may also be associated with the amount of brown versus white adipose tissue, with more physical activity favoring the presence of brown adipose tissue (Dong et al. 2023). It has been established that physical activity and exercise can stimulate brown adipose tissue by activating the sympathetic nervous system and enhancing the endocrine function of brown fat, which can enhance both cardiac and metabolic health (Garritson and Boudina 2021). One proposed pathway responsible for this observation is the activation of uncoupling protein 1 (UCP1) with physical activity, and the presence of UCP1 increases the metabolic activity of adipose tissue (Dong et al. 2023; Stanford et al. 2015). Other physical activity pathways have been identified, which include but are not limited to **exerkines** and effects on the sympathetic nervous system (Dong et al. 2023). Exerkines are humoral factors that respond to acute or chronic exercise and have been identified as key contributors to the cardiometabolic benefits of exercise (Chow et al. 2022). Through these pathways, there is a browning of white adipose tissue, referred to as beiging, in which white adipose tissue adapts to gain characteristics typically observed in brown adipose tissue (Dong et al. 2023).

Physical Activity and Liver Adiposity

Physical activity has been demonstrated to reduce liver adiposity, which may reduce the risk of nonalcoholic fatty liver disease and its associated health risks (Keating et al. 2012). A reduction in liver adiposity is observed in response to aerobic and resistance forms of physical activity when performed at a similar frequency and duration (Hashida et al. 2017). The effect of reducing liver adiposity is observed when physical activity is coupled with a reduced-energy-intake diet compared to the diet alone (Goodpaster et al. 2010). Physical activity may reduce liver adiposity through multiple pathways, including reduced delivery of free fatty acids and glucose to the liver, enhanced fatty-acid oxidation, and decreased fatty-acid synthesis (van der Windt et al. 2018).

Lean Body Mass

The converse of body adiposity is lean body mass. This component of body composition consists of subcomponents that include organs, muscle, connective tissues, bone, and water. All these components of lean mass are important for optimal body functions. However, this section will focus on total lean body mass and muscle mass.

Total Lean Body Mass

Typical clinical and health-fitness measures of body composition include a measure of total lean body mass. Within the context of overweight and obesity, lean body mass is of interest because it has been associated with the more metabolically active components involved in energy expenditure (e.g., muscle) and affects physical mechanics, strength, and body organ functions. It is important to understand that while muscle mass is a large component of lean body mass, the measure of lean body mass is not a direct measure of muscle mass.

Physical activity is associated with a greater amount of lean body mass, which would suggest that increasing physical activity will result in an increase in lean body mass. These increases in lean body mass are typically greater with higher amounts of physical activity, and inclusion of resistance training may be an important behavioral target to affect lean body mass (Bellicha et al. 2021). Physical activity, when not accompanied by a concurrent reduction in energy intake through intentional dietary restriction, will typically result in a modest increase in lean body mass (Bellicha et al. 2021).

Lean body mass decreases with weight loss–induced restriction in dietary intake, which can occur with behavior modification, MBS, or AOMs (Wadden, Chao, Moore, et al. 2023). The magnitude of the decrease in lean body mass increases as restriction in dietary intake becomes more severe. The decrease in lean body mass with behavior modification is approximately 15% to 25%, compared to a decrease of approximately 25% to 40% with MBS or AOMs (Wadden, Chao, Moore, et al. 2023). Physical activity has been added to interventions for weight loss in efforts to counter the loss of lean body mass, and these efforts have included the addition of both aerobic and resistance forms of physical activity.

Results from studies are mixed regarding whether the addition of physical activity results in preservation of lean body mass in conjunction with dietary restriction. When beneficial effects are observed, this combination typically results in an attenuation of the loss of lean body mass rather than full preservation of lean body mass (Donnelly et al. 2004). Moreover, resistance forms of physical activity may be more effective for attenuating the loss of lean body mass with weight loss when compared to aerobic forms of physical activity (Donnelly et al. 2009). Within the context of weight loss induced by MBS, resistance exercise has been shown to attenuate the loss of lean body mass in younger persons, but it becomes less effective with increasing age (Morales-Marroquin et al. 2020). There is a paucity of data to inform whether physical activity attenuates the loss of lean body mass when weight loss is induced by AOMs (Wadden, Chao, Moore, et al. 2023).

Muscle

Skeletal muscle is a key component of lean body mass. However, most studies of overweight and obesity do not include a direct measure of muscle mass but rather include a measure of lean body mass. Thus, caution is warranted when examining data from studies where muscle is not measured, because it may not be appropriate to infer that measures of lean body mass reflect muscle mass.

Some studies have used imaging techniques to quantify changes in skeletal muscle that occur with weight loss. Goodpaster et al. (1999) used computed tomography (CT) to examine changes in skeletal muscle with weight loss and reported that the decrease in skeletal muscle with diet-induced weight loss was primarily a result of low-quality rather than high-quality muscle. In simple terms, dietary-induced weight loss altered muscle composition, indicating that a moderate reduction in weight selectively depletes low-density skeletal muscle in individuals with obesity (Goodpaster et al. 1999). Other factors that reflect muscle quality, such as insulin sensitivity and mitochondrial function, are also improved with weight loss (Dubé et al. 2011; Menshikova et al. 2017). This may suggest emphasizing muscle quality rather than the volume of muscle mass within the context of overweight and obesity and subsequent weight loss. Interestingly, exercise appears to be superior to a hypocaloric diet for increasing mitochondrial function, despite similar reductions in insulin resistance among individuals with obesity (Dubé et al. 2011; Menshikova et al. 2017).

Physical activity, primarily in the forms of aerobic and resistance modes of physical activity, also contributes a vital role to enhancing muscle quality (Botella et al. 2023; Grgic et al. 2019; Helgerud et al. 2007; Konopka and Harber 2014; Short et al. 2003; Toigo and Boutellier 2006; West and Phillips 2010), and this may also apply within the context of treatment for overweight or obesity. Donnelly et al. (1993) reported that despite the significant reduction in lean body mass with diet-induced weight loss, the addition of resistance exercise training resulted in muscle hypertrophy (measured by muscle biopsies) and a concurrent increase in muscular strength.

Even within the context of weight loss induced by MBS, the addition of physical activity, primarily in the form of aerobic training, has been shown to be beneficial. Higher amounts of walking (measured by steps per day) were associated with enhanced preservation of thigh skeletal muscle as measured by a CT scan (Carnero et al. 2017). Moreover, physical activity that primarily included aerobic forms of exercise enhanced the same measures of muscle quality, such as the insulin sensitivity and mitochondrial function mentioned previously, following MBS (Coen, Menshikova, et al. 2015; Coen, Tanner, et al. 2015). Long-term aerobic exercise preserves motor units, mitochondrial function, and protein homeostasis (Crane et al. 2013). In particular, walking preserves but does not increase skeletal muscle mass among adults with overweight or obesity (Ross et al. 2024).

CHAPTER SUMMARY

Physical activity is an important lifestyle component to be included in efforts to prevent and treat overweight and obesity. Physical activity may also contribute to favorable changes in body composition that include enhanced reductions in total and regional adiposity, attenuation of lean body mass, and enhancement of muscle quality. Moreover, physical activity may contribute to factors that can assist with eating behaviors by affecting hunger and satiety. These beneficial effects warrant consideration when developing programming efforts for the treatment of overweight or obesity and justify the inclusion of physical activity in therapeutic approaches. However, the evidence does not support that one form of physical activity may be more favorable than others for all components that regulate body weight or that may be affected by overweight and obesity or weight loss. This supports the inclusion of a multimodal physical activity approach that includes aerobic, resistance, and other modes of physical activity to treat patients with overweight or obesity who may also have other concurrent chronic health conditions.

KEY POINTS

- Physical activity is associated with the prevention of weight gain and the development of obesity.
- Physical activity contributes to the regulation of eating behavior through mechanisms that may assist with the physiological control of hunger and satiety.
- Physical activity contributes to enhancing total energy expenditure.
- Physical activity without dietary modification results in modest weight loss of 1 to 7 lb (0.5-3 kg) and can enhance weight loss by approximately 20% when combined with dietary modification.
- Physical activity contributes to changes in body composition by reducing total and regional adiposity, potentially attenuating lean body mass loss with weight loss and enhancing components of muscle quality.

CHAPTER QUIZ

Quiz answers can be found in the appendix.

1. The type of adipose tissue that surrounds internal organs and is associated with a less favorable cardiometabolic risk profile but can be reduced with physical activity is
   a. visceral fat
   b. brown fat
   c. white fat
   d. subcutaneous fat

2. Which hormone is known as the hunger hormone and is temporarily suppressed after acute bouts of exercise?
   a. leptin
   b. insulin
   c. ghrelin
   d. cortisol

3. The constrained energy-expenditure model proposes that
   a. energy expenditure from different sources adds up independently
   b. the body regulates overall energy expenditure within a narrow range
   c. weight loss is easy with physical activity alone
   d. energy balance is not influenced by physical activity

4. The type of adipose tissue that contains smaller droplets of lipids and has many mitochondria that make it capable of metabolizing glucose and lipids is
   a. visceral fat
   b. brown fat
   c. white fat
   d. subcutaneous fat

5. On average, physical activity for at least 150 minutes per week, performed at a moderate to vigorous intensity and not coupled with intentional restriction of energy intake, results in
   a. no weight loss
   b. 1-7 lb (0.5-3 kg) of weight loss
   c. 11-22 lb (5-10 kg) of weight loss
   d. 22 lb (>10 kg) of weight loss

6. In what way does physical activity modify adipose tissue?
   a. It results in browning of white adipose tissue.
   b. It results in whitening of brown adipose tissue.
   c. It does not alter either brown or white adipose tissue.
   d. It results in brown adipose tissue becoming more brown and white adipose tissue becoming more white.

7. Weight loss alters muscle in which of the following ways?
   a. It reduces insulin sensitivity of muscle.
   b. It results in muscle hypertrophy without the inclusion of physical activity.
   c. It contributes to the loss of low-quality muscle.
   d. It increases muscle mass.

8. Which mode of physical activity or exercise may have the greatest influence on attenuating the loss of lean body mass during weight loss that results from a restriction in energy intake?
   a. aerobic training
   b. resistance training
   c. high-intensity interval training
   d. no mode of physical activity and exercise has a greater influence than others

9. Which is true regarding excess postexercise oxygen consumption?
   a. It contributes significantly to weight loss.
   b. It represents the elevated energy expenditure once a period of physical activity has ended.
   c. It occurs only after aerobic exercise but not resistance exercise.
   d. It occurs only after resistance exercise but not aerobic exercise.

10. Which is true regarding resting energy expenditure?

    a. With weight loss, physical activity results in a substantial increase in resting energy expenditure.

    b. Resting energy expenditure is the smallest contributor to total energy expenditure.

    c. Resting energy expenditure is strongly associated with total body adiposity but not lean body mass or muscle mass.

    d. Resting energy expenditure decreases with weight loss.

CASE STUDY

Case study answers can be found in the appendix.

An adult with obesity presents to a health-fitness facility seeking weight loss. The individual reports the presence of a few cardiometabolic risk factors, including hypertension and hypercholesterolemia, both controlled with medication. The individual does not appear to have mobility limitations and does not report skeletal muscle disorders that will limit the ability to begin a structured physical activity program. This adult has an initial goal to reduce weight by 20 lb (9 kg) within approximately 6 months of starting the weight loss program but is not seeking to initiate use of an anti-obesity medication or metabolic or bariatric surgery to facilitate weight loss. Because of family and occupational responsibilities, the individual indicates the ability to come to the health-fitness facility 3 days per week. The person reports irregular engagement in exercise and a tendency to experience muscle soreness from exercise, which causes them to not enjoy it and to stop exercising.

1. The approach that should be taken with this individual is which of the following?

    a. Only initiate an aerobic exercise program.

    b. Only initiate a resistance exercise program.

    c. Wait until the individual experiences weight loss through dietary modification before initiating an exercise program.

    d. Initiate an exercise program in combination with recommending a diet that reduces energy intake and is guided by an appropriately trained professional.

2. Because the individual can attend the health-fitness facility only 3 days per week, which of the following should be recommended?

    a. aerobic exercise only

    b. resistance exercise only

    c. a combination of aerobic and resistance exercise

    d. at-home exercise instead of health-fitness facility attendance

3. Because the individual has obesity with a few cardiometabolic risk factors, which of the following is appropriate when designing their exercise program?

    a. Never recommend resistance exercise, because it will elevate the individual's blood pressure.

    b. Periodically monitor the individual's blood pressure during exercise and assess whether any of the exercises are causing musculoskeletal discomfort.

    c. Only recommend exercises that are not weight supported (e.g., a stationary cycle) so that musculoskeletal injuries do not occur.

    d. There is no need to periodically monitor the individual during their exercise.

4. Based on the individual's history of reporting muscle soreness following exercise, which of the following is NOT an appropriate approach when designing their exercise program?

   a. Develop an exercise program with gradual progressions to assist in minimizing muscle soreness.

   b. Place no limits on how an exercise program is developed and progressed, because muscle soreness is a normal response to exercise.

   c. Assess whether there are specific exercises that may contribute to muscle soreness, and adapt or modify these exercises appropriately.

   d. Periodically assess how the individual is feeling in response to their exercise sessions, and modify the exercise prescription in an appropriate manner.

5. The individual is not experiencing weight loss after 1 to 2 months of their program. Which of the following is an appropriate approach to assist the individual to achieve their weight loss goal?

   a. Assume that the exercise is causing an increase in lean body mass and muscle, which is resulting in the scale not reflecting weight loss.

   b. Stop any resistance exercise, because this is causing increases in muscle mass that are limiting weight loss.

   c. Refer the individual to their physician, because they likely have a medical condition that is limiting their weight loss.

   d. Evaluate the individual's exercise behaviors and eating behaviors to first confirm adherence to the recommended weight loss program.

CHAPTER 4

Coaching Lifestyle Modification and Behavior Change

Rachelle Acitelli Reed, PhD, and Susie Reiner, PhD

After completing this chapter, you will be able to

- identify and explain key behavior-change theories relative to lifestyle modifications, focusing on physical activity and nutrition to improve weight loss outcomes;
- describe common evidence-based strategies coaches can use to facilitate behavior change, prevent relapse, and assist participants with achieving health- and weight-based goals; and
- explain the practical application of the concepts presented within this chapter relative to weight loss outcomes.

Theory-based behavioral interventions are an effective way to increase physical activity, encourage adoption of nutrient-dense eating patterns, and promote other health behaviors in adults. This chapter explores many of the essential elements fitness professionals and coaches should master to more effectively serve clients, promoting long-lasting behavior change based on current evidence in the field of exercise psychology. The chapter reviews key dynamics of the client–coach relationship, provides an overview of important behavioral theories, outlines several principles of lifestyle modification, and briefly covers nutritional considerations for weight management.

A Brief History of Coaching Theory

Fitness professionals and health and wellness coaches can better serve their clients by using many tools from the field of psychology, an area of science that focuses on people and how the mind and environment influence human behavior (American

Psychological Association 2023a). Psychology provides coaches with evidence-based theories, models, and tools for facilitating behavior change in their clients. A theory refers to a systematic view of a behavior that identifies relationships between variables and specific behaviors or situations (Glanz and Rimer 2015).

Coaching theory applies psychological methods to working with others. Coaching psychology is a field that applies psychological theories and concepts to the practice of coaching, while exercise psychology involves psychological factors and theories related to physical activity and exercise (Buckworth et al. 2013). In the context of fitness, health, and wellness, *coaching* can be defined as facilitating sustainable change in clients by improving their self-efficacy, internal motivation, ability to set and achieve attainable goals, and ability to adjust plans as needed (Deiorio et al. 2022). Coaches can be further categorized as practitioners of coaching psychology, helping improve well-being and physical and mental outcomes in their clients (WellCoaches 2023). For example, if a personal trainer or coach is working to help a client maintain or lose weight, the application of a theory based in exercise psychology would help the coach identify variables that may influence health behaviors and provide insight into how those variables both interact with one another and make the behavior more or less likely. In summary, exercise psychology theories provide a framework that can help coaches offer evidence-based practice to improve the health and well-being of their clients.

Defining Key Terms: Health, Wellness, and Lifestyle

Many approaches have been presented to define the concept of health over the past century. The following three definitions of *health* are currently used in various levels of health promotion (Sartorius 2006):

1. The absence of any disease or impairment
2. A state that allows an individual to adequately cope with all demands of daily life
3. A state of balance or equilibrium that individuals establish within themselves and between themselves and their social and physical environment

The third definition, in which the presence or absence of disease alone does not necessarily dictate one's health, provides a more multidimensional approach to the human condition. For instance, this definition helps to transition someone from being defined or stigmatized as a diabetic to a person who has diabetes. The World Health Organization (2005) goes on to say,

> Health is a state of complete physical, mental and social well-being and not merely the absence of disease or infirmity. The enjoyment of the highest attainable standard of health is one of the fundamental rights of every human being without distinction of race, religion, political belief, economic or social condition.

It is important to note that habitual physical activity levels may be a more critical factor affecting cardiovascular health in all individuals than is body mass index or the presence of chronic diseases. Inactive individuals who are underweight or of healthy weight experience a higher risk of cardiovascular disease morbidity and mortality than do physically active individuals with overweight or obesity (Blair 2009).

Wellness includes striving for health but is also a holistic integration of one's perceptions of physical and mental health with the surrounding environment (Adams et al. 2000). Wellness is a personalized approach to thriving in any circumstance and requires self-regulation and reflection to direct behaviors toward one's own best interests (Corbin and Pangrazi 2001). Wellness is directly linked to lifestyle factors that influence the development of chronic disease or affect other measures of health, including alcohol use, overweight and obesity, physical activity, sleep, and smoking (Centers for Disease Control and Prevention 2020). It is important for fitness professionals to foster multifaceted health- and wellness-promoting behaviors in their clients to promote long-term behavior change conducive to weight loss. Lifestyle factors, such as physical activity levels, eating habits, sleeping patterns, and stress levels, substantially affect clients' health, fitness, and wellness status. Thus, clients with excess body weight and adiposity may be characterized by inactivity, impaired mental health, physical limitations, and obesity-related illness (Buratta et al. 2021; Pataky et al. 2014).

Dynamics of the Client–Coach Relationship

The client–coach relationship establishes the foundation for all future communications, interactions, and tailored programming. Moore and colleagues (2005) describe the client–coach relationship as a "relational flow" between individuals, in which progress and behavior change are most probable when an "intuitive dance" occurs between the two. This framework of coaching suggests that coaches should strive to have more than just knowledge of programming, change adoption, and content alone; effective coaching relationships are also marked by harmony, conformity, and accord, where the coach shows a true investment in the client (Egan 2010).

Emotional Intelligence

The client–coach relationship is most professional and effective when both individuals display emotional intelligence (EI) in their interactions. The American Psychological Association (2023b) defines *EI* as the ability to process emotional information and use it in reasoning and other cognitive activities. According to Mental Health America (2023), high EI overlaps with strong interpersonal skills, because individuals with higher EI are more easily able to identify how they are feeling, what those feelings mean, and how those emotions affect their behavior (and, in turn, situations and other people). In addition, higher EI has been linked to improvements in both mental and physical well-being in adults (Bru-Luna et al. 2021). An example of using EI with a client striving for weight loss would include a deeper understanding of their history with weight loss, the emotions surrounding their thoughts and actions related to weight loss, and their situational awareness within conversations that may affect behaviors.

EI is typically broken down into four major components:

1. Self-awareness
2. Self-regulation
3. Situational awareness
4. Situational regulation

Table 4.1 briefly discusses each component (Ackley 2016).

Table 4.1 Components of Emotional Intelligence

Component	Brief description
Self-awareness	• Core and starting point of everything • Ability to recognize emotions and understand the effects of emotions in context • Knowledge of one's own strengths and weaknesses
Self-regulation	• Ability to effectively manage emotions and think before reacting and speaking • Ability to follow through and follow up
Situational awareness	• Ability to read the room and recognize others' emotions • Ability to be empathetic, picking up on cues put forth by others
Situational regulation	• Ability to influence and manage relationships and situations and to work as part of a team or partnership • Ability to effectively handle conflict

Adapted from Ackley (2016).

Although numerous factors, including client readiness to change, influence the likelihood of successful and sustainable behavior change, coaches who seek to improve—and use EI in—their client relationships may be more successful in helping clients reach their health and fitness goals (Mantell 2013). The following list offers 10 characteristics of successful, emotionally intelligent coaches:

1. Stay within their scope of practice, referring clients to other practitioners as needed
2. Understand exercise science, nutrition, and behavior-change principles
3. Practice lifelong learning, using continuing education and feedback to improve
4. Have high emotional intelligence and display it during all interactions
5. Implement a compassionate, empathetic approach to communication
6. Take an organized, evidence-based approach
7. Use active listening and motivational interviewing skills to elicit discussions about change
8. Invest in their own physical and mental health, leading by example
9. Motivate clients and see each as a unique person
10. Build rapport quickly and work diligently to maintain client trust

SWOT Analysis to Enhance Self-Awareness

A SWOT (strengths, weaknesses, opportunities, and threats) analysis is a strategic planning tool credited to Stanford University's Albert Humphrey (Brandenburger 2019). It is widely used in the business world but can also be a valuable tool for health and fitness professionals seeking to enhance their self-awareness and EI. In the context of health and fitness, a SWOT analysis involves a reflective assessment of internal factors, such as personal strengths and weaknesses, which could include skills, knowledge, or emotional traits. Additionally, SWOT analysis considers external factors, such as potential threats (which could include changes in the fitness industry or obstacles to personal growth) or opportunities to acquire more knowledge. By conducting a SWOT analysis, health and fitness professionals can gain deeper insights into themselves, allowing them to make informed decisions, set goals, and develop strategies to change weaknesses into opportunities (American Council on Exercise 2021). Table 4.2 provides example prompts that can help coaches improve their ability to work with clients who have weight loss goals.

Table 4.2 Visual of SWOT Analysis With Prompts for Coaches

Strengths	Weaknesses
• What knowledge do I have that others do not? • What education, certifications, and experiences do I have that I can use to propel me? • Do I have expertise or experience in working with clients who want to lose weight?	• What needs improvement in my work with clients who seek weight management goals? • Am I lacking confidence in one or more areas of my business? • Am I able to apply theory to practice and help clients see change in different outcomes?
Opportunities	**Threats**
• Is additional knowledge or research about weight management available? • Do I have an opportunity to expand my professional network to include other professionals who work with clients to lose weight? • Can I better use social media or marketing to build my personal business or find clients?	• What current obstacles exist for me in working with clients on various weight loss interventions? • Is the pricing structure of working with me (versus attending a big-box gym, for instance) affecting client acquisition?

DISC Model of Understanding Personality Types

According to Wilson and Dishman, personality traits represent "enduring and consistent between-person differences in predispositions for cognitions, emotions and behaviors" (2015, 230). Physical activity and personality are both dynamic constructs; therefore, personality traits should not be expected to contribute uniformly to physical activity adoption or maintenance (Wilson and Dishman 2015). This principle applies to working with clients seeking weight loss, because each person will respond differently to an intervention. However, using tools to better understand clients' personalities may help coaches to improve their communication and coaching techniques.

The DISC model is a tool for understanding personality types. Created by Dr. William Marston in 1928, it provides a helpful framework for coaches to better understand their own personality as well as that of their clients. The DISC model proposes four personality types: D (dominance), I (influence), S (steadiness), and C (conscientiousness) (DISC Profile 2023). The American Council on Exercise explains that people who fall into the Dominance quadrant may be more direct and fast-paced and better at problem solving (McCall 2016). Those who fall into the Influence quadrant may be more inspiring, interactive, and able to form relationships with others quickly (McCall 2016). People who align with the Steadiness type are more likely to be reserved, steady, and supportive, and those who fall into the Conscientiousness quadrant are more likely to be cautious and careful, following the playbook a coach provides (McCall 2016).

Communication Skills
and Motivational Interviewing Principles

A well-developed, science-based program is important, but communication is essential to facilitate health behavior change, including long-term weight loss. Communication is a skill that develops over time from working with others, and self-awareness is required to consider others' thoughts and needs while expressing information and ideas. An essential attribute of effective communication is empathy, the ability to understand and identify with others' perspectives and experiences without bias (Elliott et al. 2011). An empathetic, person-centered approach to training helps to build trust within the practitioner–participant relationship across health disciplines.

Motivational interviewing (MI) is an approach developed by Miller and Rollnick (2012) that helps an individual define their current and ideal selves and isolate the behaviors that would influence movement toward the ideal self. MI considers decisional balance and autonomous decision-making to help individuals self-regulate their behaviors. MI takes a collaborative approach and follows the strategies outlined in table 4.3 to provide support and facilitate change.

Table 4.3   Motivational Interviewing and Communication Strategies

Strategy	Definition	Application example
Express empathy	Be open and respectful of where the individual is in the change process	"What you're describing is really important. Tell me more about . . ."
Develop discrepancy	Identify the gaps between goals and behavior	"What are your goals for the future? How do you see (weight loss) fitting in with these aspirations?"
Roll with resistance	Recognize client resistance as a signal to change the strategy rather than contradict the client	"It sounds like you've tried to lose weight in the past but didn't find the long-term success you're looking for. How would you change that experience if you did it all over again?"
Support self-efficacy	Support the client's belief in their ability to change	"What do you feel is the most reasonable action you can take now to set you up for success in weight loss down the line?"

Coaches can use a variety of MI strategies to allow a client's ideas and perspective to lead the conversation. These include open-ended questions, affirmations, reflective listening, and summaries of the conversation points to ensure clients feel they have been heard and understood.

- *Open-ended questions* are questions that cannot be answered with a simple *yes* or *no*, provoking a deeper thought process about the issue. These questions normally start with *how* or *what*, such as "What have you tried before to manage your weight?"

instead of "Have previous weight loss interventions worked for you?" The former example evokes abundantly more information than the latter.

- *Affirmations* help to acknowledge positive behaviors and build a client's self-efficacy. For example, saying "You've already taken the hardest step in coming in today. You're clearly a determined and resourceful person" provides encouragement and recognizes the work the client has already accomplished toward their weight loss goal.
- *Reflective listening* is a way for coaches to show they are truly listening and understanding a client's words and actions. Eye contact, body language, nodding, and verbal cues such as "OK, I see" help clients know they are being heard.
- *Summaries* are a form of reflective listening in which a coach collects key points from the conversation and explains them back to the client to indicate understanding and correct any misunderstandings. Summarizing can also help identify probing questions that will provide a deeper exploration of a topic such as weight loss.

It is important to note that communication extends beyond verbal interactions and includes nonverbal cues that can indicate a practitioner is listening and attentive during the conversation. Nonverbal cues include an open and receptive posture, eye contact, gestures such as nodding, and facial expressions that coincide with what a participant is expressing. One of the easiest ways to observe one's own body language or nonverbal cues is to practice parts of a conversation in a mirror, observe the physical movement of the body, and adjust accordingly in interpersonal interactions.

Setting SMART Goals

Goal-setting is a fundamental and effective strategy for promoting changes in health behaviors. When defining goals, researchers tend to classify them as either objective or subjective. Objective goals focus on "attaining a specific standard or proficiency on a task, usually within a specified time" (Locke and Latham 2002, 705). Subjective goals refer to more general statements that are not as easily measurable or objective. Coaches can often facilitate the transition from subjective goals, such as "I want to lose fat mass," into smaller, more objective goals, such as "I want to increase my step count by 500 to 1,000 steps a day to increase my movement in a manageable way." Goal-setting has been widely studied in the exercise sciences, with literature reviews indicating that individuals who set specific goals perform better than those who skip goal-setting (Burton and Weiss 2008; Weinberg 2010). Additionally, goal-setting has been widely accepted in nutrition intervention studies focusing on weight-related outcomes (Pearson 2012).

Evidence suggests that goals work for changing behavior when they are energizing and promote action, when they lead people to seek out goal-relevant information, and when they influence and encourage persistent effort (Locke and Latham 2002). One widely recognized framework for setting goals within the health and wellness arena is the SMART goal framework, summarized in table 4.4.

Table 4.4   SMART Goal Framework

Letter	Description
S (specific)	Goal specificity helps clients to properly assess whether they are making progress toward a goal. Coaches should use communication skills and tools to involve their clients in the specific goal-setting process. Often, clients will need direction to transition a loftier, less-specific goal into a narrower, more objective one.
M (measurable)	Setting goals that are measurable can help clients self-monitor their progress by noting small successes week to week. Examples of self-monitoring tools to help track progress may include written diaries or records, wearable fitness trackers that track steps or active minutes, body composition assessments, and fitness testing.
A (attainable)	Setting challenging but doable goals is an important component of SMART goal-setting. Goals that are too easy may be met without much effort, but goals that are too challenging may be discouraging. Coaches should use their knowledge of exercise science and nutrition to help clients set attainable, objective goals relative to weight management.
R (realistic)	Realistic goals, sometimes also called relevant goals, are those that are realistic for clients based on their preferences, lifestyle, and environment. For instance, what is realistic for a working mom of four young children living in a suburb may differ from what is realistic for an older adult couple living in a city.
T (timely or time-bound)	Setting specific time frames with regular check-ins can help clients stay on track toward meeting their goals. For instance, weight loss or body composition goals should have evidence-based timelines that are challenging but attainable for clients. Regular check-ins also allow coaches to reassess strategies or amend goals and timelines as needed.

Key Determinants of Health Behaviors

Changing human behavior is complex, because humans interact with their environment in a dynamic way. Thus, having a well-rounded understanding of the key determinants of health behaviors is imperative for health and fitness professionals. There is strong evidence to suggest that lifestyle modifications can markedly enhance the prognosis of chronic diseases (Farhud 2015). These modifications have been shown to reduce the major metabolic risk factors for chronic diseases and premature death, including obesity. The risk of developing obesity-related illness is largely attributable to lifestyle-related factors rather than genetic predisposition, underscoring the significant potential of lifestyle modification interventions for obesity-related health complications (Michaelsen and Esch 2023). In particular, the key determinants of health behaviors are emotion, motivation, and operant conditioning.

Emotion

Emotions are a central aspect of the human experience and can influence our levels of motivation and effort, our thoughts, and our behaviors (Carver and Scheier 2001). For example, a client who feels stressed, sad, or depressed may be less likely to put effort into positive behavior change, even though this contradicts their goals (Carver and Harmon-Jones 2009; Tice et al. 2001). The good news is that coaches can help participants build self-efficacy and improve their emotional experiences relative to health behaviors such as weight loss. Some research suggests that positive feelings experienced from a single workout can be a predictor of physical activity levels a year later (Williams et al. 2008). Fitness professionals and coaches should be aware of participants' emotions so that they can positively influence emotional states and promote progress toward health-related goals (Carver and Harmon-Jones 2009).

Motivation

Motivation is central to many theories of behavior change because it is a proximal determinant of behavior (Knittle et al. 2018; Teixeira et al. 2012). *Motivation* can be defined as the intensity and direction of someone's effort, with *intensity* meaning the amount of effort expended and *direction* referring to whether someone actually seeks out a behavior (Knittle et al. 2018; Teixeira et al. 2012). Motivation is dynamic, meaning it regularly shifts along a spectrum both in the short and long term. The term *amotivation* describes a lack of motivation to engage in an activity or behavior. When learning from a client about their motivations, coaches should be aware that motivations generally fall into one of two categories (Teixeira et al. 2012):

1. *Extrinsic motivation* can be defined as doing an activity for a reward or recognition from others (National Academy of Sports Medicine 2021). For example, an extrinsically motivated client may seek out a fad weight loss diet because they are seeking approval from someone else or want to look a certain way for an event.

2. *Intrinsic motivation* can be defined as doing an activity because of inherent satisfaction with the outcome (Deci 1975). For example, a client intrinsically motivated to start an exercise program may feel personal accomplishment, enjoyment, or satisfaction after each workout.

Clients can have both intrinsic and extrinsic motivators for different behaviors simultaneously. In general, intrinsic motivation may lead to longer-term physical activity and nutrition adherence, in turn facilitating healthy weight management (Ntoumanis et al. 2018). From a coaching perspective, understanding initial motivations and reassessing them over time is an important part of providing a tailored and emotionally intelligent approach for clients.

Operant Conditioning

Operant conditioning was first introduced by B.F. Skinner in the 1950s and remains a fundamental concept in behavioral sciences (Skinner 1950). This learning theory suggests that individuals' behaviors are shaped by the consequences that follow them (Staddon and Cerutti 2003). According to this theory, reinforcement (either positive or negative) and punishment (either positive or negative) are the core tools that modify behaviors. In general, behavior followed up with a positive consequence is likely to be repeated, while behavior followed up with a negative consequence is less likely to be repeated (Staddon and Cerutti 2003; Strohacker et al 2014). Interventions based on operant conditioning have been applied to a variety of health behaviors, including physical activity, and applying key tenets of this learning theory may be appropriate in coaching scenarios (Leeder 2022; Strohacker et al. 2014). Table 4.5 defines reinforcement and punishment types, according to operant conditioning.

Table 4.5 Key Operant-Conditioning Terms

	Reinforcement	Punishment
Positive	Add something pleasant to increase the likelihood of a behavior.	Add something unpleasant to decrease the likelihood of behavior.
Negative	Remove something unpleasant to increase the likelihood of a behavior.	Remove something pleasant to decrease the likelihood of a behavior.

Theories and Models of Behavior Change

Theories and models provide a framework for better understanding adoption and maintenance of health-promoting habits such as physical activity and good nutrition. This section reviews five models and theories about which coaches and fitness professionals should develop working knowledge.

Socioecological Model

The socioecological model presents a comprehensive perspective on health, encompassing various factors that can affect an individual's well-being. How an individual relates to and perceives their environment is multifaceted. The socioecological model was introduced by Urie Bronfenbrenner in the 1970s to understand child development (Bronfenbrenner 1979) and was formalized as a theory in the 1980s. The U.S. Centers for Disease Control and Prevention has since adapted the theory for health promotion efforts to create environments conducive for convenient and economical health choices (Sallis et al. 2008). Within the framework of the socioecological model, as shown in table 4.6, health is understood to be influenced by the interplay between individual (intrapersonal) factors, social (interpersonal) factors, community dynamics, and the physical and political environment (Israel et al. 2018; Sallis et al. 2012; Sallis et al. 2008).

Focusing on multiple levels that influence behavior within the socioecological model is crucial for long-term change in health behavior. Adopting a socioecological perspective enhances interventions and enables a clearer understanding of the multitude of factors affecting one's behaviors. This approach yields solutions beyond an individual's barriers to changing physical activity and nutritional behaviors because it considers the social determinants of health that drive decision-making (Caperon et al. 2022).

Table 4.6 Multilevel Strategies Using Socioecological Theory

Socioecological level	Definition	Potential change strategy
Intrapersonal factors	Personal characteristics such as biology, age, education, income, knowledge, attitudes, beliefs, preferences, and health history	Tailor the weight loss program to include an individual's favorite exercise modalities and foods
Interpersonal factors or social environment	An individual's social connections, such as friends, partners, coworkers, and family members, who affect behavior and experiences	Create a walking club or social media group with common goals

Socioecological level	Definition	Potential change strategy
Organizational or community factors	Settings where social relationships are nurtured, such as schools, work-places, and neighborhoods, along with their characteristics affecting health	Collaborate with employers to offer healthier food choices and oppor-tunities to participate in physical activity on site
Physical environment	Weather, geography, availability of and access to facilities, and safety	Raise awareness of current health-promotion programs within the com-munity
Societal or policy factors	Broader factors, including cultural and social norms as well as health, economic, urban planning, educa-tional, and social policies, that can either foster or impede health	Advocate for budgetary allocation to build well-lit walking paths and bike lanes

Transtheoretical Model and Stages of Change

The transtheoretical model (TTM), developed by Prochaska and DiClemente in the 1980s, is one of the most popular frameworks for promoting changes in health behavior (Prochaska et al. 1992; Prochaska and Velicer 1997). The TTM is an intuitive approach because it tailors the intervention based on how ready for change an individual is at present. This structured, multidimensional model helps individuals progress through various stages of change when adopting and sustaining health-promoting behaviors.

The stages of change include precontemplation (having no intention to make a change in the next 6 mo), contemplation (intending to change within the next 6 mo), preparation (preparing to change in the next 30 d), action (currently having engaged in the change behavior for 6 mo or less), and maintenance (having regularly engaged in the change behavior for more than 6 mo). The TTM acknowledges the inherent complexities and cyclical nature of behavior change, recognizing that individuals may or may not progress linearly through the model and that relapse into earlier stages is common. See table 4.7 for further explanation.

Table 4.7   Strategies in the Transtheoretical Model (Stages of Change)

Stage of change	Definition	In simple terms	Behavioral approach
Precontemplation	Having no intention to make a change in the next 6 mo	No action	• Enhance awareness of the advantages of a physically active lifestyle and the disadvantages of a sedentary one, particularly in terms of health • Use positive reinforcement to encourage increasing physical activity • Discuss advantages and disad-vantages of initiating a regular exercise regimen

(continued)

Table 4.7 Strategies in the Transtheoretical Model (Stages of Change) *(continued)*

Stage of change	Definition	In simple terms	Behavioral approach
Contemplation	Intending to change within the next 6 mo	Considering	• Continue to provide information about the health benefits of physical activity and the detrimental health consequences of a sedentary lifestyle • Discuss resources that are available to increase exercise levels
Preparation	Preparing to change in the next 30 d	Planning	• Provide a client-centered exercise prescription aligned with the client's lifestyle, goals, and needs • Discuss potential barriers to physical activity and exercise • Give support and positive encouragement to enhance self-esteem, self-efficacy, and self-confidence
Action	Having currently engaged in the change behavior for ≤6 mo	Doing	• Assess progress through regular monitoring • Discuss exercise barriers as they arise and develop a plan to overcome them • Modify the exercise program to accommodate changes in lifestyle and goals • Provide positive reinforcement by celebrating any sign of progress and achievement of goals
Maintenance	Having regularly engaged in the change behavior for >6 mo	Continuing	• Provide instruction on the competencies required for sustained engagement in physical activity and exercise • Monitor progress but on a less regular basis • Develop a plan to overcome new or potential barriers to physical activity and exercise • Permit greater autonomy and responsibility regarding physical activity and exercise

A fundamental construct of the TTM is decisional balance, which involves weighing pros and cons of engaging in the behavior and of outcomes after changing the behavior (Plotnikoff et al. 2001). For example, when an individual understands that the advantages of their weight loss outweigh the disadvantages, they are more apt to move forward through the next stage of change. In addition, cultivating self-efficacy is an essential element in the TTM because it helps an individual to develop confidence in their ability to accomplish the change. Interventions that use the TTM framework have effectively changed smoking, exercise, nutritional, and other health behaviors (Sarkin et al. 2001; Spencer et al. 2006; Spencer et al. 2007; Velicer et al. 1998).

Social Cognitive Theory

Initially created by Albert Bandura, social cognitive theory (SCT) is one of the most popular theoretical frameworks for understanding physical activity behaviors (Bandura 1986; Trost et al. 2002). SCT has also been widely applied in randomized controlled trials for nutrition interventions (Rigby et al. 2020). SCT is based on a concept called *reciprocal determinism*, or the interaction between people and their environments (Bandura 1986). It suggests that three main factors influence and determine behavioral choices: (1) the external environment (e.g., walkability of one's neighborhood), (2) personal characteristics (e.g., a person's personality and preferences), and (3) behavioral factors. According to SCT, a person's behavior is the interplay of these three factors; the environment influences both behavior and personal factors, while personal factors and behavior also influence the environment (Bandura 1997).

Self-efficacy is a central component of SCT. Self-efficacy can be broadly defined as situation-specific self-confidence, or an individual's belief in their ability to engage in and perform a specific behavior (Bandura 1997). In theory, the more confident one feels in their ability and skills to succeed, the more likely they are to engage in a behavior. When it comes to physical activity, the following behavioral strategies can improve self-efficacy: planning action, reinforcing effort, identifying progress toward goals, engaging in self-monitoring strategies, and seeking social support (Olander et al. 2013). Additionally, research suggests that self-efficacy can be improved by mastery experience, vicarious experience, verbal persuasion, and physiological or affective states (Bandura 1977). Table 4.8 provides examples of how SCT can be applied to improve a client's self-efficacy.

Table 4.8   Sources of Self-Efficacy

Source	Client-centered application examples
Mastery experience	• Celebrate small weight loss successes on the way toward a larger goal, helping to show the client's mastery over their weight loss journey • Take a form video to show the client their improvement or progressions in push-ups
Vicarious experience	• Provide examples of others who have had success in tackling similar weight loss or body composition goals • Ask the client to recall a friend or family member whom they have seen make lifestyle changes with success
Verbal persuasion	• Remind the client of how far they have come already • Explain the reasoning—in a way that matters to the client—behind your programming plans or nutrition plans
Physiological states	• Draw awareness to how the client's body may feel after sleeping well or eating a nutrient-dense meal after a workout • Educate the client on how their mood may improve after a workout

Health Belief Model

Created in the 1950s, the health belief model (HBM) suggests that an individual's likelihood of engaging in a health behavior is based on their beliefs (Rosenstock 1974). According to the HBM, some individuals examine costs and benefits associated with a given behavior and are more likely to engage when the benefits outweigh the costs (American College of Sports Medicine 2018). This value-expectancy model has two main components that may influence a person's behaviors (Rosenstock 1974):

1. *Perceived threats.* One's perception of their susceptibility to a threat and of its severity is used to assess how much a given disease state or diagnosis may affect their quality of life.

2. *Outcome expectations.* One's assessment of perceived benefits and barriers is used to decide whether action would lead to a beneficial outcome without large barriers in the way.

The components outlined above and categorized in table 4.9 can also be visualized as an equation:

$$(\text{perceived threat}) + (\text{outcome expectation}) = \text{likelihood of action}$$

Table 4.9 Application of the Health Belief Model

CLIENT'S EVALUATION OF THE ADVANTAGES AND DISADVANTAGES OF INITIATING A CHANGE	
Perceived threats	**Outcome expectations**
The number of perceived barriers exceeds that of perceived benefits	Change is unlikely
The perceived benefits outweigh the barriers, and the perceived threat of illness is high	Preventive action is likely
Very little threat is perceived	Change is unlikely

The HBM also suggests that some individuals experience a cue to action—an event or diagnosis that has pushed them toward making a behavior change, such as weight loss (Rosenstock 1974). The cue-to-action component differentiates the HBM from other models of behavior change. Because the HBM focuses on a person's decision-making process, it may be most applicable early in the coach–client relationship. Coaches may consider applying principles of the HBM to help clients better identify their perceived threats as well as to provide education and temper the client's outcome expectations (American College of Sports Medicine 2018). It is important for exercise professionals to understand client perceptions regarding obesity-related illness, including the perceived benefits of and barriers to participating in an exercise program. This can be achieved by making the seriousness of the illness more apparent and by implementing cues to action, such as introducing health information and education (Rosenstock 1974).

Self-Determination Theory

The self-determination theory (SDT) was developed by Deci and Ryan (2008), who theorized that people have innate and universal psychological needs for autonomy, competence, and relatedness. *Autonomy* is defined as acting on one's own volition and decisions (Deci and Ryan 1985, 2008), *competence* indicates that an individual feels confident or capable in their environment (Deci and Ryan 2004; Sylvester et al. 2014), and *relatedness* refers to feelings of connection with others (Deci and Ryan 2004, 2012). An individual's perception of their experience and satisfaction within these parameters can determine their behavior (see table 4.10).

Table 4.10 Self-Determination Theory

BASIC PSYCHOLOGICAL NEEDS		
Autonomy	**Competence**	**Relatedness**
Acting on ones' own volition and decisions	Feeling confident or capable in one's environment	Feeling connected to others

The SDT is regulated by three types of motivation (amotivation, extrinsic motivation, and intrinsic motivation) and a series of behavioral regulation stages (amotivation, external, introjected, identified, and integrated). The more effectively an individual's motivation is identified and integrated, the more self-determined or autonomous their behavior will be. Applying the SDT to an exercise program that incorporates autonomous support can positively influence the client's satisfaction regarding their innate psychological needs. This can subsequently lead to more positive feelings toward the behavior of interest and better adherence to the program (Klain et al. 2015). Providing guidance and making program decisions through the lens of the SDT provides autonomy for a client by helping them feel they are in control of their environment, socially supported, and competent in their ability to perform.

Barriers to Exercise and Nutrition Behaviors

Barriers to exercise and nutrition behaviors can be separated into two categories: actual barriers and perceived barriers. Actual barriers can be objectively identified and may include factors such as not having access to child care, lacking transportation to a workout class, or not having the equipment needed to perform certain workouts. Perceived barriers, in contrast, include lack of time, self-perception of one's health status, and other factors that may influence an individual's likelihood of changing a given behavior (Herazo-Beltrán et al. 2017). Regardless of the barrier type, evidence suggests that barriers can have a profound and negative effect on one's likelihood to change behaviors (U.S. Department of Health and Human Services 2018).

Using evidence-based approaches, coaches can help clients overcome common barriers. From a weight-management perspective, helping a client identify barriers to improving physical activity and nutrition behaviors is key; if barriers can be adequately addressed through coaching, a client may have more success in managing weight and improving body composition.

CHAPTER SUMMARY

The overall purpose of this chapter was to outline the basic principles of evidence-based behavior change theories, models, and client-facing strategies that coaches can apply within the client–coach relationship. The adoption of health-promoting behaviors is no easy task, but coaches who can skillfully use evidence-based communication, with the theories and models from this chapter in mind, can make meaningful improvements in the lives of their clients. Creating a thoughtful and evidence-based exercise program while addressing key aspects of behavior change is more likely to increase participation in and adherence to health and fitness goals.

KEY POINTS

- Coaches and fitness professionals should strive to improve their emotional intelligence, communication abilities, and working knowledge of behavior-change principles to better serve clients in their weight loss goals. A SWOT (strengths, weaknesses, opportunities, and threats) analysis is one tool fitness professionals can use to generate better self-awareness and strategize an action plan.

- Developing a professional, empathetic, and trusting rapport is central to the coach–client relationship. Principles of motivational interviewing and open-ended questioning skills will enhance the relationship, making long-term adoption of behavior change more likely.

- Behavior-change theories and models from the field of psychology help coaches and fitness professionals better understand and predict both adoption and maintenance of health behaviors, including physical activity and nutrition programs designed to promote weight loss.
- While many behavior-change theories and models exist, coaches and fitness professionals can use key tenets of each as appropriate with their individual clients. Working knowledge of behavioral science and psychology allows for a more tailored approach to weight management.
- Coaches and fitness professionals should guide their clients to effectively evaluate common barriers to behavior change and maintenance, identify factors that motivate their behaviors, and improve their self-efficacy.

CHAPTER QUIZ

Quiz answers can be found in the appendix.

1. _____ refers to the ability to recognize your own emotions and to be aware of the emotions of others, using that information in various situations and contexts.
   a. Sympathy
   b. Emotional intelligence
   c. Self-awareness
   d. Perception of barriers

2. A SWOT analysis is a tool based on both self-reflection and self-awareness that coaches can use to better understand their strengths, _____, _____, and _____.
   a. weaknesses; opportunities; theories
   b. wellness choices; opportunities; threats
   c. weaknesses; opportunities; threats
   d. wellness choices; opportunities; theories

3. The _____ model proposes that individuals move through five stages of change when working to improve health-promoting behaviors.
   a. socioecological model
   b. health belief model
   c. transtheoretical model
   d. social cognitive model

4. _____ refers to an individual's belief in their ability to engage in and perform a specific behavior.
   a. Self-efficacy
   b. Reciprocal determinism

   c. Action
   d. Precontemplation

5. Knowledge, attitudes, and beliefs would fall into what level of socioecological theory?
   a. interpersonal
   b. community
   c. intrapersonal
   d. societal

6. Which of the following strategies would provide guidance to help someone progress through the transtheoretical model?
   a. finding a social connection to facilitate a behavior
   b. weighing the pros and cons of changing one's behavior
   c. incorporating autonomous decision-making
   d. focusing on perceived benefits and barriers

7. Which of the following strategies would help a participant feel more autonomous in their program?
   a. tailoring the intervention to the participant's current stage of change
   b. sharing success stories about similar participants to encourage change
   c. providing positive feedback and reinforcement about skills and abilities
   d. allowing the participant to make key decisions within the intervention

8. If a client makes a statement such as "I will start to make better eating choices,

because otherwise, I may face more health problems," which type of motivation are they displaying?

a. extrinsic motivation

b. amotivation

c. intrinsic motivation

d. energizing motivation

9. In the health belief model, _____ can be defined as one's perception of how severe and serious a given disease state or diagnosis may be and how much it may affect their quality of life.

a. outcome expectations

b. perceived barriers

c. perceived stress

d. perceived threats

10. Which of the following communication strategies would best facilitate behavior change?

a. providing educational materials on the benefits of exercise

b. having a client identify what has worked for them in the past

c. informing a client that they are not meeting the recommended guidelines for exercise

d. avoiding eye contact when a client discusses their past failures

CASE STUDY

Case study answers can be found in the appendix.

Roy and Penny are an older adult couple. After a recent wellness screening by Roy's doctor, they find out that Roy is showing signs of both prediabetes and hypertension and has a body mass index (BMI) of 30.1 kg/m^2. Roy is not currently active and has no intention of starting an exercise program in the next 6 months, but Penny would like for him to engage in regular physical activity and try to lose some weight before his next doctor's appointment. Your first coaching session with Roy and Penny is scheduled for tomorrow, so you are busy preparing your materials and strategy; answer the questions below to help you ensure a great first experience.

1. Given Penny's sense of urgency to improve both her own and Roy's physical activity behaviors and weight loss goals, you deduce that she is using key tenets of the health belief model (HBM), such as perceived threats. Based on the HBM, explain both the perceived threats and the outcome expectations that Penny may have regarding her partner's health status.

2. Based on the transtheoretical model, what would you say is Roy's present stage of change in regard to changing his health behaviors?

a. precontemplation

b. contemplation

c. preparation

d. action

3. You are strategizing about your communication approach with Roy, knowing that Penny is bringing him in to meet with you. Using the strategies of motivational interviewing, what are three examples of questions you might ask him?

4. What lifestyle behaviors could potentially be affecting Roy's blood test, blood pressure, and BMI results? How would you facilitate self-awareness and self-regulation of Roy's lifestyle behaviors?

5. Two evidence-based ways to improve self-efficacy include verbal persuasion and vicarious experiences. If you were to use these strategies to improve Roy's self-efficacy, what would that look like? Provide at least three examples of tactics that may be useful.

PART II

THE ASSESSMENT

CHAPTER 5

Exercise Preparticipation Interview and Health Screening

Deborah Riebe, PhD, and Christie L. Ward-Ritacco, PhD

After completing this chapter, you will be able to

- conduct an exercise preparticipation interview and health history screening,
- complete a cardiovascular disease risk factor analysis in a real-world setting,
- determine a course of action once a client's medical risk has been established, and
- assess a client's stage of readiness to engage in regular exercise and create a stage-matched intervention.

An important role of an exercise professional involves evaluating individuals' health before they engage in physical activity. A thorough health appraisal guides decisions about the need for medical clearance or referral to a medically supervised program and provides insight into modifications to the exercise prescription that may be appropriate for a given person based on their health status.

It is important to assess all individuals who are ready to begin an exercise program; however, particular care should be taken with clients who are obese, because they are more likely to have health challenges than are clients who are not overweight. Obesity predisposes people to health conditions including type 2 diabetes, cardiovascular disease, chronic kidney disease, certain cancers, obstructive sleep apnea, hypertension, osteoarthritis, musculoskeletal disorders, premature death, and depression (Kivimäki et al. 2022; Lin and Li 2021). For example, a recent study found that people with obesity were approximately 3, 5, and 13 times more likely to have one, two, or four or more obesity-related diseases, respectively, compared to those who maintained a healthy weight (Kivimäki et al. 2022).

A variety of health-screening tools exist; some are relatively simple, whereas others are more in depth. Exercise professionals should select the most appropriate instrument based on the characteristics of their clients, such as age, exercise history, general health status, and the type of exercise program in which the client intends to engage.

In general, there are three steps to follow when screening a client's health, each with a different purpose. First, the exercise preparticipation health screening identifies individuals who may be at high risk for adverse exercise-related cardiac events (ACSM 2022). Next, obtaining a more detailed medical history identifies health issues that may be affected by participation in exercise. Finally, a cardiovascular disease (CVD) risk factor analysis educates the client about their risk for heart disease, the leading cause of death worldwide (WHO 2020). Information from these instruments should be used by the exercise professional to make decisions about the health and safety of their client.

In addition to health screening, identifying factors that motivate or impede an individual's participation in physical activity is essential. Determining an individual's readiness to engage in regular physical activity provides important information about which behavioral strategies will be the most effective in assisting individuals to adopt a more physically active lifestyle.

Exercise Preparticipation Health Screening

Exercise preparticipation health screening, as described by the American College of Sports Medicine (ACSM), is a brief process designed to identify people who are at risk for acute myocardial infarction or sudden cardiac death during exercise (ACSM 2022; Riebe et al. 2015). It is not intended to provide a comprehensive medical history but rather to serve as a guide for the exercise professional to identify people at risk for cardiovascular complications that result directly from participation in aerobic exercise. Before initiating an exercise program or increasing exercise intensity, individuals at high risk for such complications should receive medical clearance, defined as approval from a health care professional to engage in exercise (ACSM 2022). There is an increased risk, although low, of adverse cardiovascular events during exercise, especially when previously sedentary individuals perform vigorous exercise to which they are unaccustomed (Franklin et al. 2020). Despite the rarity of exercise-related cardiovascular events, preventing them is critical because of their serious nature.

The ACSM exercise preparticipation health screening process uses four factors to determine the need for medical clearance:

1. the client's current level of physical activity;
2. the presence of signs and symptoms that suggest cardiac, peripheral vascular, or cerebrovascular disease; metabolic disease (type 1 or 2 diabetes); or renal disease (see table 5.1);
3. the presence of known cardiac, metabolic, or renal disease; and
4. the intended intensity of the exercise program (ACSM 2022; Riebe et al. 2015).

Recommendations for the initial intensity of exercise are provided in table 5.2.

An alternative to the ACSM exercise preparticipation health screening process is the self-administered Physical Activity Readiness Questionnaire for Everyone (PAR-Q+), used to determine one's readiness to exercise based on seven general health questions (PAR-Q+ Collaboration 2023). The PAR-Q+ is designed to be self-guided; however, the follow-up questions can be confusing for some individuals, so it is helpful to have an

Table 5.1   Signs and Symptoms of Cardiac, Metabolic, and Renal Disease

Disease	Signs and symptoms
Cardiac	• Discomfort (e.g., pressure, tingling sensation, pain, heaviness, burning, tightness, squeezing, or numbness) in the chest, jaw, neck, back, or arms • Light-headedness, dizziness, or fainting • Temporary loss of visual acuity or speech • Temporary numbness or weakness on one side of the body • Ankle swelling • Shortness of breath • Rapid heartbeat or palpitations, especially if associated with physical activity, eating a large meal, emotional upset, or exposure to cold (or any combination of these) • Burning or cramping in the legs when walking a short distance • Shortness of breath at rest or during light-intensity activity
Metabolic (presence of diabetes)	• Frequent urination • Excessive thirst • Extreme hunger • Fatigue • Blurred vision • Unexpected weight loss • Numb or tingling hands and feet
Renal	• Changes in urination frequency or blood in the urine • Swelling of the feet or ankles • Loss of appetite, nausea, or vomiting • Fatigue and weakness • Difficulty sleeping • Dry, itchy skin • Muscle cramps

Adapted from National Kidney Foundation; Centers for Disease Control and Prevention (2023); and American Heart Association (2023).

Table 5.2   Exercise Preparticipation Health Screening Recommendations

	MEDICAL CLEARANCE	
	Recommended	**Not necessary**
Client is physically active	Clients who report signs or symptoms of cardiovascular, metabolic, or renal disease should discontinue their exercise program and seek medical clearance. Asymptomatic clients with cardiovascular, metabolic, or renal disease who have not received medical clearance within the past 12 months should seek medical clearance before engaging in vigorous-intensity exercise.	Clients who do not have cardiovascular, metabolic, or renal disease and report no signs or symptoms of these diseases can continue with moderate- or vigorous-intensity exercise. Clients with cardiovascular, metabolic, or renal disease who are asymptomatic can continue with moderate-intensity exercise. Asymptomatic clients with cardiovascular, metabolic or renal disease can engage in vigorous-intensity exercise if they received medical clearance within the past 12 months.
Client is inactive	Clients with cardiovascular, metabolic, or renal disease who are asymptomatic and clients who report signs or symptoms of these diseases can begin light- to moderate-intensity exercise following medical clearance.	Clients who do not have cardiovascular, metabolic, or renal disease and report no signs or symptoms of these diseases can begin a light- to moderate-intensity exercise program.

Adapted from Riebe et al. (2015).

exercise professional assist with the questionnaire when needed. When a client answers *yes* to any of the follow-up questions on the second or third page of the PAR-Q+, they should speak with a qualified exercise professional or complete the electronic Physical Activity Medical Examination (ePARmed-X+) (Warburton et al. 2014). The ePARmed-X+ is more detailed than the PAR-Q+ and asks questions about specific health conditions. This screening tool also provides advice about the need to visit a health care provider or to seek advice from an exercise professional prior to engaging in exercise (Health Link British Columbia n.d.; Warburton et al. 2014).

Medical History

A medical history provides the exercise professional with additional information regarding the health and well-being of a client. Readily available medical history forms can range from brief to comprehensive and should be selected based on the best fit for the population being evaluated. Because individuals with obesity are at higher risk for chronic diseases, orthopedic issues, and other health conditions compared to individuals who are not overweight, a more detailed health history may be helpful (see table 5.3). The additional information gained during the medical history can help the exercise professional identify people who need medical clearance for reasons other than being at high risk for having an exercise-related cardiovascular event (e.g., they have active cancer) and can further help in individualizing and modifying the exercise prescription.

Table 5.3   Suggested Contents of a Medical History

Demographics	Age, sex, race, and ethnicity
Physical activity and exercise history	Current activity levels and past attempts at regular exercise; discussion of barriers to being regularly active
Medical conditions	Cardiovascular diseases, pulmonary diseases, metabolic diseases, blood disorders, cancer, neuromuscular diseases, neurologic conditions, and other medical conditions
Musculoskeletal and orthopedic conditions	Arthritis, osteoporosis, low-back pain, joint pain and swelling, previous orthopedic injuries, and surgical procedures
Mental health conditions	Depression, anxiety, and other mental health conditions
Family history	Family history of cardiovascular, pulmonary, metabolic, or renal disease; cancer; and neurologic conditions
Current medications, vitamins, and supplements	Over-the-counter and prescription medications, vitamins, or supplements taken regularly
Medication allergies	Adverse reactions to medication may be classified as predictable side effects of the drug or individual sensitivity to the drug

Adapted from ACSM (2022).

Cardiovascular Disease Risk Factor Analysis

Cardiovascular diseases are the leading cause of death worldwide (WHO 2021). Globally, an estimated 17.9 million people died of CVDs in 2019, with 85% of these deaths due to heart attack and stroke and 33% occurring in people under the age of 70 years

(WHO 2021). Because the risk of CVD can be reduced by changing lifestyle behaviors, including increasing physical activity, a CVD risk factor analysis is a useful step in the health screening process. The presence of CVD risk factors increases the likelihood that an individual will develop a CVD, and having multiple risk factors exponentially increases the risk for CVDs (WHO 2021). A CVD risk factor analysis can be used for educational purposes and to help clients understand how improved lifestyle choices can affect their health.

Risk factors that are associated with CVD include age, family history, high blood pressure, physical inactivity, smoking, high body mass index or waist circumference, and high cholesterol and high blood glucose levels (ACSM 2022). Clinical cut points for each risk factor have been established to help practitioners classify individuals as having or not having a risk factor. The clinical cut points described in table 5.4 are based on recommendations made by the ACSM (2022).

Table 5.4 Clinical Cut Points for Cardiovascular Disease

Factor	Risk level
Age	Men older than 45 y and women older than 55 y
Blood glucose	1. Fasting plasma glucose level ≥100 mg/dL (5.5 mmol/L), 2. 2-h plasma glucose value ≥140 mg/dL (7.77 mmol/L) in an oral glucose tolerance test, or 3. Glycated hemoglobin (HbA$_{1c}$) level ≥5.7%
Blood pressure	1. Systolic blood pressure ≥130 mm Hg or diastolic blood pressure ≥ 80 mm Hg or 2. Currently taking antihypertensive medication
Body mass index or waist circumference	1. Body mass index ≥30 kg/m^2 or 2. Waist girth >40 in. (101.6 cm) for men and >38 in. (96.5 cm) for women
Cigarette smoking	1. Current cigarette smokers, 2. Those who have quit smoking cigarettes in the past 6 mo, or 3. Individuals regularly exposed to environmental smoke
Family history	An individual whose father, brother, or son experienced a myocardial infarction, coronary revascularization, or sudden cardiac death before 55 years of age or whose mother, sister, or daughter experienced a myocardial infarction, coronary revascularization, or sudden cardiac death before 65 years of age
Lipids	1. Low-density lipoprotein (LDL) cholesterol level ≥130 mg/dL (3.37 mmol/L), 2. High-density lipoprotein (HDL) cholesterol level <40 mg/dL (1.04 mmol/L) in men and <50 mg/dL (1.30 mmol/L) in women, 3. Non-HDL cholesterol level <130 mg/dL (3.37 mmol/L), or 4. Taking lipid-lowering medication (additionally, if total serum cholesterol level is the only lipid level available, a total cholesterol level ≥200 mg/dL [5.18 mmol/L] would also be considered a positive risk factor related to lipid levels)
Physical inactivity	Individuals who do not meet the minimum 75 min/wk of vigorous or 150 min/wk of moderate physical activity or an appropriate combination of moderate-to-vigorous physical activity

Adapted from ACSM (2022).

Currently, there is one blood variable associated with a decreased risk for CVD. Individuals with high levels of high-density lipoprotein (HDL) cholesterol, defined as greater than 60 mg/dL (1.55 mmol/L), have a lower risk of developing CVD.

While age and family history are nonmodifiable risk factors for CVD, other factors are considered modifiable through changes in lifestyle. Increasing physical activity is associated with lowering one's CVD risk in addition to positively affecting other CVD risk factors, including blood pressure and blood glucose levels.

There is an online resource that can help individuals who do not currently have a CVD to estimate their 10-year risk for developing heart disease or stroke. The Atherosclerotic Cardiovascular Disease Risk Estimator Plus uses an algorithm developed by the American Heart Association (Lloyd-Jones et al. 2019) and the American College of Cardiology (2023). A 10-year risk assessment is provided to the individual by providing information related to age; sex; race; current resting systolic and diastolic blood pressure; recent levels of total, high-density lipoprotein, and low-density lipoprotein cholesterol; smoking status; diabetes diagnosis; use of aspirin therapy; and use of medication for treating high cholesterol or high blood pressure.

One of the challenges associated with completing a risk factor analysis is that not all clients will have recently visited their health care provider or may not be aware of their lipid and glucose levels. In those cases, it may be prudent for the exercise professional to advise the client to visit a health care provider and become more informed about these aspects of their health.

Physical Activity Readiness

The transtheoretical model (TTM) of behavior change proposes that people are in different stages of readiness for making behavioral changes, including becoming physically active. The TTM includes five stages of change (Prochaska and Velicer 1997):

1. Precontemplation (no intention of becoming physically active in the next 6 months)
2. Contemplation (intending to become physically active within the next 6 months)
3. Preparation (preparing to become physically active in the next 30 days)
4. Action (regularly active for 6 months or less)
5. Maintenance (regularly active for more than 6 months)

The most effective interventions for promoting physical activity occur when the exercise professional uses behavior-change strategies that are matched to the client's stage of change (Prochaska and Velicer 1997).

The TTM can guide the exercise professional when counseling clients about engaging in a regular physical activity by providing stage-matched strategies to help clients move through the stages of change. In the early stages (precontemplation, contemplation), the strategies are cognitive in nature. As individuals move further along in the change process (preparation, action, and maintenance), behavioral processes that require the client to take actual steps toward change are more effective. Weighing the pros and cons of being physically active, along with self-efficacy (defined as confidence in one's ability to be active), are also related to stages of change. Typically, in the earlier stages, the cons of being active outweigh the pros, whereas the pros outweigh the cons in the action and maintenance stages. Exercise self-efficacy is lowest in the precontemplation and highest in the maintenance stage.

Table 5.5 presents the behavioral strategies that match each stage, along with examples of how to apply the strategies to clients in different stages of change.

Table 5.5   Transtheoretical Model Stages of Change and Associated Strategies and Examples for Exercise Professionals

Stage	Strategy and examples

Precontemplation (PC) Contemplation (C)	• Help the client increase their physical activity knowledge.
	  – Visit a website that discusses physical activity (PC, C).
	  – Have the client think about and talk to other people who are overweight and have made exercise a part of their life (PC, C).
	• Help the client consider how the consequences of their current behavior may affect others in their life.
	  – Have them think about how being inactive may affect their family and friends (PC, C). For example, does the client worry about setting an example for their children?
	• Increase the client's awareness of the health risks of physical inactivity.
	  – Help them learn how physical activity can help prevent and treat chronic diseases (PC, C).
	  – Provide information to help them learn about the negative consequences of physical inactivity (PC, C).
	• Assist the client in increasing the pros of physical activity.
	  – Ask the client to think about the benefits associated with physical activity (PC).
	  – Show how the pros outweigh the cons by contradicting the cons. For example, if someone says that they do not have time for exercise, show them how physical activity can be incorporated into any lifestyle throughout the day (C).
	• Help clients to think differently.
	  – Work with clients to improve their self-image using visualization, such as visualizing how life might be different if they were physically active (C).
	• Target the client's exercise self-efficacy.
	  – Have the client think about a time in the past when they accomplished a goal, including the barriers they overcame and the worthwhile feeling of accomplishment (C).

Preparation	• Help the client to gain self-efficacy for exercise.
	  – Clients should take small steps toward regular exercise. For example, suggest that they buy new walking shoes, take a walk around the block, or make plans to exercise with a friend.
	• Assist the client in publicly committing to change.
	  – Clients can make a public statement that they intend to become active or create and sign an exercise contract, witnessed by a friend or family member.
	• Help the client to increase their exercise awareness.
	  – Have them assess their surroundings to identify opportunities to be active that exist in the community.

(continued)

Table 5.5 Transtheoretical Model Stages of Change and Associated Strategies and Examples for Exercise Professionals *(continued)*

Stage	Strategy and examples

Action (A) Maintenance (M)	• Encourage clients to create a system for reminders (A, M).
	  – Use their calendar to schedule time for exercise.
	  – Set a daily alarm to remind them that it is time to move.
	  – Post inspirational messages on their mirror or refrigerator.
	• Encourage clients to eliminate unhealthy thoughts (A, M).
	  – Establish a list of positive responses to any thoughts or worries that come up (e.g., "I am too tired to exercise" can be replaced with "Think about how much energy I will have when my workout is over").
	• Encourage clients to reward themselves for being active (A).
	  – Reinforce good physical activity habits with personal rewards.
	• Remind clients to enlist social support (A, M).
	  – Create a physical activity plan that includes others.
	  – Use social media networks or apps that offer encouragement and opportunities to share one's progress with others.
	• Encourage clients to rely on increased self-efficacy (M).
	  – Clients should regularly remind themselves of how far they have come.
	  – Keep a running tally of things the client has done in the past that helped them be and stay active.
	• Remind clients to reevaluate themselves (A, M).
	  – Clients should enjoy and embrace their new self-image as physically active people.

Adapted from Prochaska and Velicer (1997).

Additional Screening Topics

The entire screening process provides the exercise professional with the opportunity to discuss the effect of excess weight on health and the health-related benefits of regular exercise. These conversations provide an opportunity to learn more about the client so that their program is individualized and targeted to their needs, because a one-size-fits-all approach to exercise programming rarely produces consistent results for clients. The screening process is also a great time to discuss behavior-based issues, such as the client's perceived barriers to participation in regular physical activity, which may provide a starting point for interventions to make physical activity an enjoyable and regular part of the client's daily life.

Discussing a client's health, including their weight history, should be done in a nonjudgmental and compassionate manner, and it should be emphasized that any information shared will be useful for designing an effective and engaging exercise prescription. If sensitive health matters arise, it will be pertinent that the client understands the confidentiality policies outlined in the informed consent.

Most importantly, a comprehensive screening process provides the exercise professional with information essential to making decisions about medical clearance before the client begins an exercise program and gives important information for developing a safe and effective exercise prescription. The recommendations provided in this chapter are a guide; exercise professionals are encouraged to use their clinical judgment when making decisions about the need for medical advice or clearance. The overall goal of the screening process is to help exercise professionals maximize success and minimize risk when assisting a client to get started with a regular program of physical activity.

CHAPTER SUMMARY

This chapter reviewed steps that exercise professionals should take to evaluate the health status of a client prior to engagement in physical activity. It is essential to carefully assess each client and identify those who need medical clearance before engaging in an exercise program. At the same time, it is important to avoid referring individuals to their health care providers if they can safely engage in physical activity, as this can be a barrier to adopting a program. The tools reviewed in this chapter and the clinical judgment of the exercise professional can both be used to make prudent decisions about medical referral. Information gained in the process should also inform and individualize the exercise prescription.

KEY POINTS

- The overall exercise preparticipation interview and health screening process provides the exercise professional with essential information about factors that might influence the exercise prescription.
- Although acute myocardial infarction or sudden cardiac death during exercise are rare, the ACSM exercise preparticipation health screening is a brief process designed to help identify people who are at risk for these events.
- A thorough medical history and a CVD risk factor analysis can be used to educate clients about their risk for heart disease and how lifestyle changes, including regular exercise, can lower their risk.
- Determining a client's stage of change when starting an exercise program allows the exercise professional to tailor intervention strategies to the individual's readiness to become active.

CHAPTER QUIZ

Quiz answers can be found in the appendix.

1. Excessive thirst is a sign or symptom of which medical condition?
   a. cardiovascular disease
   b. hypertension
   c. renal disease
   d. diabetes

2. According to the ACSM's list of cardiovascular risk factors, what is the defining criterion for high levels of low-density lipoprotein cholesterol?
   a. ≥100 mg/dL
   b. ≥130 mg/dL
   c. ≥150 mg/dL
   d. ≥200 mg/dL

3. What is the purpose of the ACSM's exercise preparticipation health screening procedure?
   a. Identify people who are at risk for acute myocardial infarction or sudden cardiac death during exercise.

   b. Identify the 10-year risk of having a myocardial infarction.
   c. Identify all medical conditions that should be considered when designing an exercise program.
   d. Identify cardiovascular disease risk factors.

4. Which of the following best describes an individual who is in the preparation stage for exercise?
   a. They are thinking about starting an exercise program within the next 6 months.
   b. They have no intention of beginning an exercise program.
   c. They are thinking about starting an exercise program within the next 30 days.
   d. They are thinking about starting an exercise program with no specific start date identified.

5. What is the leading cause of death worldwide?
   a. influenza
   b. diabetes
   c. cancer
   d. heart disease

6. A client who has been physically active for the past 10 years reports that they are having palpitations during exercise. What should you tell them?
   a. Discontinue exercise and seek medical advice.
   b. Continue with your normal exercise routine and seek medical advice.
   c. Do not worry; having palpitations during exercise is normal.
   d. Decrease exercise intensity and continue with regular workouts.

7. What is a good strategy to use with someone in the precontemplation stage for exercise?
   a. Set a date to exercise with a friend.
   b. Add reminders to exercise into your phone.
   c. Think about the benefits of exercise.
   d. Buy new walking shoes.

8. According to the ACSM's list of cardiovascular risk factors, what is the defining criterion for high blood pressure?
   a. systolic blood pressure ≥130 mm Hg or diastolic blood pressure ≥80 mm Hg
   b. systolic blood pressure ≥140 mm Hg or diastolic blood pressure ≥90 mm Hg
   c. systolic blood pressure ≥120 mm Hg or diastolic blood pressure ≥80 mm Hg
   d. systolic blood pressure ≥160 mm Hg or diastolic blood pressure ≥100 mm Hg

9. Your client's sister was diagnosed with hypertension at age 42 years, her father had a heart attack at age 61 years, and her mother takes medication for high cholesterol. Does the client have a family-history risk factor for cardiovascular disease?
   a. Yes, because her sister was diagnosed with hypertension at age 42.
   b. Yes, because her father had a heart attack at age 61.
   c. Yes, because her mother takes medication for high cholesterol.
   d. No, she does not have a family-history risk factor.

10. During which stage of change is self-efficacy the highest?
   a. contemplation
   b. preparation
   c. action
   d. maintenance

CASE STUDY

Case study answers can be found in the appendix.

Andre, a 47-year-old nonsmoking man, reports that he has not exercised in over 10 years. He is interested in starting a brisk walking program, because he finds himself getting winded after climbing the stairs in his house. His only significant medical history is a torn anterior cruciate ligament that occurred 20 years ago. Other characteristics include height of 5 ft 11 in. (1.8 m); weight of 222 lb (100.7 kg); body mass index of 32.0 kg/m^2; resting heart rate of 72 beats per minute; resting blood pressure of 136/84 mm Hg; LDL cholesterol level of 120 mg/dL^2; HDL cholesterol level of 44 mg/dL^2; and fasting blood glucose level of 118 mg/dL^2. Andre's father was diagnosed with type 2 diabetes at age 41 years and died of lung cancer at age 66 years. His mother has been taking medication for hypertension since she was 44 years old but has no other health challenges.

1. According to the ACSM preparticipation guidelines, should Andre get medical clearance before starting an exercise program?
2. Which cardiovascular disease risk factors does Andre have?

CHAPTER 6

Health-Related Physical Fitness Assessments

Meir Magal, PhD, and Kathleen S. Thomas, PhD

After completing this chapter, you will be able to

- administer health-related physical fitness assessments to clients with obesity,
- select appropriate field tests for clients with obesity based on their functional abilities,
- explain physical fitness assessment results to clients with obesity, and
- describe the value of conducting physical fitness assessments in program design.

Overweight and obesity increase the risk of certain chronic diseases, including but not limited to cardiovascular disease, diabetes, cancer, and musculoskeletal disorders, regardless of age and ethnicity (NHLBI and NIDDK 1998). Effective bodyweight management relies on maintaining a balance between energy intake and energy expenditure, especially when aiming for weight loss among individuals with overweight or obesity (Lang and Froelicher 2006; Wadden et al. 2020). Research has demonstrated that, as a weight loss intervention, reductions in energy intake combined with increases in energy expenditure through physical activity and exercise lead to greater weight loss than relying solely on energy-intake restriction, often resulting in an initial 5% to 10% reduction in body weight (DeLany et al. 2014; U.S. Preventive Services Task Force 2018). Such a reduction in body weight may also have a favorable effect on cardiovascular disease risk. Other research has shown that even a modest weight reduction of 2% to 5% can significantly decrease triglyceride levels, blood glucose, hemoglobin A_{1c} percentage, and the risk of developing type 2 diabetes (Donnelly et al. 2009; Jensen et al. 2014).

Achieving clinically meaningful weight loss for individuals who are overweight or have obesity can be challenging due to low fitness levels (Liguori et al. 2022). Therefore, combining a moderate reduction in energy intake with a well-designed exercise prescription to increase energy expenditure is an effective way to manage body weight in this population (DeLany et al. 2014; Lang and Froelicher 2006; U.S. Preventive Services

Task Force 2018; Wadden et al. 2020). Using field tests to assess physical fitness before prescribing exercise is a common and effective practice in many exercise programs. These tests must be reliable, precise, easy to conduct, and affordable. The information gathered from these tests and from the client's medical and exercise background informs the exercise professional about the client's fitness and health status, aids in the process of creating and customizing workout plans (i.e., the exercise prescription), and helps to set achievable weight, health, and fitness goals for the client (Feito and Magal 2022; Liguori et al. 2022).

Anthropometric Measurements

Before conducting any fitness assessments, the exercise professional should assess several resting measures. Anthropometric measurements are noninvasive, quantitative measurements that assess various body parameters, including but not limited to height, weight, body mass index (BMI), and waist circumference (Casadei and Kiel 2022). In adults, these measures can be used to assess health, identify potential risk factors for several medical conditions, assess nutritional status, and aid in diagnosing specific diseases, such as anorexia and obesity (Gavriilidou et al. 2015). The resulting data should be interpreted and explained to the client clearly and concisely. This information can be used to educate the client about their current condition and establish a baseline for future visits.

Height Measurement

Height is usually measured with a stadiometer mounted to a wall or integrated into a scale with a height-measuring rod. Regardless of the type of instrument used, it is essential for exercise professionals to ensure that the stadiometer is calibrated and to measure height precisely by asking the client to follow a set of routine steps:

1. Remove footwear and headwear.
2. Stand upright, with both feet placed flat on the floor and the heels touching each other.
3. Maintain a neutral head position by looking straight ahead.
4. Inhale normally and hold your breath.

If a wall-mounted stadiometer with a horizontal headboard is used, the client should stand against the wall, with both heels, the midbody, and the upper body in contact with the wall. The horizontal headboard must be lowered until it touches the top of the client's head to ensure precise measurements.

Weight Measurement

There are various methods to measure weight using a scale. Each uses different mechanisms. An eye-level mechanical beam scale, commonly found in health care facilities, uses a system of springs to display weight and provides a zero-point calibration method. Alternatively, electronic or digital scales can also be used. Some electronic scales allow for calibrating a standard amount of weight to ensure accuracy. However, if there is any deviation in accuracy, professional service may be required to restore the scale's calibration. It is also important to note that most scales have weight limits and may not be suitable for individuals who are overweight or have obesity. A bariatric scale with an appropriate weight capacity and stability features, such as one with a handrail or seat, should be used in such cases (figure 6.1).

Several steps must be taken to improve the accuracy of the weight measurement:

1. Ask the client to wear minimal clothing, remove shoes, and empty pockets to obtain accurate measurements.

2. Take measurements in the morning, or at least at a consistent time of day, when the client has had no recent meal or drink consumption.

3. The client should empty their bladder within an hour before the measurement.

Body Mass Index

The Quetelet index, or BMI, is a measure obtained by dividing the client's weight in kilograms by their height in meters squared to assess the risk of obesity. The following ranges have been used by the National Heart, Lung, and Blood Institute (NHLBI) to describe the BMI classifications (NHLBI and NIDDK 1998):

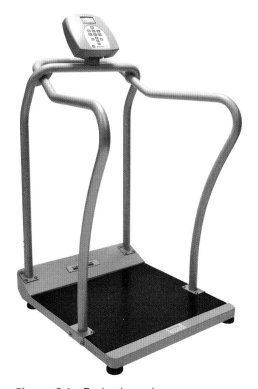

Figure 6.1   Bariatric scale.

Photo by [Pelstar LLC / Health o meter® Professional Scales, www.homscales.com]

- Underweight: BMI less than 18.5 kg/m^2
- Healthy weight: BMI of 18.5 to 24.9 kg/m^2
- Overweight: BMI of 25.0 to 29.9 kg/m^2
- Class 1 obesity: BMI of 30.0 to 34.9 kg/m^2
- Class 2 obesity: BMI of 35.0 to 39.9 kg/m^2
- Class 3 obesity: BMI of 40.0 kg/m^2 or greater

Numerous studies have indicated that individuals with an overweight classification are at elevated risk for various chronic health conditions; however, indication of the risk of premature death based on overweight alone is not as strong, and risk of death seems to be more related to fat accumulated in the abdominal area (Cameron et al. 2013; Klein et al. 2007; Kyrou et al. 2015; Lewis et al. 2009). Individuals with an obesity classification, however, are at higher risk of a number of health concerns and also of premature mortality (Ehrampoush et al. 2017; Lukaski 2013). Exercise professionals can easily perform the BMI calculation using a spreadsheet. In addition, numerous BMI calculators are available online, such as the one provided by the Obesity Education Initiative of the NHLBI (2023).

Waist Circumference and Waist-to-Hip Ratio

Although BMI is an accepted measure for assessing the relationship between height and weight and for classifying cardiovascular and metabolic disease risks, it does not account for body fat distribution, as discussed in chapter 3. The distribution of fat is a crucial indicator of health and chronic disease risk; therefore, waist circumference and the waist-to-hip ratio (WHR) can be used to further specify the type of obesity. Android obesity, or apple-shaped obesity, is characterized by fat accumulation in the abdominal region, whereas gynoid obesity, or pear-shaped obesity, is characterized by fat accumulation in the hips and thighs (Kyrou et al. 2015). Android obesity is associated with increased risk of developing various chronic conditions and premature death. Conversely, gynoid obesity is typically less damaging and may even offer protection against cardiometabolic complications (Cameron et al. 2013; Klein et al. 2007; Kwon et al. 2017; Manolopoulos et al. 2010).

When measuring waist and hip circumference, the client should stand upright. The measurements should be done over the bare skin while the client stands with their hands held freely to their sides. Measurements should be taken using a spring-loaded (Gulick) tape measure while the tester stands at the client's side and should be recorded to the nearest 0.2 in. (0.5 cm), taken in duplicates, and reported as a mean.

Measuring Waist Circumference

1. Have the client stand with the feet together and the arms folded across the chest.
2. Measure the waist circumference while the client's abdominal muscles are relaxed.
3. Position the measuring tape in a horizontal plane around the abdomen at the narrowest part of the torso, below the xiphoid process (the lowest part of the breastbone) and above the umbilicus (the belly button).
4. Keep the plane of the tape parallel to the floor. Hold the tape snug but without compressing the skin.
5. At the client's normal minimal respiration, take the measurement to the nearest 0.2 in. (0.5 cm) in duplicates, and report the mean.

Measuring Hip Circumference

1. Have the client stand with the feet together and arms folded across the chest.
2. Measure the hip circumference horizontally at the widest part of the buttocks, using a spring-loaded (Gulick) tape measure while standing at the client's side.
3. Keep the plane of the tape parallel to the floor. Hold the tape snug but without compressing the skin.
4. Take the measurement to the nearest 0.2 in. (0.5 cm) in duplicates, and report the mean.

Waist and hip circumference are typically interpreted together with the BMI. There is a direct relationship between age, WHR, and health risk. For example, for those who are 20 to 29 years of age, a WHR greater than 0.94 in men and greater than 0.82 in women indicates a very high health risk. More detailed information for men and women of different ages is presented elsewhere (Bray and Gray 1988).

Cardiovascular Hemodynamics

The cardiovascular system consists of the heart (pump) and blood vessels (conduits) and is responsible for circulating blood to different body parts. *Cardiovascular hemodynamics* refers to the flow of blood through the body, and both blood pressure (BP) and heart rate (HR) play a critical role in the process. BP quantifies the force of blood on arterial walls during the systole, or contraction, phase and the diastole, or relaxation, phase of the cardiac cycle. Systolic blood pressure (SBP) is the higher number (the top number of the BP ratio), and diastolic blood pressure (DBP) is the lower number (the bottom number of the ratio). The HR is the number of times the heart contracts per minute. Collecting BP and HR values before conducting any fitness assessments is important for establishing baseline measures.

Blood Pressure Measurement

Exercise professionals typically measure BP through auscultation, which involves listening to internal sounds of the body using a stethoscope. The American College of Cardiology (ACC) and the American Heart Association (AHA) provide recommended standardized procedures for measuring and classifying BP (Whelton et al. 2018). To commence the BP measurement, a cuff is applied to the upper arm and inflated with air, eventually leading to a complete occlusion of blood flow at the brachial artery. Upon the slow release of air pressure from the BP cuff, the pressure inside the cuff will eventually be lower than the driving pressure of the blood in the artery, and the first sound will be heard in the stethoscope. The release of air from the blood pressure cuff establishes blood flow at the brachial artery. However, it causes a pressure differential, which leads to turbulent blood flow and the generation of Korotkoff (pulsating) sounds. Korotkoff sounds occur in five phases, which are heard in sequence when the blood pressure cuff is deflated (Beevers et al. 2001).Typically, the first sound heard is the SBP, and the last is the DBP. As the pressure in the blood pressure cuff subsides, blood flow within the brachial artery returns to normal (Pickering et al. 2005).

Equipment for Measuring Blood Pressure

Measuring BP through auscultation requires a stethoscope (a listening device), a cuff with an inflatable bladder that wraps around and applies pressure to the upper or lower limb, and a manometer to measure and display pressure (figure 6.2). A sphygmomanometer is a complete unit that includes a BP cuff and a manometer.

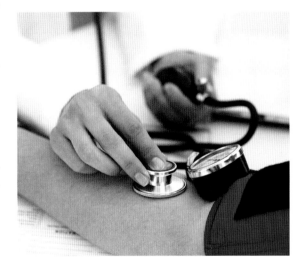

Figure 6.2   A sphygmomanometer is a complete unit that includes both a blood pressure cuff and a manometer.

Ivan-balvan/iStockphoto/Getty Images

Originally, BP was measured using a mercury sphygmomanometer, but because mercury is toxic to the environment and cleaning protocols are stringent, aneroid sphygmomanometers, which operate without fluid, are now more common (Buchanan et al. 2011; O'Brien 2000). Compared to a mercury sphygmomanometer, aneroid sphygmomanometers contain many more working parts. In addition, aneroid sphygmomanometers tend to be less accurate, especially with heavy use, and therefore require calibration against a standard mercury manometer twice yearly.

Small, medium, and large BP cuff sizes are typically available. Exercise professionals should be aware of the index line on the sphygmomanometer cuff, which helps with determining the correct cuff size. For appropriate size accuracy, the index line must fit within the range lines when it is encircling the client's arm. Using the wrong cuff size may result in either overestimating or underestimating BP (Bailey et al. 1991; Canzanello et al. 2001). An additional option, typically found at a medical facility or office or at a client's home, is an electronic BP machine. This system is filled with fluid instead of air and uses the oscillatory method for measuring BP. One shortcoming of electronic BP devices is that they are difficult to calibrate (Feito and Magal 2022).

Blood Pressure Assessment and Interpretation

When assessing BP, exercise professionals should be aware of psychological factors, such as white-coat syndrome and masked hypertension, that may affect BP measurements (Whelton et al. 2018). White-coat syndrome is a condition in which an individual experiences increased BP due to anxiety or stress that arises from being in a doctor's office. Masked hypertension, on the other hand, is a condition in which blood pressure readings appear normal in a doctor's office, but higher blood pressure levels are detected when taken at home.

In addition, the measurement of BP in individuals who are overweight or have obesity presents physical challenges. As mentioned earlier, an appropriately sized cuff is critical for obtaining valid BP measurements. Because individuals with overweight or obesity often have a large arm circumference, an extra-large cuff may be needed, although measurements may be less accurate if the arm circumference is greater than 16.5 in. (41.9 cm) (Stergiou et al. 2018). Another challenge the exercise professional may encounter is that arms with a greater circumference often have a conic shape. Cone-shaped BP cuffs are available for these situations, but another alternative exists. When a large cuff is unavailable for brachial artery BP measurements, a validated wrist device held at heart level may be more accurate (Irving et al. 2016). The procedures for assessing resting blood pressure involve multiple steps that are detailed elsewhere (Feito and Magal 2022).

According to the ACC and AHA guidelines, blood pressure levels below 120 mm Hg systolic and 80 mm Hg diastolic are classified as normal. Levels between 120 and 129 mm Hg systolic and below 80 mm Hg diastolic are classified as elevated. Levels between 130 and 139 mm Hg systolic or between 80 and 89 mm Hg diastolic are classified as stage 1 hypertension, and levels above 140 mm Hg systolic or 90 mm Hg diastolic are classified as stage 2 hypertension (Whelton et al. 2018). Several studies have suggested that obesity may be responsible for 40% to 70% of hypertension (Forman et al. 2009; Garrison et al. 1987; Huang et al. 1998). Furthermore, data from four longitudinal studies among adolescent to middle-aged individuals demonstrated that being obese or developing obesity during these years increases the risk of developing hypertension by almost threefold. However, returning to a healthy weight reduces the risk to normal levels (Juonala et al. 2011).

Heart Rate Measurement

The HR is the number of times the heart contracts in 60 seconds, measured as beats per minute (bpm). Resting HR has no known or accepted standards but has traditionally been regarded as a gauge for cardiovascular endurance. As aerobic fitness improves, resting HR typically decreases. There are also no standards for HR during exercise; however, the response of HR to a standard amount of exercise is central to numerous cardiovascular endurance field tests. Several methods exist to measure HR at rest and during exercise in a fitness setting, including manual palpation and the use of wearable technology.

Traditionally, palpation for a pulse has been measured at the radial or carotid arteries. The radial pulse can be measured by lightly pressing the index and middle finger against the radial artery in the groove on the lateral wrist (figure 6.3), and the carotid pulse can be measured by pressing the fingers lightly along the medial border of the sternomastoid muscle in the lower neck (figure 6.4). When palpating the carotid artery, the exercise professional should be aware of the carotid sinus area to avoid causing a slowed HR or a drop in BP by stimulating the baroreceptor reflex.

The simplest way to measure HR through palpation is to count the number of heartbeats for 15 to 60 seconds. If a shorter measurement period is used, it is necessary to multiply the HR reading by a factor to obtain the bpm. For instance, if the HR is counted for 30 seconds, the number of heartbeats should be multiplied by two. Exercise professionals should be aware that a shorter measurement time is associated with a higher likelihood of calculation errors (Kobayashi 2013).

Wearable devices may serve as a viable alternative to manual palpation; however, the accuracy of these devices can vary. While some HR monitors appear to be more precise during rest, their accuracy during exercise is inversely related to the intensity of the exercise (Boudreaux et al. 2018; Cadmus-Bertram et al. 2017; Horton et al. 2017). Additionally, research indicates that wearable devices are more reliable when used during tests on a treadmill than on a stationary cycle ergometer or elliptical trainer (Gillinov et al. 2017). Specifically related to field testing, exercise professionals should be mindful that using a chest strap instead of a wrist-worn sensor for HR monitoring

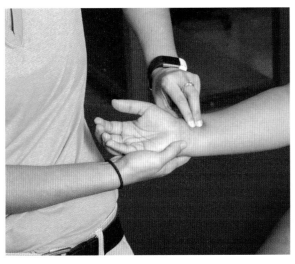

Figure 6.3   Palpating for a radial pulse.

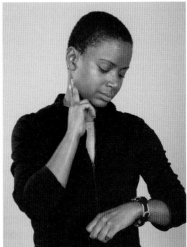

Figure 6.4   Palpating for a carotid pulse.

increases accuracy (Boudreaux et al. 2018; Cadmus-Bertram et al. 2017; Horton et al. 2017). Furthermore, while wearable technology can aid in the real-time display of HR data during exercise, the technology may be less accurate when the test calls for measuring recovery HR (Magal et al. 2023).

Rate Pressure Product

The rate pressure product (RPP), or double product, represents the oxygen demands of the heart muscle and is a measurement often used during exercise. The RPP is particularly useful when comparing different submaximal exercises and when training or testing individuals with cardiovascular disease. Additionally, the RPP is often reproducible; as such, it may serve as a valuable guide for the onset of unwanted symptoms related to heart disease, such as chest pain and shortness of breath. The RPP can be easily calculated by multiplying the HR by the SBP during a given exercise.

$$RPP = (HR \times SBP) \div 100$$

The resultant product, the RPP, is typically a large number and therefore is divided by 100. For example, if a client's HR is 140 and their SBP is 150, then the RPP will be 210:

$$RPP = (140 \times 150) \div 100 = 210$$

Muscular Strength

Muscular strength is defined as the amount of force produced by a specific muscle or muscle group at one time. This is referred to as the 1-repetition maximum (1-RM) and is the standard for assessing muscular strength (Bohannon 2015; Levinger et al. 2009). Muscular strength is measured both statically and dynamically using a variety of field tests. Static, or isometric, strength is specific to the joint angle and muscle groups being tested, but it has been reliably measured with instruments such as handheld dynamometers or cable tensiometers (Chamorro et al. 2021; Lee et al. 2020). Grip strength, measured with a handheld dynamometer, is a good indicator of overall body strength and muscle mass (Bohannon 2015; Chamorro et al. 2021; Wong 2016). When assessing muscular strength in individuals who are overweight or have obesity, it is important to understand the different types of field tests that will provide the most appropriate data for the population.

For example, individuals who are overweight or have obesity may have significantly greater grip strength compared to individuals who are not overweight or obese, but when using assessments requiring load bearing through the arms (e.g., pull-ups, flexed-arm hangs, or push-ups), these results may be reversed (Alaniz-Arcos et al. 2023). Therefore, load-bearing assessments may not be appropriate for this population of clients, and handheld dynamometry should be used instead.

Upper-Body Strength Assessments

When assessing grip strength, the use of a pretest and posttest would be the best way to measure improvement for clients in this population and is a more appropriate individual outcome. The following are the steps to measure overall static strength using a handheld dynamometer or a 1-RM bench press.

Handheld Dynamometer Assessment

1. Instruct the client to stand with their feet shoulder-width apart and to hold the dynamometer to their side with their dominant hand.

2. Set the dynamometer to zero.

3. Have the client squeeze the handle of the dynamometer as hard as possible without holding their breath.

4. Have the client repeat this twice, then switch to the nondominant hand.

5. Use the highest value recorded from either hand as the maximal grip strength.

Before testing upper-body strength, ensure the client has properly warmed up by performing low-weight, submaximal repetitions of the exercise that is to be used for assessment. Once the client has received the appropriate instructions and become familiarized with the techniques, they should perform the 1-RM bench press to measure upper-body dynamic strength.

1-RM Bench Press

1. Align the client in the machine or onto the bench appropriately for a free-weight press.

2. Be sure to use proper spotting techniques, particularly when using the free-weight bench press.

3. Determine the 1-RM within four trials, with substantial rest periods (up to 5 min) between trials.

4. Select an initial weight that the client feels is within their capacity to lift.

5. Increase the resistance by 5% to 10% with each trial until the client can no longer complete the repetition with control and within the entire range of motion (ROM).

Lower-Body Strength Assessments

As with the upper-body assessment of strength, when testing lower-body strength, make sure that the client has had a proper warm-up prior to the testing session by performing low-weight, submaximal repetitions of the exercise that is to be used for assessment. Once appropriate instruction and familiarization have been conducted, the following are the steps to measure lower-body dynamic strength by having the client perform the 1-RM leg press.

1-RM Leg Press

1. Align the client in the machine properly.

2. Be sure to give the client proper safety instructions.

3. Determine the 1-RM within four trials, with substantial rest periods (up to 5 min) between trials.

4. Select an initial weight that the client feels is within their capacity to lift.

5. Increase the resistance by 10% to 20% each trial until the client can no longer complete the repetition with control and using the entire ROM.

6. Express scores as a ratio of the weight pushed in pounds divided by the client's body weight in pounds. For a beginner, a good ratio for which to strive is the ability to lift about 75% of one's body weight. Exercise professionals should take into account the comparison between measurements during pretests before and

posttests following a specific intervention (i.e., exercising three times a week for 12 weeks). This would consider the percentage of increase from the baseline 1-RM to the postintervention 1-RM.

As with the handheld dynamometer or 1-RM bench press, the best way to determine improvement in lower-body strength is to conduct pretests and posttests for clients.

Trunk Strength Assessments

Field tests used to measure trunk strength assess muscular endurance. Tools used to clinically assess the strength of the trunk muscles are designed to measure peak rotational force and torque within a joint's ROM at a constant angular velocity (Hall 2022). However, the machines for these assessments are very expensive, and the results are not replicated by a particular field test. Field tests for muscular endurance of the trunk will be discussed in the next section, which will also address the appropriateness of these tests for individuals who are overweight or have obesity.

Muscular Endurance

Muscular endurance is defined as the ability to produce submaximal forces over repeated exertions before reaching muscle fatigue. Muscular endurance can be measured in absolute values by counting the number of times an activity, such as push-ups or pull-ups for the upper body or squats for the lower body, can be repeated (Liguori et al. 2022). Muscular endurance can also be expressed as a percentage of a 1-RM. For example, an individual's ability to perform 6 to 8 repetitions at 70% of the 1-RM would denote relative muscular endurance. While muscular strength is the amount of force (single muscular contraction) produced in a very short period, muscular endurance is the ability to produce lower amounts of force (multiple muscular contractions) over an extended period. In fitness assessments, the 1-RM value can be used to calculate the values for muscular endurance testing. For example, if an individual performs a 1-RM lift at 85 lb (39 kg), then that value can be used to calculate their submaximal lift weight at 60% to 85% of the 1-RM (51-72 lb [23-33 kg]) to improve muscular endurance and contribute to an increase in muscular strength in the long run.

Pull-ups and push-ups require lifting one's body weight, and they are generally very limiting for individuals who are overweight or have obesity (Sizoo et al. 2021). Instead, having the client perform wall push-ups, repetitions of a percentage of the 1-RM bench press, or the YMCA bench press test (described in the next section) would be more appropriate than using assessments for athletes and individuals of healthy weight but would still provide the information needed to create an exercise program that effectively addresses the needs of the client (Kim et al. 2002; Ronai 2020).

Upper-Body Endurance Assessments

The YMCA bench press test has been widely used as a reliable and valid field test for upper-body muscular endurance and is appropriate for all body types. A bar weight of 80 lb (36 kg) for men or 35 lb (16 kg) for women is used (Kim et al. 2002; Ronai 2020). As with the upper-body assessment of muscular strength, the exercise professional should make sure that the client has had a proper warm-up prior to the testing session by performing a few low-weight, submaximal repetitions of the exercise after appropriate instruction and familiarization have taken place. The following are the steps to measure the YMCA bench press.

YMCA Bench Press

1. Align the client on the bench properly.
2. Be sure to use proper safety instructions and a spotter.
3. Set a metronome (or a metronome app) to 60 clicks per minute.
4. The test begins with the bar positioned on the client's chest. Ask the client to move the bar through the full range of motion to the metronome beat (about 30 lifts per minute).

The test is terminated when proper form, full range of motion, or metronome cadence cannot be maintained or if the client requests to stop (Golding 2000).

Lower-Body Endurance Assessments

Traditional lower-body tests for muscular endurance include timed isometric wall sits (hips and knees at 90° angles), the 60-second squat test, 5- to 10-repetition sit-to-stand tests, and the timed stair-ascent test. All of these have high test–retest reliability (Cuenca-Garcia et al. 2022; Kjaer et al. 2016). These tests are very simple to conduct and have been used for all ages and body types (Hansen et al. 2013; Kjaer et al. 2016). It is not necessary to perform all of these tests; they are simply provided here as options for assessing lower-body muscular endurance.

The 5- to 10-repetition sit-to-stand test has been used in healthy adults aged 18 to 64 years with and without back pain and has been shown to have high test–retest reliability. It is simple to administer.

The 5- to 10-Repetition Sit-to-Stand Test

1. The required equipment includes a stable chair (this can be placed against a wall) to use as a guide for depth and a stopwatch to time how long it takes to go from sitting to standing either 5 or 10 times.

2. Have the client place their hands across their chest while performing the test, as shown in figure 6.5.

3. The client should begin in a seated position and stand straight up, then immediately sit back down. Record the amount of time it takes the client to complete either 5 or 10 repetitions.

The 60-second squat test is used for a variety of populations, although it may be more challenging for older, untrained adults. The following are the steps to conduct this test.

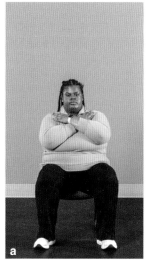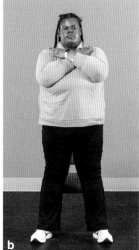

Figure 6.5   The 5- to 10-repetition sit-to-stand test.

60-Second Squat Test

1. As with the 5- to 10-repetition sit-to-stand test, use a stable chair as the guide for depth and have the client place their hands across their chest.

2. Set a timer for 60 seconds. Have the client begin in a seated position and move from seated to standing as many times as possible for the 1-minute period.

3. Record the number of repetitions completed.

Trunk Endurance Assessments

Although several tests have been designed to measure trunk muscle endurance (full sit-ups, curl-ups, and the Biering-Sørensen test, to name a few), these assessments have little test–retest reliability (Castro-Pinero et al. 2021; Cuenca-Garcia et al. 2022), and often, they can exacerbate existing back problems. For that reason, trunk assessments were left out of the American College of Sports Medicine's *Guidelines for Exercise Testing and Prescription*, 11th Edition (Liguori et al. 2022). For individuals who are overweight or have obesity, these assessments would be challenging and may not be accurate; therefore, they are not recommended (Deforche et al. 2003).

Cardiorespiratory Fitness

Cardiorespiratory fitness refers to the ability of the circulatory and respiratory systems to provide oxygen to working muscles during physical activity. It is essential to measure cardiorespiratory fitness, because it has been linked with mortality risk and several adverse health conditions, including cardiovascular disease, hypertension, stroke, type 2 diabetes, obesity, certain cancers, depression, and cognitive dysfunction (Feito and Magal 2022; Liguori et al. 2022).

Several field tests can determine cardiorespiratory fitness levels in the general population. The more common assessments include the Rockport 1 mi (1.6 km) walk test, the 6-minute walk test (6-MWT), the Cooper 12-minute run test, and the 22 yd (20 m) shuttle run for a variety of ages (Bohannon et al. 2015; Castro-Pinero et al. 2021; Cuenca-Garcia et al. 2022; Cooper Institute 2007; Evans et al. 2014; Manttari et al. 2018; Mayorga-Vega et al. 2016; Weiglein et al. 2011). These tests are valid and reliable alternatives to a formalized laboratory test for the maximal rate of oxygen consumption during physical exertion ($\dot{V}O_2$max) and would be useful for assessing cardiovascular fitness in individuals who are overweight or have obesity (Mayorga-Vega et al. 2016).

Rockport 1-Mile Walk Test

The Rockport 1 mi (1.6 km) walk test, which has been shown to be a valid predictor of outcomes in the 1.5 mi (2.4 km) run test in moderately to highly fit men in the U.S. Air Force (Weiglein et al. 2011), is also considered a reliable test for individuals who are overweight or have obesity.

1. The Rockport walk test is conducted by establishing a pathway 1 mi (1.6 km) in length. The client walks the entire flat distance as quickly as possible (Weiglein et al. 2011).

2. Record the amount of time required to complete the distance, along with heart rate.

3. Also record the client's $\dot{V}O_2$max. To calculate this value, obtain the following information from the client, then use the formula provided:

   - Age (years)
   - Sex (male = 1, female = 0)

- Body weight (lb; 2.2 lb = 1 kg)
- Time to complete the walk, in minutes and seconds (expressed in minutes and hundredths of minutes)
- Final heart rate (bpm)

Formula: $\dot{V}O_2max = 132.853 - (0.0769 \times \text{body weight}) - (0.3877 \times \text{age}) + (6.315 \times \text{sex}) - (3.2649 \times \text{time}) - (0.1565 \times \text{heart rate})$

6-Minute Walk Test

The 6-MWT was originally used for frail older adults to assess both cardiorespiratory fitness and functional movement. However, it has recently been shown to be beneficial for all ages and body shapes, with a high test–retest correlation, and it is commonly used as a clinical field test in physical therapy practices (Bohannon et al. 2015; Castro-Pinero et al. 2021; Cuenca-Garcia et al. 2022; Hansen et al. 2013; Jalili et al. 2018; Kaminsky et al. 2015; Kline et al. 1987; Nolen-Doerr et al. 2018).

1. Instruct the client about the rating of perceived exertion (RPE) scale (how hard the client feels they are working on a scale from 6 to 20, with 6 being extremely light and 20 being maximal exertion; see table 6.1), then have them walk for 6 minutes as quickly as possible.
2. After each minute, ask the client how they feel according to an RPE chart. Allow them to rest if they need to, but continue recording the time during any rest periods.
3. Calculate the distance (in meters) covered in 6 minutes by multiplying the number of full laps completed by the distance per lap, then adding the distance of any partial lap completed by the end of the test.

Table 6.1   Sample Rating of Perceived Exertion (RPE) Scale

Rating	Description
1	Nothing at all (lying down)
2	Extremely little
3	Very easy
4	Easy (could do this all day)
5	Moderate
6	Somewhat hard (starting to feel it)
7	Hard
8	Very hard (making an effort to keep up)
9	Very, very hard
10	Maximum effort (cannot go any further)

Reprinted by permission from D.H. Fukuda and K.L. Kendall, "Fitness Evaluation Protocols and Norms," in *NSCA's Essentials of Personal Training*, 3rd ed., edited for the National Strength and Conditioning Association by B.J. Schoenfeld and R.L. Snarr (Human Kinetics, 2022), 204.

To interpret the 6-MWT, calculate the normal distance (in meters) for the client's sex, age, height, and weight using the following equations established by Enright and Sherrill (1998) among 290 healthy adults aged 40 to 80 years:

Men: distance = $(7.57 \times \text{height in cm}) - (5.02 \times \text{age}) - (1.76 \times \text{weight in kg}) - 309$

Women: distance = $(2.11 \times \text{height in cm}) - (2.29 \times \text{weight in kg}) - (5.78 \times \text{age}) + 667$

Motor Function, Functional Mobility, and Flexibility

Functional mobility pertains to one's capacity to move autonomously and securely while performing activities of daily living (ADLs) and engaging in everyday life at home and in the community. Functional mobility is often regarded as a critical gauge of a person's overall health status (Bouça-Machado et al. 2018).

Flexibility has also been used to assess one's capacity to perform ADLs and is defined as the ability to move a joint through its complete ROM without pain or discomfort; however, methods of assessing flexibility have been controversial in the literature, and there are mixed results on their validity (Castro-Pinero et al. 2021; Cooper Institute 2007; Cuenca-Garcia et al. 2022; Hansen et al. 2013; Liguori et al. 2022). The most common flexibility assessments are the original and modified sit-and-reach tests, the toe-touch test, and the use of goniometers to assess the ROM of an individual joint (Cooper Institute 2007; Cuenca-Garcia et al. 2022; Kjaer et al. 2016).

Several field tests also assess motor function (i.e., tasks that require voluntary control over movements of the joints and body segments to achieve a goal), including the timed up and go (TUG) test (Centers for Disease Control and Prevention 2017; Cuenca-Garcia et al. 2022).

TUG Test

The TUG test is designed to measure motor function and is a common assessment used for lower-limb injuries and for physical function in a variety of populations. It is effective in recognizing dynamic balance and physical mobility problems (Castro-Pinero et al. 2021; Cuenca-Garcia et al. 2022; Montgomery et al. 2020).

1. Direct the client to stand from a seated position in a chair, walk forward 10 ft (3.0 m), turn around, walk back to the chair, turn around, and sit down (Centers for Disease Control and Prevention 2017).

2. On average, most healthy adults complete the TUG test in 10 seconds or less. Individuals who require 12 or more seconds to complete it are considered at high risk for falls (Montgomery et al. 2020).

Sit-and-Reach Tests

Several different protocols have been used to conduct the sit-and-reach test. All are designed to measure the maximal amount of trunk flexion. Both the original sit-and-reach test and the modified chair sit-and-reach version have been shown to have high test–retest reliability (Cuenca-Garcia et al. 2022) when conducted as shown in figure 6.6. It is important to instruct the client to focus on smooth and proper form rather than on the number of centimeters reached while performing the test. Mobility may factor into the type of protocol you will use with clients who are overweight or have obesity. These individuals may have difficulty sitting on the floor and getting up from the floor, so the modified chair sit-and-reach version of the test may accommodate this population more appropriately (Kjaer et al. 2016).

Original Sit-and-Reach Test

1. This test requires a box designed to measure the distance the client can reach in centimeters. The test can be performed bilaterally or unilaterally; unilateral performance seems to reduce the amount of lumbar curvature to provide a more accurate measurement (Miñarro et al. 2007).

2. Have the client sit on a mat on the floor with one foot extended forward, the knee straight, the ankle flexed 90°, and the whole foot in contact with the box. The other leg is off to the side in a relaxed position.

3. Have the client overlap their hands with their nondominant hand on top of their dominant hand, reach their hands to the front of the box, and place their fingertips on the slider.

4. Instruct the client to reach forward as far as possible, and record the distance reached in centimeters.

Chair Sit-and-Reach Test

1. The chair sit-and-reach test may be more comfortable than sitting on the floor for individuals who are overweight or have obesity.

2. Have the client sit on a chair and outstretch one leg with the knee straight, keeping the other leg to the side with the knee flexed and the foot on the floor.

3. Instruct the client to overlap their hands with their nondominant hand on top of their dominant hand and reach forward as far as possible toward the toes of the outstretched leg (figure 6.6).

4. If the client cannot reach their toes, record the distance in centimeters between their fingertips and toes as a negative score. If their fingertips overlap their toes, record the overlapping distance in centimeters as a positive score.

Similar to the other assessments of physical fitness, the results of pretests and posttests should be compared to determine any changes in flexibility.

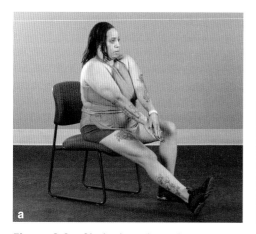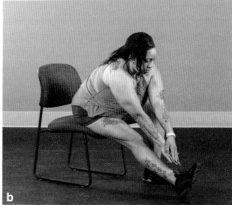

Figure 6.6   Chair sit-and-reach test.

CHAPTER SUMMARY

When considering health-related physical fitness assessments in individuals who are overweight or have obesity, be sure that you have taken the necessary precautions for them to participate safely and at a level that is appropriate for their body size. Common vital signs should be within normal limits, and when they are not, it may be appropriate to have the client obtain a thorough examination from their physician. Some fitness assessments that are appropriate for an individual with an athletic build or lower body weight may not be appropriate for clients who are overweight or have obesity. Remember that assessments requiring lifting one's body weight (such as push-ups, pull-ups, or flexed-arm hangs) may be difficult or even impossible for someone with overweight or obesity. Therefore, this chapter offers alternatives to allow a more accurate account of fitness levels.

KEY POINTS

- Effective weight management depends on the balance of energy intake and energy expenditure.
- Increasing physical activity with reductions in energy intake can produce a significant reduction in body weight.
- Before conducting fitness assessments, the exercise professional should collect resting measures, including height, weight, waist circumference, waist-to-hip ratio, blood pressure, and heart rate.
- Effective and reliable field tests inform the exercise professional and the client about health and fitness status and provide important information to create appropriate workout plans.
- Some physical fitness tests may not be appropriate for individuals who are overweight or have obesity; alternatives should be considered for reliable results among this population.

CHAPTER QUIZ

Quiz answers can be found in the appendix.

1. Which of the following is NOT one of the steps for measuring height with a stadiometer?
   a. The client must remove footwear and headwear.
   b. The client must stand upright, with both feet placed flat on the floor and the heels touching each other.
   c. The client must maintain a neutral head position by looking straight ahead.
   d. The client must exhale completely.

2. Which of the following is NOT one of the steps for measuring weight on a bariatric scale?
   a. The client should wear minimal clothing.
   b. The client can choose whether to remove shoes.
   c. The client should empty their bladder within an hour before the measurement.
   d. The client should empty their pockets.

3. Using the body mass index classification, which of the following is considered class 2 obesity?

   a. 25.0-29.9 kg/m^2
   b. 30.0-34.9 kg/m^2
   c. 35.0-39.9 kg/m^2
   d. ≥40.0 kg/m^2

4. Which of the following describes android obesity?
   a. pear-shaped physique
   b. apple-shaped physique
   c. fat accumulation around the abdominal area
   d. both b and c

5. Which of the following is NOT used in the measurement of blood pressure?
   a. stethoscope
   b. blood pressure cuff
   c. sphygmomanometer
   d. pulse oximeter

6. Which variable or variables make up the rate pressure product, or double product?
   a. heart rate
   b. diastolic blood pressure
   c. systolic blood pressure
   d. a and b
   e. a and c

7. Which of the following is an INCOR-RECT step in the measurement of static strength with a handheld dynamometer?

   a. The measurement is completed only with the dominant hand.

   b. The dynamometer should be set to zero prior to starting the measurement.

   c. The client should stand with their feet shoulder-width apart.

   d. All of the above are incorrect.

8. Which of the following definitions describes muscular endurance?

   a. the amount of force produced by a specific muscle or muscle group at one time

   b. the ability to produce submaximal forces over repeated exertions before reaching muscle fatigue

   c. a given muscular force production over a short period

   d. none of the above

9. Which of the following is an example of a cardiorespiratory fitness assessment?

   a. 60-second squat test

   b. 1-repetition maximum bench press

   c. timed up and go test

   d. 6-minute walk test

10. Which of the following is an example of a motor and functional mobility assessment?

   a. 60-second squat test

   b. 1-repetition maximum bench press

   c. timed up and go test

   d. 6-minute walk test

CASE STUDY

Case study answers can be found in the appendix.

Mrs. Penelope has never been involved in a formalized exercise program and has struggled with excess weight her entire life. At age 40, she has recently been informed by her physician that her blood glucose and hemoglobin A_{1c} values are at prediabetic levels and that she needs to make some lifestyle changes to reduce the chance of developing type 2 diabetes. She is 5 ft 6 in. (168 cm) tall and weighs 240 lb (109 kg), with a BMI of 38.7 kg/m^2. Her resting blood pressure is borderline high at 130/85 mm Hg, and her resting heart rate is 70 bpm. There are no other documented health concerns. Mrs. Penelope's mother has had type 2 diabetes since age 52, and her father was diagnosed with high blood pressure at age 40. Mrs. Penelope has trouble walking up and down stairs but can walk without aid for an extended period on level ground. She says that she is strong in her upper body, but her legs get fatigued by the end of the day just working and running errands. She knows that she needs to lose weight and perform some planned physical activity, but she doesn't know where to start. She was referred to you by her family physician to begin an exercise program.

1. What health-related assessments would you perform on Mrs. Penelope?

2. Which field test would best accommodate Mrs. Penelope to measure her cardiorespiratory fitness? Explain why you chose this test.

3. Does this client have any contraindications that would preclude you from conducting certain fitness tests on her? If so, what tests should be avoided, and why might they be unsafe for this individual? If not, indicate why you would be comfortable with conducting any of the fitness assessments.

4. How would you assess Mrs. Penelope's muscular endurance? Which test, or tests, would you use and why?

5. Would you prescribe cardiorespiratory exercise, resistance training, or both? Provide a rationale for your answer.

PART III

THE APPLICATION

CHAPTER 7

Warm-Up Concepts

Amy Bantham, PhD, Rachele Pojednic, PhD, and Alexios Batrakoulis, PhD

After completing this chapter, you will be able to
- explain the rationale and psychophysiological responses to warm-up,
- describe the structure of a warm-up routine tailored to clients with obesity,
- provide detailed instructions and tips for implementing engaging warm-up drills, and
- use feasible fitness games to provide positive exercise experiences in various settings.

Physical exercise is an essential component of obesity management. Although exercise traditionally has been used to help individuals reduce body weight and improve body composition (O'Donoghue et al. 2021), even in the absence of weight loss, exercise helps improve overall health and enhance the quality of life for individuals with obesity (Pojednic et al. 2022). However, for individuals with excess weight, exercise can be more challenging, and specific considerations must be taken into account to ensure a safe and effective workout. One such consideration is the warm-up, a critical element in any exercise program (Franklin et al. 2022). Clients with excess weight are prone to injury when participating in various exercise activities, with or without supervision. Thus, an individualized warm-up regimen is a pivotal aspect of any type of workout for people with an unhealthy weight, aiming to provide real-world results in an efficient, safe, and pleasant manner (McGowan et al. 2015).

Benefits of a Warm-Up Routine

The warm-up is an essential preparatory phase that precedes the main exercise session (Franklin et al. 2022). Engaging in warm-up routines helps transition tissues and systems from a state of rest to the appropriate intensity of exercise. Preparatory exercises should target key muscles and enhance blood circulation, which allows for proper fuel use and metabolism while also potentially minimizing the chances of injury or cardiovascular issues during the workout. A warm-up will serve several key purposes when working with clients with obesity, as described in the following sections.

Temperature Regulation

A warm-up gradually increases the core temperature, which is particularly important for individuals with obesity. An elevated core temperature leads to improved muscle metabolism, oxygen uptake, muscle fiber performance, and rate of conduction velocity, resulting in overall improvements in exercise performance while reducing the risk of injury. Also, an increased core temperature is beneficial for reducing tissue viscosity, improving elasticity of muscles and tendons, increasing synovial fluids within the joints, and dilating blood vessels within the active body regions (McGowan et al. 2015).

Cardiovascular Preparedness

Clients with obesity often have underlying cardiovascular issues (Powell-Wiley et al. 2021). A well-structured warm-up helps to gradually increase the heart rate (Horia-Daniel at al. 2018), preparing the cardiovascular system for the demands of exercise and reducing the risk of sudden cardiac events. A progressive warm-up activates the body's cardiopulmonary, motor, and energy-producing systems (Barnard et al. 1973), facilitating energy transfer to activities at a greater intensity and complexity during the workout. From a safety perspective, this an important element for people with a high body mass index, because several cardiovascular complications and metabolic dysfunction are common among such populations.

Improved Muscle Function

For clients with obesity, achieving proper muscle activation can be challenging due to potential restrictions of movement (Wearing et al. 2006). A warm-up helps activate dormant muscles and improve muscle coordination, making exercises more effective and safer at the planned intensities (McGowan et al. 2015). Importantly, middle-aged and older adults with obesity tend to develop sarcopenia, a condition characterized by loss of lean body mass, strength, and function and contributing to frailty, osteoporosis, and cardiovascular disease. A progressive, multicomponent warm-up routine in conjunction with muscle-strengthening activities (see chapter 8) may potentially prevent major symptoms of several sarcopenia-related, noncommunicable diseases and promote physical independence (Polyzos et al. 2023).

Psychophysiological Responses to Warm-Up

In addition to the physiologic responses by muscle tissues and whole-body systems, the warm-up period is also recognized as an opportunity to mentally prepare for exercise and to focus on the workout ahead. Many individuals engage in psychological preparation before exercise (Rumeau et al. 2023; Tod et al. 2005), which can include strategies such as mental visualization, repetition of cue words, and motor imagery (Weinberg and Gould 2023). Understanding the psychophysiological responses to a warm-up is crucial for tailoring it to the specific needs of clients with obesity.

Psychological Preparation

Individuals with obesity may experience anxiety and fear related to exercise (Hamer et al. 2021). A warm-up provides an opportunity to build confidence and reduce exercise-related stress (Weinberg and Gould 2023), making the main workout more effective and enjoyable. A progressive and customized warm-up routine may also improve concentration and arousal levels, which is a major benefit for people who tend to be inexperienced in the gym and are currently sedentary. A smart warm-up could be the magic bullet for clients with excess weight who seek to engage in regular, structured, movement-based programs under an exercise professional's supervision.

Neuromuscular Activation

Progressive activation of the sympathetic nervous system is one of the priorities when conducting a warm-up routine for clients with obesity. Neuromuscular connections improve during a warm-up, enhancing muscle coordination (McGowan et al. 2015). This is particularly important for individuals who may struggle with proper movement patterns due to obesity, given that this population often has difficulty engaging in activities of daily living due to limited range of motion in all joints, poor functional capacity, postural dysfunction, and various musculoskeletal health issues related to obesity (Wearing et al. 2006). Hence, integrated movements that synchronize the muscles and joints and promote movement efficiency are needed as part of a comprehensive warm-up routine for individuals with overweight or obesity.

Safe and Effective Warm-Ups for Individuals With Obesity

Several factors need to be considered when designing a warm-up for a client with obesity, including an individual's training experience and the intensity of the exercise bout. It is essential to tailor warm-up routines to the specific needs and preferences of each individual. Such an approach will create unique and positive exercise experiences through feasible, injury-free bodily activities adapted for the person with overweight or obesity.

Understanding Clients' Needs and Preferences

The warm-up provides an opportunity for fitness professionals to take the time to ask about their client's motivations and preferences for the exercise session. It allows professionals to understand their clients' experience with exercise, their favorite warm-up drills, and even their least favorite warm-up drills. This helps professionals deliver an individualized, client-centered exercise session that best sets their clients up for success. This point is critical, given that individuals with greater body mass are likely to be an underserved population due to the lack of a personalized approach in a commercial gym setting (Bantham et al. 2021).

Building Rapport With Clients

Fitness professionals can use the warm-up time to build rapport with their clients. It allows them to open the communication channels and demonstrate that they can meet their clients where they are in terms of interests and motivations. This helps professionals establish themselves as a trusted, empathetic resource who can help grow their clients' confidence in exercising. Considering that emotional connection is critical when serving physically inactive populations characterized by poor mental health, such as many individuals with excess weight, the warm-up time may be a beneficial tool for building clients' self-confidence, self-efficacy, and self-esteem (Gilyana et al. 2023).

The Optimal Warm-Up Concept

For individuals with overweight or obesity, a well-designed warm-up should be a short (15-minute), multicomponent session, combining both general and specific drills within any type of workout and aiming to enhance physical performance and body functionality, reduce the risk of injury, and diminish the potential for muscle soreness after exercise (Abad et al. 2011; McGowan et al. 2015). In particular, a feasible, effective, and enjoyable warm-up routine consists of a gradual increase in movement and exercise intensity, involving a series of drills primarily aiming to improve joint mobility and prepare the client for the workout both physically and mentally. In simple terms, a dynamic warm-up is an optimal concept regarding the implementation of this introductory workout phase for people with overweight or obesity (Horia-Daniel and Georges 2018). This appropriate and progressive warm-up strategy integrates the following key components, incorporating exercises that are suitable for any setting with no need for equipment:

1. cardiopulmonary load
2. mobility
3. static and dynamic stretching
4. movement preparation and remediation
5. neuromuscular activation

Cardiopulmonary Load

Various low-intensity, whole-body, repetitive activities are recommended to previously inactive individuals with excess weight to increase core temperature and activate the body's cardiopulmonary, motor, and energy-producing systems. In a traditional gym setting, treadmill walking with no elevation, seated stationary biking, and recumbent stepping are suggested as the optimal modalities for this particular phase of a warm-up routine adapted for individuals with overweight or obesity. In general, almost any other low-impact, non-weight-bearing activity that is simple to execute, induces slow stress on the joints, and creates the desired effects mentioned previously could be a suitable option to prepare the body for exercise.

Taking this into account, upright stationary bikes, ellipticals, steppers, and row machines do not seem to be user-friendly cardiorespiratory exercise equipment for beginners with overweight or obesity, who commonly have poor functional capacity and reduced physical fitness levels. However, weight-bearing aerobic exercise training, such as walking or jogging, has been reported as an effective training modality for improving bone metabolism among people with overweight or obesity during weight loss (Hinton et al. 2006). Importantly, traditional, equipment-based modalities may be boring for inexperienced clients with unhealthy weight, leading to low adherence and high attrition rates (Burgess et al. 2017).

In a personal training studio or home gym setting, access to a variety of cardio equipment is limited. Therefore, alternative aerobic-based activities are necessary during the introductory phase of a comprehensive warm-up session. Simple, low-intensity bodyweight movements can be performed in either a standing or seated position using a chair or stability ball. In any case, cardiopulmonary load should be conducted using a short (3- to 5-min), low-intensity (40%-50% of maximal effort or a rating of perceived exertion [RPE] of 9-11 on a scale of 6-20), and low-skill exercise protocol.

WARM-UP EXERCISES TO BUILD CARDIOPULMONARY LOAD

Seat Marching

Instructions

1. Sit tall on a chair, bench, or stability ball with the back off the backrest and the feet together and flat on the floor.
2. Moving from the hip, slightly lift the knees alternately while marching in place (*a*).
3. Prevent low-back rounding or excessive shifting to either side (*b*).

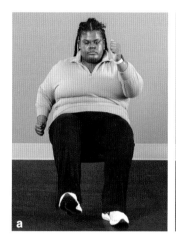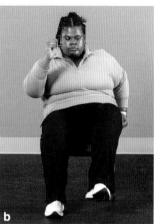

Training Tip

- Seat marching is recommended for deconditioned persons with overweight or obesity to increase heart rate, enhance hip mobility, and improve balance.

Standing Marching

Instructions

1. Stand with the feet hip-width apart.
2. Lift the knees alternately while marching in place, forward, backward, and side to side (*a*, *b*).

Training Tip

- Marching increases the heart rate, hip mobility, and balance.

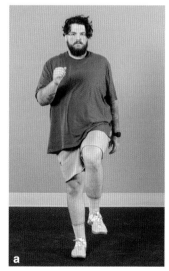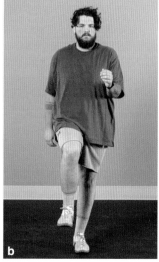

Stepping

Instructions

1. Stand with the feet hip-width apart in front of a low step platform (*a*).
2. Step up and down on the platform (*b*).

Training Tip

- This exercise is recommended for individuals with overweight or obesity who have no musculoskeletal health issues in the lower extremities.

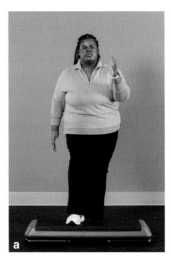
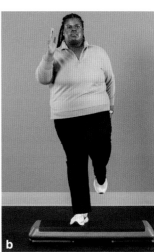

Mobility Exercises

Mobility work generally begins with activities involving the smaller joints and gradually progresses to larger, full-body motions. When working with a client with excess weight, this may be particularly important to understanding movement patterns and joint restrictions and encouraging appropriate intensities. Given that individuals with overweight or obesity often have poor spinal mobility due to prolonged sitting and inactivity (Heneghan et al. 2018), the overactive muscles should be highlighted after postural and functional movement assessments.

Each of the following mobility exercises should be performed for 15 to 20 seconds (8-12 repetitions) with a work-to-rest ratio of 1:1. All mobility exercises can be performed in either a standing or seated position (seated exercises are recommended for deconditioned persons or older adults with overweight or obesity). Also, myofascial release techniques, such as with a foam roller or massage ball and performed independently or with assistance from an exercise professional, can be very helpful within a dynamic warm-up routine, especially for deconditioned clients with overweight or obesity who struggle with chronic pain, stiffness, or any other dysfunctions in specific muscle groups. These techniques can also be used during a cool-down for pain relief, relaxation, and recovery.

Ideally, a few techniques targeted to specific muscle groups can help in addressing specific muscle hypertonicity and improving body functionality. Typically, two to three foam roller exercises (20-30 s per side or position) can be included in a comprehensive warm-up session at the beginning of the mobility work before static and dynamic stretching exercises. Such an approach can inhibit overactive muscles and improve flexibility, muscle recovery, and movement efficiency (Glänzel et al. 2023; Xiaoting et al. 2020).

Myofascial release may be painful for clients with excess weight, and therefore, it should be used with discretion for sedentary beginners with excess weight. A cautious approach may promote pain-free workouts with minimal discomfort and emotional stress, aiming to create positive exercise experiences for clients with overweight or obesity and with poor mental health or impaired functional capacity. Further details and suggested myofascial release exercises can be found in chapter 11.

WARM-UP EXERCISES TO IMPROVE MOBILITY

NECK EXERCISES

Neck Half Rotations

Instructions

1. Sit on a chair or bench with the feet shoulder-width apart.
2. Place the hands on the thighs (a).
3. Rotate the neck slowly to the left, looking over the shoulder (b).
4. Take the neck to a comfortable end of the range of motion.
5. Repeat to the right.

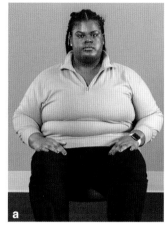
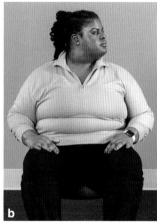

Neck Side Flexion

Instructions

1. Sit on a chair or bench with the feet shoulder-width apart.
2. Place the hands on the thighs (a).
3. Slowly draw the left ear toward the left shoulder, stopping for 1 to 2 s (b).
4. Take the neck to a comfortable end of the ROM.
5. Repeat to the right.

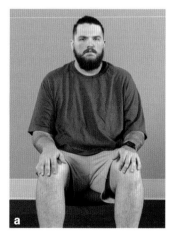
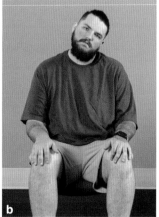

Training Tip

- Neck movements promote cervical spine mobility, enhancing activities of daily living and postural control.

JOINT EXERCISES

Wrist Circles

Instructions
1. Stand with the arms in the goalpost position.
2. Make small circles with the wrists, moving first in one direction (*a*) and then in the other (*b*).
3. Gradually increase the size of the circles.

Training Tip
- Wrist circles can help improve wrist mobility and reduce the risk of strains during exercises.

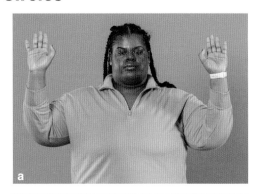

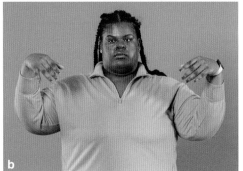

Ankle Rolls

Instructions
1. Stand with one foot slightly off the ground supported by a high chair.
2. Rotate the ankle in a circular motion, first clockwise (*a*) and then counterclockwise (*b*).
3. Perform 10 to 15 rotations with each ankle.

Training Tip
- Ankle rolls are essential for enhancing ankle mobility.

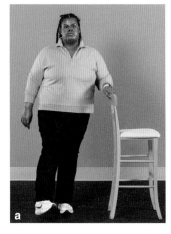

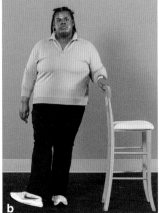

Shoulder Rolls

Instructions

1. Stand with the feet shoulder-width apart.
2. Let the arms hang by the sides.
3. Slowly roll the shoulders forward (*a*) and then backward (*b*).

Training Tip

- Perform 10 to 15 rolls in each direction to enhance shoulder mobility and reduce stiffness.

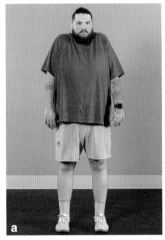
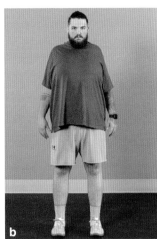

SHOULDER EXERCISES

Shoulder Circles

Instructions

1. Stand with the arms extended to the sides (*a*).
2. Move the arms in a circular motion, first forward and then backward (*b*).
3. Gradually increase the size of the circles.

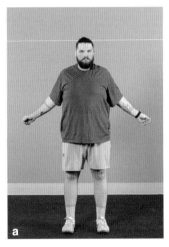
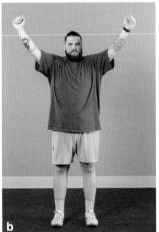

Arm Hugs

Instructions

1. Stand in an upright position, with the arms outstretched at the sides of the body at shoulder height (*a*).
2. Keeping the arms straight, embrace the upper body with both arms (*b*).
3. Repeat this motion, bringing the arms behind the back with each repetition.
4. Gradually increase the speed of movement, but always ensure a controlled tempo.

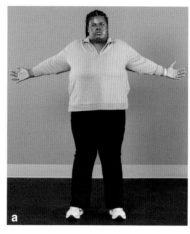
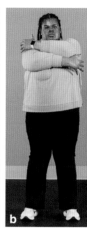

Arm Raises

Instructions

1. Stand with the arms down at the sides (*a*).
2. Move the arms in all directions, performing front raises (*b*), lateral raises (*c*), full-side lateral raises (*d*), and overhead presses (*e*).
3. Gradually increase the range of motion and speed of movement, but always ensure a controlled tempo.

Training Tips

- Shoulder moves help activate and prepare the glenohumeral joint for exercise.
- To avoid joint discomfort or blood pressure elevation, explosive execution is not recommended.

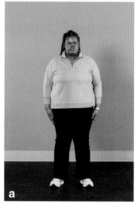
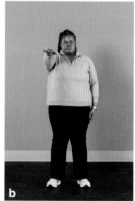
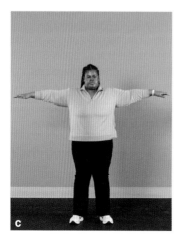
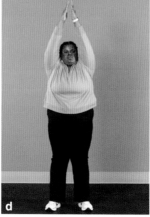
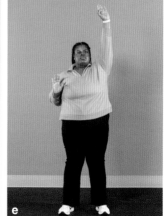

<u>CORE MOVES</u>

Torso Rotations

Instructions

1. Stand with the feet shoulder-width apart and the arms extended out to the sides.

2. Rotate the torso to the right (*a*) and then to the left (*b*) in a controlled manner.

Training Tip

- Torso rotations enhance thoracic spine mobility and prepare the core for exercise.

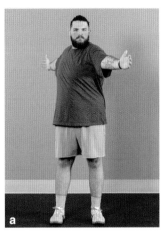
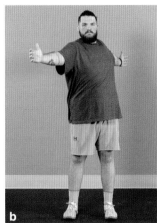

Torso and Hip Rotations

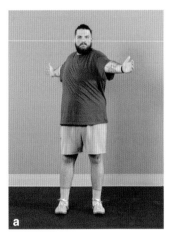
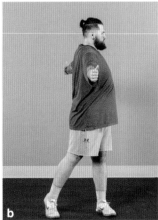
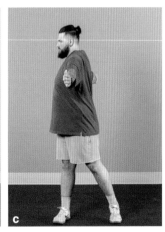

Instructions

1. Stand with your feet shoulder-width apart and the arms extended out to the sides (*a*).

2. Rotate the torso and hips to the left (*b*) and then to the right (*c*) in a controlled manner.

Training Tip

- Torso and hip rotations enhance thoracic spine and hip mobility and prepare the core for exercise.

Hip Rotations

Instructions

1. Stand with the feet shoulder-width apart.
2. Grasp a stick and extend the arms out to the front (*a*).
3. Rotate one hip to the left and then to the right in a controlled manner (*b*).
4. Repeat with the opposite leg.

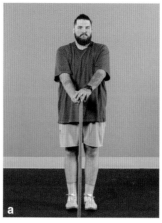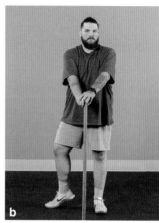

Training Tip

• Hip rotations enhance hip mobility and prepare the core for exercise.

Diagonal Chop

Instructions

1. Stand with the feet shoulder-width apart.
2. Hold a Pilates mini ball or lightweight object with both hands.
3. Perform diagonal chopping motions from the shoulder down to the opposite hip (*a*) and back up (*b*).

Training Tip

• This exercise engages the core and helps prepare for functional movements.

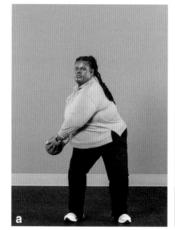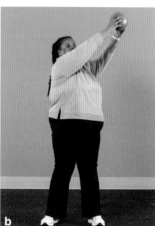

Static and Dynamic Stretching

Stretching precautions for individuals with excess weight should be carefully considered. Exercise professionals should start by implementing easy stretches that can be performed in either a standing or seated position. Additionally, stretches on the ground may often be challenging and uncomfortable, and thus, a padded mat or alternative positions are highly recommended. Typically, after reducing tension in overactive muscles using foam rolling, it is time to implement a mixture of static and dynamic stretches. For static stretching, using short holds lasting 15 to 30 seconds is appropriate for lengthening some overly tight muscles. Although research shows that static stretching during a warm-up decreases physical performance among athletes (Chaabene et al. 2019), previously inactive individuals with obesity can benefit from the use of some static stretches in combination with dynamic stretches. Hence, short-duration static stretching (2-3 targeted exercises) should be conducted before dynamic stretches, and this is a critical part of the warm-up routine before activating the underactive muscles to prepare them for exercise. Further details and recommended static stretches for clients with overweight or obesity are presented in chapter 11. For dynamic stretching, a back-and-forth motion to the end range of a stretch that targets specific overactive muscles (2-3 targeted exercises for 15-30 s per side or position) is highly recommended for all clients with excess weight. One example of the many dynamic exercises professionals could choose is quadruped cat–cow.

Quadruped Cat–Cow

Instructions

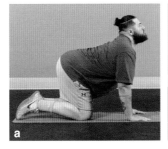
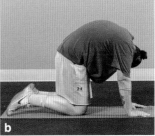

1. Begin on the hands and knees in table pose, with a neutral spine and the knees in line with the hips.
2. While inhaling, lift the sit bones upward, press the chest forward, and drop the belly while lifting the head, relaxing the shoulders away from the ears, and gazing straight ahead (*a*).
3. While exhaling, round the spine outward, tuck in the tailbone, draw the pubic bone forward, and release the head toward the floor (*b*).

Training Tips

- This exercise promotes spinal mobilization without the joint compression that regularly occurs during standing movements.
- The exercise can be included in both the warm-up and cool-down phases of a workout.

Movement Preparation and Remediation

After performing the mobility exercises for specific joints and muscles using foam rolling and stretching, the next phase of a warm-up routine is to enhance the functional kinetic chain by activating postural muscles. To do this, specific movements designed to remedy faulty movement patterns should be correctly performed. Such an approach improves dysfunctional movement patterns commonly observed among inactive individuals with obesity, who may be negatively affecting their movement and performance when engaging in activities of daily living. In this phase of the warm-up, more focus needs to be placed on the exercise selection and movement quality and less focus on choosing the most appropriate exercise training scheme (i.e., sets and repetitions). Typically, 1 to 2 sets of 8 to 12 repetitions per exercise, with a work-to-rest ratio of 1:1, is recommended.

EXERCISES FOR MOVEMENT PREPARATION AND REMEDIATION

Abdominal Hollowing

Instructions

1. Sit on a chair, bench, or stability ball with the feet shoulder-width apart.
2. Place the hands on the thighs.
3. Draw in the belly button to activate the deep abdominal muscles.
4. Maintain a neutral spine for 2 to 3 s. The head should remain level, with the eyes focused ahead.

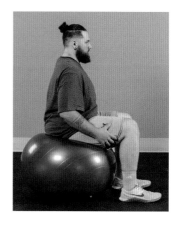

Training Tips

- This exercise engages the core and is recommended to improve performance of low- or moderate-intensity activities, such as daily tasks, Pilates classes, or rehabilitation sessions.

- Hollowing can also be performed in a quadruped position (i.e., on all fours) or while standing (close to a wall). A supine (lying) position may be uncomfortable for clients with excess weight.

Abdominal Bracing

Instructions

1. Sit on a chair, bench, or stability ball with the feet shoulder-width apart.
2. Place the hands on the thighs.
3. Contract both the deep and superficial trunk muscles isometrically, as if expecting to be punched in the belly.

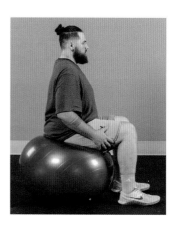

Training Tips

- This exercise provides core stiffness, creates lumbar spine stability, prevents chronic low-back pain, and is recommended for complex movements and high-intensity activities such as weight training.

- Bracing can also be performed in a quadruped position (i.e., on all fours) or while standing (close to a wall). A supine (lying) position may be uncomfortable for clients with excess weight.

Glute Bridge

Instructions

1. Lie supine, with the knees bent and the feet flat on the ground.
2. Squeeze the glutes and lift the hips off the ground (*a*).
3. Lower the hips back to the ground (*b*).

Training Tip

- Glute activation enhances hip stability and prepares the core for stabilization.

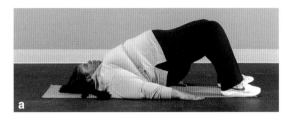

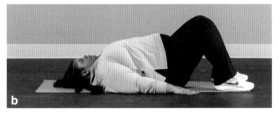

Bird Dog

Instructions

1. Start in a quadruped position (i.e., on all fours) and keep the spine neutral (*a*).
2. Extend one arm straight out, keeping it in line with the torso (*b*).
3. Straighten the opposite leg and raise it, maintaining a neutral spine (*c*).
4. Pause for one count at the top.
5. Return to the start position and repeat with the other arm and leg.

Training Tips

- This exercise generates shoulder and hip mobility as well as lumber spine stability during movement of the upper and lower extremities.
- Deconditioned clients with excess weight may perform this exercise partially (i.e., raising only one arm or leg at a time) to gradually master the whole movement.

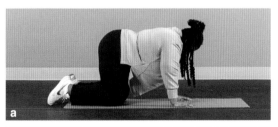

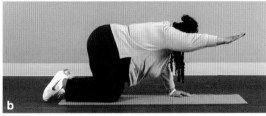

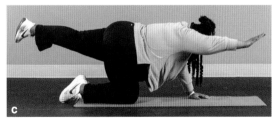

Quadruped Thoracic Rotations

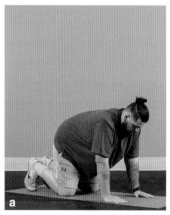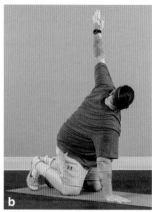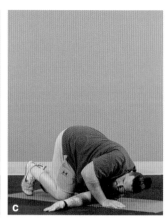

Instructions

1. Start in a quadruped position (i.e., on all fours), keeping the spine neutral (*a*).
2. Lift one arm, then externally rotate the chest (*b*).
3. Slide the lifted hand underneath the supporting hand, turning the ribcage to reach through (*c*).
4. Lift the elbow to turn the ribcage away from the support arm.
5. Repeat on the other side.

Training Tip

- This exercise increases thoracic spine and glenohumeral mobility in a user-friendly position for individuals with excess weight.

Back-to-Wall Shoulder Flexion

Instructions

1. Stand with the back pressed against a wall and the feet shoulder-width apart (*a*).
2. Lift one arm overhead while keeping it straight. Try to touch the thumb to the wall without needing to arch the back (*b*).
3. Keep the core engaged throughout the movement.

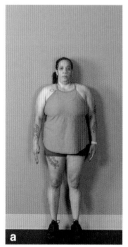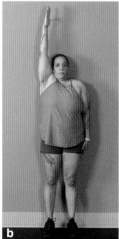

Training Tips

- This exercise promotes overhead shoulder mobility and lumbar spine stability.
- The lying version (supine shoulder flexion) is not recommended for individuals with excess weight, because it may put them into an uncomfortable position due to a larger waist circumference that can impede breathing patterns.

Wall Slides

Instructions

1. Stand facing a wall with the feet hip-width apart.
2. Flex the elbows to 90°, and press the forearms into the wall (*a*).
3. Lift the arms overhead, sliding them along the wall (keep the elbows against the wall throughout the movement) (*b*).
4. Engage the core throughout the exercise.

Training Tips

- This exercise promotes overhead shoulder mobility, scapular stability, and lumbar spine stability.
- The lying version (supine floor slides) is not recommended for individuals with excess weight, because it may put them into an uncomfortable position due to a larger waist circumference that can impede breathing patterns.

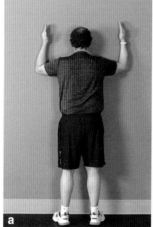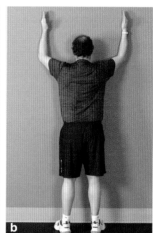

Reverse Elbow Push-Up

Instructions

1. Stand against a wall with the feet shoulder-width apart.
2. Put a foam roller at the middle of the back and push it against the wall.
3. Keep the elbows out and the chest lifted, and push off the elbows (*a*).
4. Squeeze the shoulder blades together, holding the contraction for 2 or 3 s (*b*).

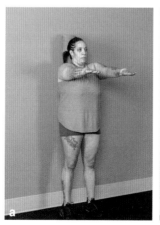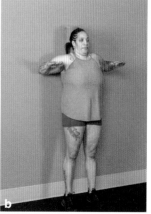

Training Tips

- This exercise promotes scapular and lumbar spine stability.
- The lying version (supine elbow push-ups) is not recommended for individuals with excess weight; it may put them into an uncomfortable position due to instability, and a larger waist circumference can impede breathing patterns.

Standing Leg Swings

Instructions

1. Stand next to a support at the side (a wall or chair) for balance.
2. Swing one leg forward and backward (*a*), maintaining a straight posture (*b*).
3. Complete the swinging motion for the desired number of repetitions, then switch to the other side.

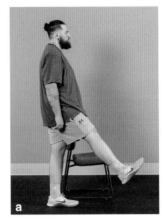 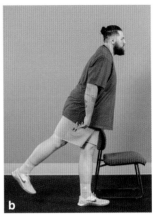

Training Tip

• Keep the swinging leg relaxed, and move it within a comfortable range of motion.

Supported Bodyweight Half Squats

Instructions

1. Stand with the feet shoulder-width apart in front of a support (such as a chair) for balance (*a*).
2. Slowly lower the body by bending the knees and hips, keeping the back straight (*b*).
3. Go as low as mobility allows without feeling discomfort or pain.
4. Push through the heels to return to the starting position.

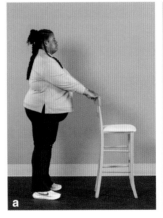 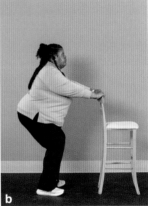

Training Tip

• Focus on proper form and alignment. Ensure optimum coordination of the kinetic chain.

Neuromuscular Activation

A comprehensive warm-up routine should include a phase targeting the central nervous system and muscular activation as well as cognitive processing for engagement. This phase should occur at the end of the dynamic warm-up and before entering the conditioning phase (main part) of an exercise session. Among people characterized by poor functional capacity, low-intensity and low-skill drills should be provided in this phase, aiming to promote agility, balance, coordination, and reactivity (Pataky et al. 2014).

Fitness games are excellent options for this purpose, delivering smart, innovative, movement-based opportunities for a warm-up experience that enhances recreation and positively contributes to the development of cognitive function (Mandolesi et al. 2018). Such a strategy mixes fun with appropriate intensity and complexity for long-term fitness success and engagement in body movement. Many people considering an exercise program mistakenly believe that recreation and exercise cannot be connected. For these individuals, turning fitness into games reconnects elements of fun and play with physical exercise. User-friendly fitness games incorporate feasible, nontraditional drills into a real-world exercise setting adapted for people with excess weight. This is crucial, given that these individuals often present with cognitive decline or poor mental health and have high dropout and low adherence rates (Quaye et al. 2023; Viester at al. 2013).

Ideally, fitness games are used as an extension of a dynamic warm-up in preparation for cardiorespiratory, muscle-strengthening, and neuromotor activities. Fun, movement-based drills improve motor skills in people with unhealthy weight, increasing functional capacity levels. In addition, these activities promote the emotional connection between exercise professionals and clients in various fitness settings. Fitness games should involve short (3-5 min), low- to moderate-intensity drills (50%-60% of maximal effort or an RPE of 10-12 on a scale of 6-20). The principal goals of fitness games are to activate the central nervous system and to learn new movement patterns without inducing fatigue.

Engaging clients who have obesity in fitness games can make the warm-up more enjoyable and motivating by mixing fun with a suitable intensity. This is important because fun appears to be one of the primary missing elements of fitness programs for clients with excess weight in the health and fitness industry worldwide. Exercise professionals should not underestimate their role in playing short fitness games with their clients; partner- or team-based warm-up drills may be an effective exercise engagement strategy, promoting inclusion and gamification that result in positive fitness experiences in either a personal or small-group training setting.

Special Considerations for Fitness Games

- Very simple drills should be implemented at first. Most games can be modified to be played with two or more clients while providing enough challenges for progress.

- Fitness games can be used in either a personal training setting, where the exercise professional is the client's partner, or in small-group training (two or more clients).

- For deconditioned clients, exercise professionals should select games primarily focusing on fun and interaction rather than physical demands. Once the client's physical fitness levels rise, more physically challenging games can be incorporated.

- To avoid boredom and lack of enthusiasm among clients, fitness games should not be the same in every session. Exercise professionals should periodically rotate and gradually advance their selections.

- Fitness games should be a short part of a dynamic warm-up (i.e., 30-60 s per game, totaling 2-3 min per session). Such an approach maintains exercise intensity and pleasure in a safe environment adapted for previously inactive clients with physical limitations and impaired functionality.

- Fitness games may make some clients feel uncomfortable or afraid of looking foolish if they make a mistake. Thus, exercise professionals should explain that such movement-based drills help improve motor skills and support body functionality, not only in gym-based exercises but also in activities of daily living.

- Asking clients to perform one easy movement while having to do something else is an excellent physical multitasking solution for improving functional capacity.

FITNESS GAMES FOR NEUROMUSCULAR ACTIVATION

Toe Touch

Instructions

1. This game is played in pairs. Two people begin by facing away from each other and trying to touch their opponent's toes.
2. The person who touches their partner's toes first wins.
3. Once the pair plays three rounds, mix up the pairs to provide clients with the opportunity to challenge other members in the session.

Training Tip

- This partner warm-up game and team-building exercise improves agility, balance, and coordination. For safety reasons, it should not be played very competitively.

Hit the Target

Instructions

1. This game is played in pairs. Two people begin by facing away from each other.
2. One person tries to touch their partner's hand; the opponent continuously moves their hand, aiming to challenge and surprise their partner.
3. The person who hits the target gets one point.
4. Once the allotted time (30 s) is up, the pair switches roles.
5. Once the pair plays two or three rounds, the person with the highest number of points wins.

Training Tip

- This is a partner warm-up game encouraging agility, reactivity, stamina, and hand–eye coordination. To allow clients to react properly and safely, the game should not be played too fast.

Pizza Delivery

Instructions

1. Create a medium-sized activity area, using four cones or weight plates to mark boundaries.
2. Give each client a flying disc or exercise balance pad.
3. Ask clients to walk throughout the activity area while balancing their "pizza" on the palm of their hand without allowing it to be knocked to the floor by another player.
4. At the same time, clients will work to knock other players' pizzas to the ground.
5. When a client's pizza falls to the floor, that client gets one point, moves to the perimeter and speed walks laps or performs 10 chair squats, then rebalances their pizza and continues playing.
6. Once the allotted time (30 s) is up, the client with the lowest number of points wins.

Training Tip

- This game is an individual physical challenge encouraging cardiovascular activity and improving agility and hand–eye coordination.

Balloon Volleyball

Instructions

1. Set up a net using a rope or a piece of fabric.
2. Use a balloon as the volleyball.
3. Pairs or teams take turns batting the balloon over the net, trying to score points.

Training Tip

- This game encourages cardiovascular activity and improves hand–eye coordination.

Balloon Party

Instructions

1. A group of clients forms a circle by facing in toward the center. Each client is given one balloon.
2. All clients hit their balloons, then try to keep all the balloons in the air.
3. Any balloon can be hit by any participant.
4. The goal is to maintain all balloons in the air throughout the game.

Training Tip

- This group-based game encourages agility, reactivity, and hand–eye coordination.

Musical Chair Squats

Instructions

1. Place a few chairs in a circle.
2. Play music and have clients walk around the chairs.
3. When the music stops, clients must quickly find a chair and perform squats until the music starts again.

Training Tips

- This game adds an element of fun, incorporates squat exercises, and improves balance and reactivity.
- Alternatively, stability balls on a base can be used instead of chairs.

Catch or Crash

Instructions

1. Two people face each other a good distance apart. Each holds a stability ball.
2. One player says "One, two, three, shoot," at which point each player throws their stability ball to the other person in one of three ways: overhead pass, chest pass, or bounce pass.
3. If the players choose the same method of toss, the balls will collide and bounce back toward the thrower, and each person will have to chase their ball down.
4. If the players choose different methods for the toss, they should try to catch the ball that was thrown by the other player.

Training Tip

- This game promotes cardiovascular activity and improves agility and reactivity.

Kneeling Side-Plank Circle

Instructions

1. A group of people forms a circle by facing in toward the center, with everyone lying on the same side (i.e., their right or left).
2. Depending on the size of the circle and number of people, use two or three stability balls.
3. Have everyone lift themselves into a kneeling side-plank position, and ensure they use proper form.
4. Roll the stability balls toward people in the circle. They will use their top arm or top leg to punch or kick the ball back into the circle and toward other players.

Training Tip

- This team-building and muscle-activation exercise enhances core stability in a fun way.

Two Butts and a Ball

Instructions

1. Client A and client B (or the trainer) sit back-to-back on a stability ball.
2. Client A stands up and sits back down.
3. When client B (or the trainer) feels the impact of client A sitting on the ball, client B (or the trainer) immediately stands up and sits back down.
4. Both individuals continue doing alternating squats on the stability ball.

Training Tip

- This partnered, muscle-activation exercise promotes reactivity, balance, and coordination.

Teamwork Wall Ball

Instructions

1. Client A and client B (or the trainer) stand next to each other facing a wall.
2. Using a stability ball or light medicine ball, client A performs a wall-ball throw and slides to the left immediately after releasing the ball.
3. Client B (or the trainer) simultaneously steps to the left in time to catch the ball, immediately performing a wall ball throw and sliding to the right as client A slides to the right in time to catch the ball.

Training Tip

- This partnered, muscle-activation exercise encourages agility and coordination.

Walk and Carry

Instructions

1. This game is played in groups of two or more people. Place a few cones or weight plates on the ground, spaced every 9 to 16 ft (3-5 m).
2. On the count of three, the first person of each group walks forward, carrying a stability ball or light medicine ball (4-11 lb [2-5 kg]), places the ball on the first point, and returns to the starting point.
3. The next person from each team walks to the first point and brings the stability ball back.
4. This continues until each team member completes a turn and returns all stability balls to the starting point.
5. The fastest team wins.

Training Tip

• This team-building game encourages stamina, reactivity, and coordination in a fun way.

Exercise Add-On Memory Game

Instructions

1. One person chooses a bodyweight exercise (exercise 1) and performs one repetition.
2. The next person chooses a different bodyweight exercise (exercise 2) and performs one repetition each of exercises 1 and 2.
3. The next person (or the first person, if only two people are playing) chooses another bodyweight exercise (exercise 3) and performs one repetition each of exercises 1, 2, and 3.
4. This continues until someone forgets one of the exercises in the sequence.

Training Tip

• This team-building game promotes cognitive function through a feasible physical challenge.

Physical Multitasking Game

Instructions

1. The client goes for a walk, bringing along a tennis ball and tossing it back and forth, playing catch with a small stick, kicking a pebble down the street, or hitting a balloon.
2. The additional movement must be performed while the client is walking in the fitness room or outdoors.

Training Tip

• This warm-up game enhances cognitive abilities while recreationally promoting body movement.

CHAPTER SUMMARY

Incorporating an appropriate warm-up routine is a fundamental aspect of any exercise program for clients with obesity. It helps prepare the body physically and psychologically for exercise, ensuring a safe and effective workout. By implementing general and dynamic warm-up drills and incorporating user-friendly fitness games, exercise experiences for clients with obesity can be enhanced, promoting better adherence to their fitness goals. It is essential for a knowledgeable exercise professional to tailor warm-up routines to the specific needs and preferences of each individual, promoting their long-term success in managing obesity through inclusive exercise strategies. This chapter equips professionals with the skills and knowledge they need to deliver a warm-up routine that builds up to a safe and effective exercise session. By providing drills, instructions, and tips, the chapter serves as a step-by-step guide for professionals to help clients with excess weight achieve their exercise goals while having fun.

KEY POINTS

- A warm-up routine at the beginning of an exercise session helps clients with obesity to prepare physically, improving exercise performance while reducing injury risk.
- A warm-up routine also helps clients prepare psychologically, becoming more comfortable with movement patterns while gaining confidence.
- Fitness professionals can use the warm-up to build rapport with their clients and can take this time to understand clients' goals and preferences.
- A library of general and dynamic warm-up drills helps fitness professionals progress clients from smaller joint activities to larger, full-body movements.
- Real-world applications can help professionals understand how to implement these detailed instructions and training tips in practice.

CHAPTER QUIZ

Quiz answers can be found in the appendix.

1. The warm-up is primarily about increasing the intensity of exercise quickly.
   a. true
   b. false

2. Gradually increasing the heart rate during a warm-up can help reduce the risk of cardiovascular issues in clients with obesity.
   a. true
   b. false

3. The warm-up phase is NOT essential for psychological preparation, particularly for individuals with obesity.
   a. true
   b. false

4. A warm-up improves muscle coordination, which is NOT critical for obese clients' exercise safety.
   a. true
   b. false

5. A well-structured warm-up can help activate dormant muscles, making exercises more effective.
   a. true
   b. false

6. What is one of the primary purposes of a warm-up routine?
   a. rapid weight loss
   b. psychological stress
   c. temperature regulation
   d. decreased muscle function

7. Why is temperature regulation important during the warm-up?
   a. to make the client sweat excessively
   b. to prevent the client from feeling cold
   c. to improve muscle function and flexibility
   d. to reduce heart rate

8. Which of the following is an example of a general warm-up drill?
   a. bench press
   b. bodyweight squats
   c. deadlifts
   d. pull-ups

9. What is the primary goal of dynamic warm-up drills using the joint-by-joint approach?
   a. increasing muscle size
   b. enhancing joint mobility and stability
   c. reducing heart rate
   d. decreasing flexibility

10. Which fitness game can be used to improve hand–eye coordination and encourage cardiovascular activity in clients with obesity?
    a. musical chair squats
    b. balloon volleyball
    c. weightlifting contest
    d. tug of war

CASE STUDY

Case study answers can be found in the appendix.

Meg, a professional who specializes in working with clients with obesity, meets Beth for an introductory session. During the warm-up routine, Meg takes a client-centered approach to understanding Beth's needs and preferences. She asks about Beth's previous experience with exercise and learns that Beth used to belong to a nearby health and fitness center but left because she did not feel comfortable there. Beth mentions that she had trouble moving between the tightly packed treadmills and the stationary bikes—her favorite pieces of cardio equipment—and disliked all the mirrors on the walls. Meg also asks about Beth's exercise goals and learns that Beth is interested in working with a professional to increase stamina and reduce fatigue. When Meg digs a little deeper, she learns that Beth's granddaughter just turned 2 years old, and Beth wants to be able to keep up with the increasingly mobile toddler when she is babysitting her. Meg finds out that Beth suffers from arthritis in her wrists, which can make certain exercises particularly painful.

1. A _____ approach helps professionals understand their clients' needs and preferences and meet them where they are.
   a. professional-centered
   b. client-centered
   c. judgmental
   d. motivational

2. All of the following are ways professionals can build rapport with clients with obesity EXCEPT
   a. asking them about their goals and motivations
   b. asking them about their exercise likes and dislikes
   c. checking whether they feel comfortable in the physical space
   d. telling them to lose 20 lb

3. Name three ways Meg can build Beth's comfort level with her and the facility.

4. Based on what you know of Beth's experience with exercise and her limitations, what is one warm-up drill you would recommend that Meg avoid?

5. Based on what you know of Beth's experience with exercise and her likes and dislikes, what is one warm-up drill you would recommend that Meg include?

CHAPTER 8

Muscular Fitness

Alexios Batrakoulis, PhD, Michael Stack, BS, and Kia Williams, MS

After completing this chapter, you will be able to

- describe psychophysiological adaptations to resistance training,
- explore myths and misconceptions linked to resistance training,
- demonstrate how to use gym equipment, body weight, and partner-assisted manual resistance training exercises,
- administer progressions and modifications of fundamental movement patterns, and
- conduct muscular fitness activities in various exercise settings.

According to the current exercise prescription guidelines with respect to resistance training for people with impaired cardiometabolic health, metabolic dysregulation, and other health complications, muscle strengthening is considered a vital tool for inducing beneficial alterations in numerous health and fitness indicators (Jensen et al. 2014; Lopez et al. 2022; Paluch et al. 2024). In many respects, the acute and chronic responses to resistance training are similar for individuals with obesity compared to their counterparts with healthy weights (Redinger 2007). However, due to the pathophysiology of obesity, subtle but important differences exist (Sale 1988). The following sections will explore the acute and chronic responses to resistance training and the role obesity plays in modifying these responses.

Physiological Responses to Resistance Training

Broadly, there are two types of responses to exercise: acute and chronic. Acute responses occur immediately during or shortly after a single exercise session, involving changes such as increased heart rate, muscle swelling, and hormonal fluctuations. In contrast, chronic responses develop over time (weeks to months to years) with consistent training and lead to long-term adaptations, such as increased muscle mass, strength gains, and enhanced metabolic capacity.

Acute Physiological Responses

Multiple body systems are necessary to successfully produce the immediate muscular contractions characteristic of resistance training. The central nervous system plays a prominent role in initiating muscle contraction through the motor cortex; efferent motor pathways carry signals from the motor cortex to individual motor units that recruit muscle fibers to produce force (Williams et al. 2007).

The cardiovascular system provides another level of systemic acute responses to resistance training. Increases in heart rate, stroke volume, and cardiac output are common during resistance training and become particularly pronounced in higher-repetition or circuit-based resistance training (Kraemer et al. 2020). These increases are in part driven by a surge in catecholamine levels in response to the homeostatic disruption brought about by resistance training. Moreover, the cardiovascular system shunts blood flow away from nonessential areas to the active muscle mass, resulting in a modest amount of local edema in that muscle. In addition to the catecholamine response, there is a robust, acute steroid hormone response to resistance training, with both testosterone and cortisol levels rising during the resistance training bout (Fortunato et al. 2018). Insulin levels modestly decrease during resistance training, in part due to the influence of increased catecholamines.

Increased levels of anaerobic glycolysis generate the adenosine triphosphate (ATP) needed to fuel muscle contraction. This not only increases muscle temperature via the release of excess metabolic heat but also decreases pH (resulting in a more acidic internal environment within the muscle) while depleting glycogen stores. Mechanical damage to muscle fibers occurs due to the tension caused by the external load. This mechanical damage results in a significant immunological response, increasing levels of inflammatory cytokines to repair the damaged tissue (Škarabot et al. 2021).

Chronic Physiological Responses

In response to resistance training over time, the central nervous system lowers the threshold for activation of the motor cortex and motor units at the local level of the muscle (Ozaki et al. 2013). Improved recruitment and synchronization of motor units increase force production. Reduced sensitization of the Golgi tendon organs and increased sensitization of muscle spindles improve the reflexive response to resistance training, allowing for greater force production.

Although resistance training is not often associated with cardiovascular adaptations, such chronic adaptations do also occur. Improvements in stroke volume (and, therefore, cardiac output) take place as a result of left ventricular hypertrophy. Improvements in cardiac output, along with increased capillarization and greater oxygen difference between arteries and veins, drive improvement in the maximal rate of oxygen consumption ($\dot{V}O_2max$) (Kraemer and Ratamess 2005). This response is even more pronounced with circuit-based resistance training.

Resistance training also leads to chronic hormonal adaptations. Testosterone and growth hormone levels tend to increase over time in resistance-trained individuals (Kraemer and Ratamess 2005). Research on long-term changes in resting cortisol levels in response to resistance training is mixed, with some studies suggesting no change and other studies suggesting a decrease (Oppert et al. 2021). One of the hallmark chronic adaptations to resistance training on an endocrine level is improved insulin sensitivity

(Damas et al. 2016). This is a very important chronic adaptation for individuals with obesity, because research shows these individuals tend to have impaired insulin sensitivity.

The adaptation most commonly associated with resistance training is increased muscle fiber size, or myofibrillar hypertrophy (Bellicha et al. 2021). When increased muscle size is coupled with the aforementioned neurological adaptations, the result is increased levels of muscular force and power production. Increasing muscle fiber size, strength, and power is particularly important for individuals who are undergoing active obesity treatment with calorie restriction. In calorie-restricted states, significant amounts of muscle mass and strength can be lost. Using resistance training to minimize these reductions in muscle mass and function can increase the likelihood of maintaining weight loss and can improve overall functional capacity following a calorie-restriction intervention (Edge et al. 2006). Regular engagement in muscle-strengthening activities can also play an important role in reversing sarcopenia (loss of muscle tissue). This is important, because sarcopenia, commonly observed in people with obesity, is associated with poor functionality, low quality of life, and premature aging (Sorace et al. 2024).

From a metabolic perspective, at the local muscle level, hydrogen ion buffering capacity increases with resistance training over time. This leads to an improved physiological ability to tolerate the anaerobic production of lactic acid (Walowski et al. 2020).

Obesity's Influence on Physiological Responses

Obesity can have some important effects on the physiological responses to resistance training. Initially, individuals with higher body weight tend to have greater levels of muscle mass and strength, due to the need to support excess fat mass (Kulkarni et al. 2016). While this is positive, to some degree, in terms of the ability to produce additional force, care should still be taken by people with obesity when performing novel resistance training. Furthermore, excess weight can cause issues with biomechanics, proprioception, balance, and general motor control. Likewise, excess weight on load-bearing joints can result in deterioration of articular cartilage, joint pain, and reductions in range of motion (Zorena et al. 2020).

Hormonally, obesity is characteristically associated with insulin resistance, which can alter glucose metabolism and impair energy production during exercise. Increased levels of adiposity due to obesity have been shown to pathologically increase inflammatory cytokines, referred to as adipokines (Speakman et al. 2018). These adipokines can blunt positive physiological adaptations to resistance training (of note, adipokines differ from myokines, the positive inflammatory cytokines that are released from muscle tissue during resistance training). Obesity has also been shown to depress testosterone and growth hormone levels. The net effect of increased adipokine activity, along with decreased testosterone and growth hormone, can result in impaired recovery and an impaired overall adaptive response from resistance training.

Obesity can also impair the thermoregulatory ability to dissipate increased levels of metabolic heat generated during exercise. This impaired thermoregulatory response can acutely limit resistance training performance (Elkington et al. 2017). In addition, obesity is associated with numerous chronic diseases and comorbidities that can have wide-ranging physiological effects. When prescribing a resistance training routine, practitioners are encouraged to understand the indications and contraindications associated with these chronic conditions and how they affect a particular individual.

Psychological Responses to Resistance Training

Psychological responses to resistance training encompass a broad range of mental and emotional changes that occur during regular participation in resistance exercise. These responses can include improved mood, increased self-esteem, and a reduction in feelings of depression and anxiety. Whereas the physiological responses to resistance training are quite predictable and fairly consistent between individuals, psychological responses can vary considerably (Schwarz and Kindermann 1992). This variation exists irrespective of body weight or body composition, but as discussed in the following section, obesity can certainly complicate psychological factors. It is important to keep this significant interindividual variation in mind when reading the subsequent section.

Acute Psychological Responses

Much like acute physiological responses, acute psychological responses occur during and immediately after exercise and can last for minutes to a couple of hours. These acute responses can be either positive or negative, with individual perception driving the specific connotation.

One hallmark of an acute psychological response to resistance training is an increase in levels of endogenous opiates. Endogenous opiates can result in feelings of euphoria (the so-called runner's high) as well as improvements in mood and in overall affect (Ten Hoor at al. 2017). Endogenous opiates likely cause the reduction in anxiety and depressive feelings that is often reported following resistance training. Resistance training may also distract individuals from worrisome and anxiety-provoking thoughts. Other positive, acute psychological responses to resistance training include mental and cognitive clarity, increased focus and concentration, a sense of accomplishment, improved confidence, and better self-image (Levinger et al. 2009).

Conversely, for some individuals, resistance training can result in a negative psychological response (Stone et al. 2007). Fatigue associated with a taxing resistance training session can result in a negative response. Performance anxiety before and during a resistance training session can also occur, particularly if the session is performed in a high-stress situation (e.g., a new workout or one taking place at a new gym or in front of peers). Frustration or disappointment can occur if performance during a resistance training workout does not meet the individual's expectations. In addition, individuals with body dysmorphia can experience reduced or worsened body image. This can be exacerbated by exercising in revealing clothing, in front of mirrors, or with other individuals.

Chronic Psychological Responses

Much like chronic physiological responses, chronic psychological responses occur over time (weeks to months to years) with prolonged training. There is also variation in the chronic psychological responses to resistance training. However, one would expect these responses to be more psychologically favorable, because individuals who derive negative acute psychological responses to resistance training likely would not persist with it long enough to accumulate more chronic adaptations. Chronic responses to resistance training vary with individual perception but mostly carry a positive connotation. Keeping that in mind, research (Rajan and Menon 2017) shows that resistance training can chronically

- reduce depression, anxiety, and other mental health disorders;
- reduce age-related cognitive decline;
- reduce risk of Alzheimer's disease and dementia;
- improve energy levels and mood;
- improve self-confidence and self-esteem;
- improve memory, concentration, focus, and cognitive performance; and
- improve body image.

Obesity's Influence on Psychological Responses

The psychology of obesity is complex. Lower levels of mental health, higher prevalence of diagnosable mental illness (Puhl and Heuer 2010), and weight stigma (Carraça et al. 2021) are very real factors that can exacerbate the negative psychological effects previously mentioned while minimizing the positive effects. As always, significant interindividual variability will exist, but research suggests that obesity complicates the psychological effects of resistance training (Carraça et al. 2021).

Although current evidence indicates that many of the positive acute and chronic responses mentioned previously are as prevalent, if not more so, for individuals with obesity as for those with healthy weight, individuals with obesity also have an increased risk of a negative psychological response. Primary areas of caution are anxiety, self-confidence, self-esteem, and body image. Obesity, when coupled with lower levels of physical activity, may result in significant anxiety about resistance training due to a lack of experience and technical competence (Carraça et al. 2021). Furthermore, those who have not engaged in resistance training before can lack confidence and self-efficacy.

Poor body image due to weight stigma, as well as persistent negative thoughts, can compound the negative psychological effects of resistance training (Pedersen 2010). However, the psychological story is not all doom and gloom. Obesity can result in high levels of muscle mass and more strength. As a result, an individual with obesity may be stronger than peers, which could improve self-confidence. Additionally, because resistance training typically has a lower cardiovascular response than aerobic exercise, it may be more psychologically enjoyable for individuals with obesity, resulting in a more positive affective response.

Debunking Obesity-Related Myths and Misconceptions Linked to Resistance Training

Many myths and misconceptions persist around resistance training and its role in obesity and weight management. Often, these myths have been propagated by fit individuals who lack knowledge of the evidence base, yet they gain credibility due to their aesthetics. In other cases, these myths have their roots in the misunderstanding or evolution of the research over time. In either case, resistance training has been significantly linked to myths and fallacies regarding its impact on body composition and physical performance among individuals with excess body weight and adiposity.

Myth 1: Resistance training turns fat into muscle, while muscle turns into fat after a person stops exercising.

Fact: Fat and muscle are distinct and different tissues. They are structurally and functionally different. They are also synthesized and degraded through different physiological pathways. The loss or gain of one is independent of the loss or gain of the other. Many individuals perceive a reduction in muscle tone and definition when they cease regular exercise, which is a largely aesthetic phenomenon. When exercise is discontinued, there is a noticeable shift in body composition and muscle cells undergo atrophy. In the absence of sufficient calorie expenditure, fat cells proliferate, resulting in a softer physique (Bavaresco Gambassi et al. 2024; Encarnação et al. 2022).

Myth 2: Aerobic exercise, not resistance training, is best for individuals with obesity.
Fact: Resistance training can assist in maintaining muscle size and strength during periods of significant energy-intake restriction. Through resistance training, individuals can better maintain their metabolic rate and functional capacity after weight loss. Fitness professionals should not view the choice of aerobic versus resistance exercise as mutually exclusive; rather, they should view these modes of exercise as equally important and complementary (Etchison 2011).

Myth 3: Building muscle supercharges metabolism.
Fact: Muscle mass is, indeed, metabolically active tissue. It is a big driver of basal (resting) metabolism. Research suggests that one additional pound of muscle burns an additional 7 to 10 calories per day (Etchison 2011). That said, given the challenge (and required time) of building even 5 to 10 lb of muscle, metabolism should not be expected to significantly increase based on muscle tissue alone.

Myth 4: Muscle mass equals bulk.
Fact: Bulk is not a scientific term but rather a term that has been created to anecdotally describe individuals who gain significant amounts of fat and muscle mass simultaneously. Since muscle is 15% denser than fat (Harrison and Leinwand 2008), for an individual with obesity, losing fat and gaining (or maintaining) muscle tissue will only serve to make them denser (leaner), not bulkier (Piercy et al. 2018).

Myth 5: Resistance training is harmful.
Fact: Research continually demonstrates that resistance training, when performed properly with qualified supervision, is safe and effective for individuals with obesity. As a result, the Centers for Disease Control and Prevention (Mazur et al. 1993) and American College of Sports Medicine (Donnelly et al. 2009) recommend resistance training in their guidelines for exercise among this population.

Myth 6: Resistance machines are safer than free weights.
Fact: When performed with correct technique and loading progressions, training with resistance machines confers no different risk of injury than free weight training. Research suggests that the greatest likelihood of injury occurs not as a result of modality but of inappropriate technique or loading (Damas et al. 2018).

Myth 7: Delayed-onset muscle soreness (DOMS) indicates progress.
Fact: DOMS occurs as a result of muscle damage, subsequent swelling, and nociceptor (pain receptor) activation. While this is a subjective indication of muscle damage, research does not indicate a strong relationship between DOMS and a beneficial adap-

tive response to resistance training (Drenowatz et al. 2015). In fact, in some cases, DOMS can be counterproductive, resulting in a compensatory reduction in nonexercise thermogenesis (Swift et al. 2018).

Myth 8: A low-calorie diet should come first and resistance training after.
Fact: Research consistently demonstrates that a combination of calorie restriction and exercise is more effective for weight loss than calorie restriction alone (Plotkin et al. 2022). As mentioned earlier, adding resistance training to a hypocaloric diet increases the likelihood of maintaining muscle mass during the period of caloric restriction. Much of the exercise traditionally used to support weight reduction, in combination with a hypocaloric diet, has been aerobic in nature. As research and clinical paradigms have evolved, it is becoming increasingly clear that resistance training plays an important role in mitigating loss of muscle mass and preserving quality of life and function during weight reduction.

Myth 9: High numbers of repetitions are better than low numbers of repetitions.
Fact: The repetition range selected for resistance training is based on the desired adaptation. Higher repetitions (8-15 per set) tend to favor more of a hypertrophic response, whereas lower repetitions (2-7 per set) result in more of a maximal strength adaptation (Schoenfeld et al. 2017). Particularly, there is no evidence supporting the statement that low-load training with high repetitions (8-15 per set) is more effective for body composition improvements compared to high-load training with low repetitions (2-7 per set). In contrast, both high- and low-load training have been demonstrated to induce substantial increases in lean body mass among well-trained young men (Schoenfeld et al. 2015). Individuals with excess weight or adiposity should commence training with a low load and subsequently increase the intensity of their training gradually to achieve a wide range of muscular fitness adaptations.

Myth 10: Training to muscle failure is the way to success.
Fact: Most research indicates that training to a point short of muscle failure is safer and more effective than training to complete muscle failure (Grgic et al. 2022). The need to train to muscle failure is a myth that largely grew out of the professional bodybuilding culture, because continually training to muscle failure is often necessary to achieve the significant muscle growth associated with pharmacologically enhanced professional bodybuilding. In contrast, research suggests that training until one has 2 to 4 repetitions in reserve is adequate to stimulate hypertrophy and improve strength. Generally, when training with low loads (8-15 repetitions per set), training with a high level of effort is of greater importance than total training volume in the process of increasing muscle size. In contrast, for high-load training (2-7 repetitions per set), muscle failure does not result in any additional benefits (Lasevicius et al. 2022).

Creating Positive Muscle-Strengthening Experiences

Due to myths and misconceptions, reluctance to engage in regular resistance training programs is common among people with excess weight, despite the role of resistance training as a key component of a multifaceted exercise plan with numerous health and fitness parameters. Traditional weight training routines have low attractiveness to individuals with overweight or obesity; current evidence reveals high dropout and low adherence rates in this population (Burgess et al. 2017). This amotivation for resistance training may be explained by the physical limitations and poor functionality commonly observed in clients with excess weight, which may play a negative role in using conventional stationary weight machines in a gym setting. The machines do not always accommodate individuals with a larger body size, making them feel embarrassed and possibly creating a negative response to training experiences. In addition, given that negative body image is common among unfit individuals with excess body weight or adiposity when viewing fitter individuals in a gym environment, a traditional resistance training workout in crowded surroundings may not be appealing to this population.

However, muscle-strengthening is considered a vital piece of the exercise training puzzle addressing obesity, and thus, exercise professionals should create person-centered, weight-inclusive resistance training approaches, aiming to support their clients with good practices and engaging exercise options.

Partner-assisted manual resistance using isometric holds may be an effective and alternative tool for exercise professionals serving populations with overweight or obesity in various exercise settings. Manual resistance seems to be as effective as traditional resistance training with free weights (Behringer et al. 2016). Isometric exercise refers to a static muscle contraction (with little movement or no change in muscle length). This adjunct muscle-strengthening method provides beneficial, long-term musculoskeletal fitness adaptations and may be particularly useful for beginners, deconditioned individuals, and older individuals with overweight or obesity who lack previous exercise experience in resistance training (Oranchuk et al. 2019a; Oranchuk et al. 2019b). An isometric approach may help clients get familiar with resistance-based exercise regimens before progressing the training stimulus and incorporating further variety into supervised muscle-strengthening exercise sessions.

Considering that individuals with overweight or obesity should engage in at least two full-body muscle-strengthening sessions weekly (Donnelly et al. 2009), partner-assisted manual resistance could be applied as an adjunct or preparatory training tool for inducing favorable changes in muscular fitness among previously inactive persons with excess weight (Baffour-Awuah et al. 2023; Lum and Barbosa 2019). Collectively, the primary psychophysiological advantages of using partner-assisted manual resistance through isometric holds are as follows (Dorgo et al. 2009; Oranchuk et al. 2019a, 2019b):

- *Proper exercise intensity:* Moderate-intensity isometrics (50%-70% of maximum voluntary isometric contraction) work well for beginners with excess weight, even for those with complications (e.g., raised blood pressure or impaired musculoskeletal health).

- *Pain-free stimulus:* Manual resistance appears to be an injury-free and appropriately intense workout without stress on the joints, promoting favorable alterations in muscular fitness among clients with overweight or obesity.

- *Emotional connection:* Partner exercises are an excellent engagement strategy for inexperienced individuals, allowing exercise professionals to connect with their clients physically, mentally, and emotionally.

- *Unique fitness experience:* Manual resistance may help to overcome common stereotypes and myths related to resistance training for people with overweight or obesity, providing an engaging muscle-strengthening experience.

EQUIPMENT-BASED EXERCISE TECHNIQUES
LOWER BODY

Horizontal Leg Press Machine

Instructions

1. Sit in a reclined position with the feet hip-width apart on the platform.
2. Exhale and push against the platform, causing the seat to slide backward (*a*).
3. Once the legs are extended, inhale and lower the weight toward the body until the knees are flexed at a 90° angle (*b*).
4. Keep the motion slow and controlled, and exhale while pushing against the platform.

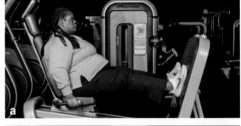

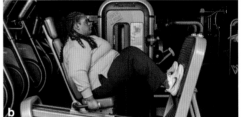

Variation

- Even a 100° to 120° angle is efficient for beginners with limited hip mobility and knee sensitivity.

Training Tip

- The horizontal type of leg press machine is preferred for clients with overweight or obesity. The diagonal (incline) type of leg press is not user-friendly for this population due to their larger waist size and potentially poor mobility.

Leg (Knee) Extension

Instructions

1. Sit on the machine with a weighted pad on top of the lower legs, and grip the handles.
2. Exhale and extend the knees while lifting the lower legs (*a*).
3. Once the legs are extended, inhale and lower the weight in a slow and controlled motion (*b*).

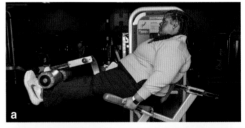

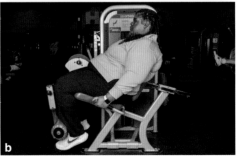

Seated Leg (Knee) Curl

Instructions

1. Sit down and engage the core while positioning the legs out in front, and grip the handles (*a*).
2. The thigh pad should rest just above the knees with the lower leg pad directly below the calves.
3. Exhale and flex the knees as far as possible, bringing the lower legs back toward the body (*b*).
4. Once the knees are fully flexed, inhale and extend the legs to the front.

Training Tip

- The seated leg curl is preferred for clients with overweight or obesity. Lying and standing versions are not user-friendly options for these individuals due to their larger waist size and potentially poor mobility.

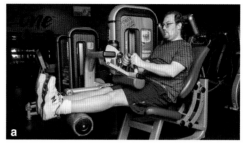

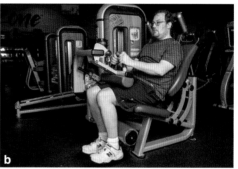

Seated Hip Adduction Machine

Instructions

1. Sit down with the legs outside the pads, and grip the handles (*a*).
2. Exhale and push the pads toward each other by bringing the legs together (*b*).
3. Inhale and return the legs to the starting position with control.

Variation

- This exercise can also be performed in a standing position, either using a stationary machine or a resistance band.

Training Tip

- For beginners with poor functionality and physical limitations, the seated version is preferred to the cable standing hip adduction machine, which requires good ankle and hip mobility as well as lumbar spine and knee stability.

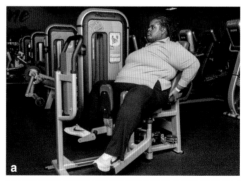

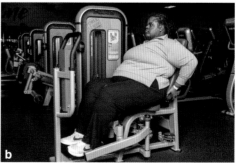

Seated Hip Abduction Machine

Instructions

1. Sit down with the legs inside the pads, and grip the handles (*a*).
2. Exhale and push the pads out by moving the legs as far apart as possible (*b*).
3. Inhale and return to the starting position with control.

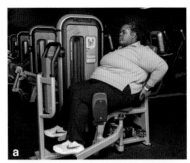

Variations

- This exercise can also be performed in a standing position, either using a stationary machine or a resistance band (banded side kick).
- If there is no access to a seated hip abduction machine, the motion can be performed against a band in a seated position.

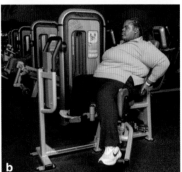

Training Tip

- For beginners with poor functionality and physical limitations, a seated machine is preferred to the cable standing hip abduction machine because the latter requires good ankle and hip mobility as well as lumbar spine and knee stability.

Cable Standing Hip Extension

Instructions

1. Attach an ankle strap to the bottom of the cable machine, face the machine, and place the working leg in back and the nonworking leg in front.

2. Grab a comfortable place on the machine for stability, and keep the posture upright and the working leg straight at all times (*a*).

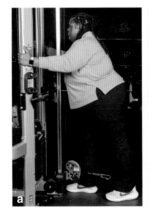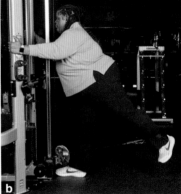

3. Exhale and swing the working leg back until the foot is just beneath the level of the glutes (*b*).

4. Squeeze the glutes at the finish position, then inhale while slowly returning the leg to the starting position.

5. Repeat with the opposite leg.

Variation

- This exercise can also be performed using machine glute kickbacks.

Training Tip

- Keep the spine neutral, squeeze the glutes at the upper position, and maintain constant tension throughout the movement.

Leg Press Calf Raise

Instructions

1. Sit down and rest the feet so just the toes are resting at the bottom of the platform.
2. Push back with straight legs as far as possible while keeping the feet against the platform.
3. Plantarflex the foot (extend the toes away from the body) (*a*), then dorsiflex the foot (allowing the toes to move back toward the body) (*b*) to return under control to the start position. Repeat.

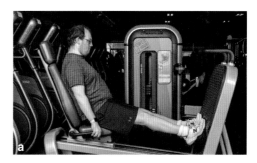

Training Tip

- The seated version is preferred to standing calf raises for beginner clients because standing raises require greater functionality.

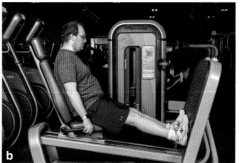

Back Squat

Instructions

1. Place the bar on the upper back, keeping the feet shoulder-width apart (*a*).
2. Inhale, brace the core slightly, and squat as deeply as possible with good form and no pain (*b*).
3. Exhale while returning to standing, or exchange air in the top position.

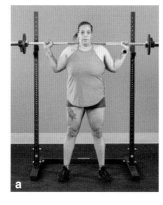
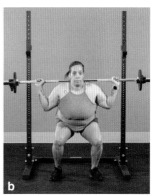

Variation

- Instead of a straight bar, the handles of a safety squat bar provide lower mobility requirements for clients with overweight or obesity.

Front Squat

Instructions

1. Standing with the feet hip-width apart, hold the barbell on the front of the shoulders with crossed lower arms to ensure an upright position and alleviate strain on the lower back (*a*).
2. Inhale, brace the core slightly, and squat as deeply as possible with good form, trying to achieve a pain-free and comfortable range of motion (*b*).
3. Reverse the movement by extending the hips and legs again.
4. Exhale on the way up or exchange air in the top position.

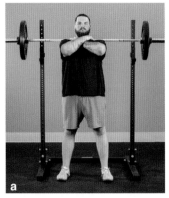

Training Tip

- The crossed-arm barbell front squat is a client-friendly option for individuals with overweight or obesity because of the decreased mobility demands in the shoulders and wrists.

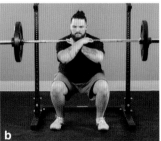

Dumbbell Lunge

Instructions

1. Stand in a split stance with the front foot 2 to 4 ft (0.5-1.0 m) in front of the back foot.
2. Hold a dumbbell in each hand and stand with the feet about shoulder-width apart.
3. Raise the back heel to place weight evenly across the ball of the back foot (*a*).

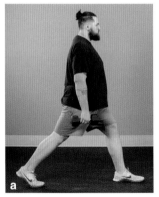
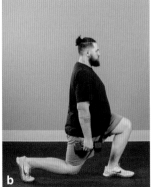

4. Inhale and sink as deeply as possible into a lunge position without letting the knee of the back leg touch the floor (*b*).
5. Return to the starting position by pushing up with the front leg while exhaling.
6. Complete the desired number of repetitions on one side, then switch sides.

Variation

- A harder way to perform this exercise is to take either a step backward or forward (dynamic lunge).

UPPER BODY

BACK

Neutral-Grip Lat Pull-Down

Instructions

1. Sit on the bench and place the thighs under the thigh pads to secure the legs.
2. Hold the V-bar so that the palms face each other.
3. Extend the arms, keeping the back straight and the chest up (*a*).
4. Exhale, and contract the lats by pulling the shoulders down and back while pulling the handle toward the chest (*b*).

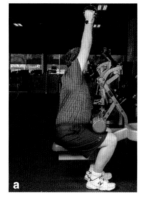 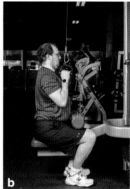

5. At the end of the movement, the shoulder blades should be pulled together, the chest should be up, and the V-bar should be against the chest.
6. Hold this position for a second, then slowly let the arms extend to the starting position while inhaling.

Variation

- This exercise can be also performed using a pronated or supinated grip. However, the neutral grip appears to be the most shoulder-friendly option for clients with overweight or obesity who have poor shoulder mobility.

One-Arm Dumbbell Row

Instructions

1. Stand facing a bench or chair and place the left hand and left knee on top of it.
2. Keep the back flat and parallel to the ground, with a slight flex in the standing leg.
3. Grip the dumbbell with the right hand, inhale, and pull the dumbbell toward

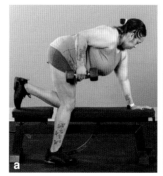 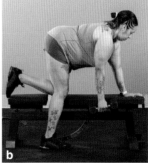

the body by driving the elbow toward the ceiling while exhaling (*a*).
4. Inhale and lower the dumbbell back to the starting position with control (*b*).
5. Complete the desired number of repetitions on one side, then switch to the opposite arm and leg.

Wide-Grip Seated Resistance Band Row

Instructions

1. Grip a resistance band with the hands slightly more than shoulder-width apart and assume the starting position (*a*).

2. Inhale and pull the handle toward the chest while leaning back slightly (*b*).

3. Exhale and slowly return to the starting position by extending the arms and leaning forward.

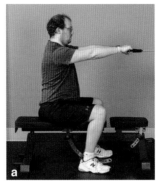
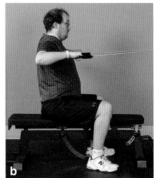

Straight-Arm Lat Pull-Down

Instructions

1. Stand facing the machine and grip the bar with a pronated grip (palms facing away from the body), slightly more than shoulder-width apart (*a*).

2. Exhale and push the bar down in front of the body with straight arms by contracting the lats (*b*).

3. Inhale and slowly return the bar to the starting position.

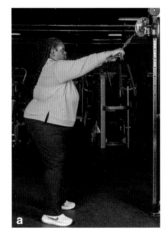
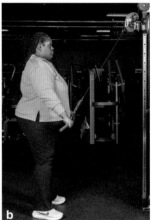

CHEST

Vertical Chest Press Machine

Instructions

1. Adjust the back support, sit down, and grip the handles.
2. Exhale and press the handles forward until the arms are straight (*a*).
3. Inhale and bring the handles back to the starting position with control (*b*).

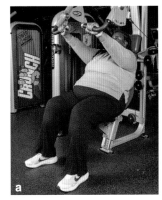
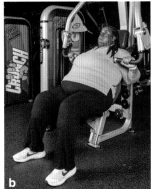

Training Tips

- This exercise avoids positions required by flat and incline chest press machines that may be uncomfortable for clients with overweight or obesity due to a larger waist size.

- This exercise option is beginner-friendly, offering more stability and requiring less balance and coordination than chest presses with free weights (dumbbells or a barbell).

Chest Fly Machine (Butterfly)

Instructions

1. Sit in the machine and grip the handles at shoulder height.
2. Exhale and use the chest muscles to push the handles forward until they meet in front of the body, keeping a slight flex in the arms (*a*).
3. Inhale and let the handles go back to the starting position with control (*b*).

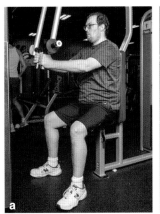
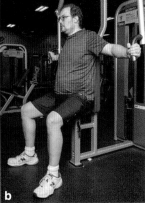

Training Tip

- Compared with pec deck and dumbbell chest flies on a flat or incline bench, this exercise is more convenient and shoulder-friendly for clients with overweight or obesity, a population commonly characterized by poor shoulder mobility and scapula stability.

Standing Cable Chest Fly (Crossover)

Instructions

1. Grip the handles in the top position of a cable cross, face away from the machine, take a split stance, and lean slightly forward (*a*).
2. Exhale and push the handles forward until they meet in front of the body, keeping a slight flex in the arms (*b*).
3. Inhale and let the handles return to the starting position with control.

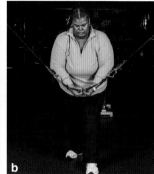

Training Tip

- This exercise engages the core more than the chest fly machine; however, it should be performed with caution if beginner clients with obesity feel uncomfortable with the range of motion due to insufficient shoulder mobility and lumbar spine stability.

SHOULDERS

Cable Front Raise

Instructions

1. Facing away from the cable machine, grip the straight bar connected to the lower position on a cable pulley, using a pronated grip (palms facing downward) (*a*).
2. Exhale, brace the core, and begin the lift by sweeping the bar upward in an arc direction until the arms and the bar are at shoulder height (*b*).
3. Inhale and reverse the movement by slowly lowering the bar until it has returned to the beginning position.

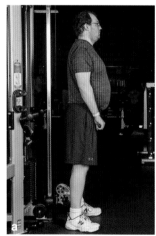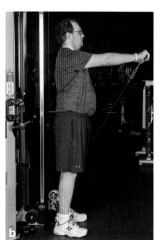

Variation

- This exercise can also be performed using a dumbbell in each hand, either in a standing or seated position.

Dumbbell Lateral Raise

Instructions

1. Stand with the feet hip-width apart and hold a dumbbell in each hand, with the arms almost straight and hanging at the sides of the body (*a*).
2. With control, lift the dumbbells out to the sides while exhaling, until the upper arms are horizontal (*b*).
3. Inhale and lower the dumbbells with control.

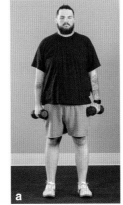
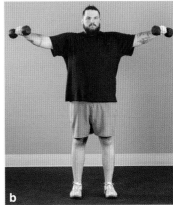

Variation

- This exercise can also be performed using handles on a dual-cable pulley.

Seated Cable Rear Delt Fly

Instructions

1. Sit with the chest lifted and keep the core braced.
2. Adjust the handles so that they can be gripped at shoulder height while facing the machine and a long range of motion can be achieved (*a*).
3. Exhale and pull the handles backward by bringing the arms out to the sides, keeping a slight flex in the arms (*b*).

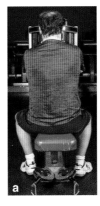
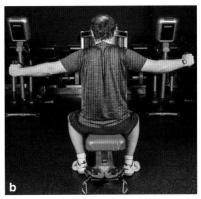

4. Inhale and reverse the movement, letting the handles go back to the starting position.

Training Tip

- This exercise is more convenient than the reverse cable fly and reverse dumbbell fly for clients with overweight or obesity, allowing them to avoid uncomfortable and challenging body positions.

ARMS

Standing Cable Triceps Push-Down

Instructions

1. Stand one step away from the cable pulley, facing the machine, and grip the bar with the hands about shoulder-width apart in a pronated grip (palms facing downward) (*a*).

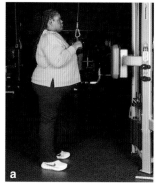
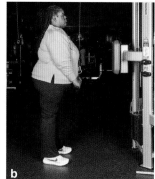

2. Pull the bar down until the upper arms are perpendicular to the floor and the lower arms are parallel to the floor. Keep the upper arms stable against the sides of the body throughout the exercise.

3. Exhale while extending at the elbows. Push the bar down until the arms are fully extended (*b*).

4. Inhale and let the bar come up, controlling the movement, until the lower arms are again parallel to the floor.

Variation

- This exercise can also be performed using a rope with a neutral grip (palms facing each other) or a bar with a supinated grip (palms facing upward).

Seated Triceps Dip Machine

Instructions

1. Sit in the triceps dip machine. Engage the core throughout the exercise.

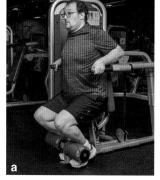
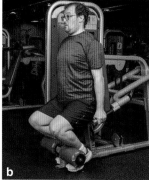

2. Place the hands on the bars with a neutral grip (palms facing each other) and the elbows pointing backward (*a*).

3. Ensure the elbows are flexed at a 90° angle and press down on the bars (*b*).

4. When extending the elbows, keep them from locking out, and pause for a second while exhaling.

5. Inhale and reverse the movement slowly, preventing the weight from touching the stack.

Standing Cable Biceps Curl

Instructions

1. Stand facing the machine. Grip the bar with a supinated grip (palms facing upward) and the hands about shoulder-width apart (*a*). Take a step back.
2. Exhale and lift the bar by flexing the elbows with control (*b*).
3. Keep the elbows at the sides of the body, inhale, reverse the movement, and lower the bar back to the starting position.

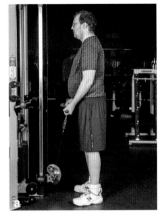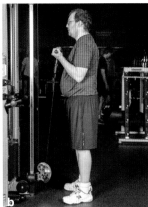

Standing Dumbbell Alternating Biceps Curl

Instructions

1. Hold a pair of dumbbells with a supinated grip (palms facing upward), with the arms hanging by the sides of the body (*a*).
2. Exhale and lift one dumbbell by flexing the elbow (*b*).
3. Keep the elbow at the side, inhale, reverse the movement, and lower the dumbbell back to the starting position.
4. Repeat with the opposite arm.

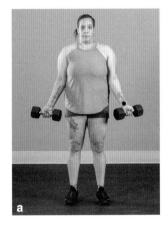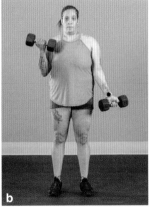

WHOLE BODY

Dumbbell Squat to Press

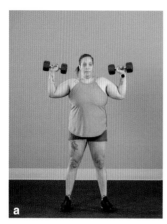 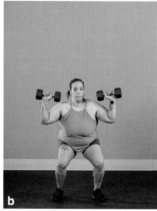 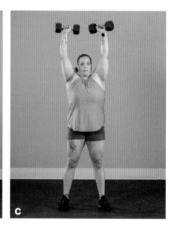

Instructions

1. Stand with the feet hip-width apart.
2. Hold a dumbbell by each shoulder, with the elbows flexed at 90° and the palms facing forward (*a*).
3. Inhale and lower into a half or full squat (depending on hip mobility) (*b*). Drive back up explosively and press the weights overhead while exhaling, until the arms are fully extended (*c*).
4. Lower the weights back to the shoulders and lower into a squat for the next repetition.

Kettlebell Sumo Squat to High Pull

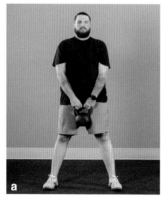 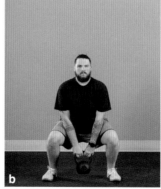 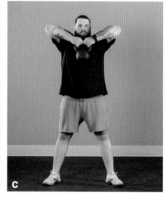

Instructions

1. Stand with the legs wider than shoulder-width apart and place a kettlebell (or dumbbell) on the floor between them. Place both hands on the weight (*a*).
2. Inhale and lower the body into a half or full squat position (depending on hip mobility) (*b*).
3. Exhale, extend the legs, and raise the weight to the chin (*c*). The flexed elbows should be in line with the top of the head.
4. Squat down to lower the weight to the floor and repeat, holding the weight throughout the exercise.

Kettlebell Swing

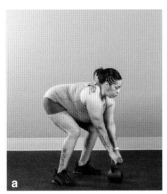 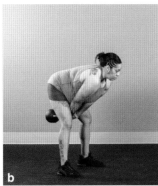 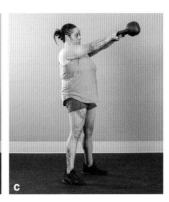

Instructions

1. Stand with the feet shoulder-width apart while holding a kettlebell with both hands (palms facing the body), keeping the arms straight down.
2. Inhale and hinge the hips, pushing them back (*a*); slightly flex the knees to bring the kettlebell between the legs (*b*).
3. Keep the back straight and engage the core.
4. Exhale, contract the glutes, and push the hips forward to lift the body into a standing position.
5. Allow the arms to swing the kettlebell as far as it will naturally go (*c*).
6. Inhale and lower the kettlebell between the legs by pushing the hips back and slightly flexing the knees.

PARTNER-ASSISTED MANUAL RESISTANCE (ISOMETRIC HOLDS)

Special Training Considerations

- Normal breathing patterns should be used, avoiding the Valsalva maneuver.
- Isometric holds should be of moderate intensity.
- The duration of isometric tension should range from 3 to 10 s.
- The work-to-rest ratio between repetitions should range from 1:2 to 1:1.

LOWER BODY

Seated Leg (Knee) Extension

Instructions

1. Have the client sit on a surface with adequate height (a bench or chair).
2. Place your hand over the client's shins to apply resistance.
3. Instruct the client to keep their leg at a 90° angle, resisting your force.

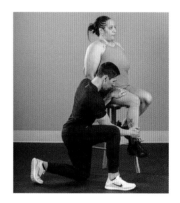

Training Tip

- This exercise could be also performed in a supine lying position; however, this may not be a comfortable body position for clients with excess weight.

Standing Leg (Knee) Curl

Instructions

1. Have the client stand and use a chair for support, flexing one knee at a 90° angle with the foot behind them.
2. Drive your hand into the client's lower calf, maintaining consistent, steady tension throughout each rep.
3. Ensure that the client keeps their leg at a 90° angle, resisting your force.

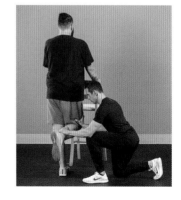

Training Tip

- This exercise could be also performed in a prone lying position; however, this may not be a comfortable body position for clients with excess weight.

Side-Lying Hip Abduction

Instructions

1. Have the client lie on the floor on their side, resting their head on the lower arm.
2. The client's lower leg should be flexed at the knee and their top leg should be straight, with the hips joints stacked.
3. Press your hands against the shin of the client's upper leg while they lift the leg upward. Maintain consistent, steady tension throughout each rep.
4. Repeat on the other side.

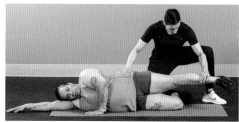

Quadruped Hip Extension

Instructions

1. Have the client take a quadruped position with a neutral spine.
2. The client raises one straight leg, maintaining a neutral spine and resisting your force applied on the ankle.
3. Have the client return to the starting position, and repeat on the other side.

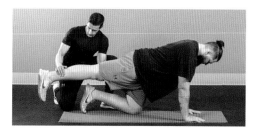

UPPER BODY

BACK

Seated Lat Pull-Down

Instructions

1. Have the client sit on a chair and hold a stick with straight arms, adopting a wide, pronated grip overhead.
2. The client flexes their arms at a 90° angle, resisting your force on the stick.
3. Instruct the client to keeps their chest up while holding this position.

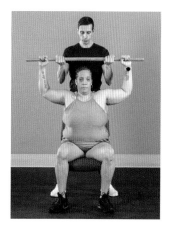

Standing Close-Grip Row

Instructions

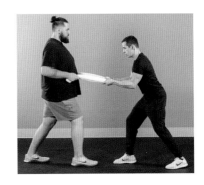

1. You and the client take a split stance, facing each other.
2. Each of you holds one end of a towel in both hands. Have the client pull the towel, flexing their elbows to a 90° angle and keeping the hands close together (supinated or neutral) in a close grip.
3. Instruct the client to engage their core while holding this position.

Standing Wide-Grip Row

Instructions

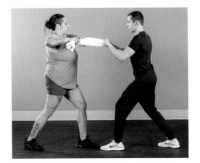

1. You and the client take a split stance, facing each other.
2. Each of you holds one end of a towel in both hands. Have the client pull the towel, flexing their elbows to a 90° angle and keeping their hands in a wide, pronated grip.
3. Instruct the client to engage their core while holding this position.

CHEST

Standing Chest Press

Instructions

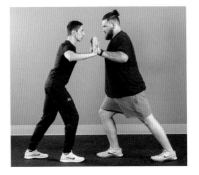

1. You and the client take a split stance, facing each other.
2. Push against each other, using your palms and keeping the elbows flexed to a 90° angle.
3. Instruct the client to engage their core while holding this position.

Seated Chest Fly

Instructions

1. Have the client sit on a chair with their arms extended straight out to the sides at shoulder height.
2. Stand behind the client as they push forward, making a circle with their arms as if preparing to hug someone.
3. Resist the client's force by pushing outward on their forearms.
4. Instruct the client to engage the core, keep their chest up, and hold the position.

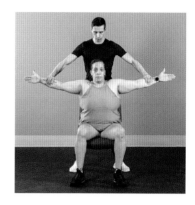

Variation

- This exercise can also be performed in a standing position to engage the core further.

Elevated Push-Up

Instructions

1. Have the client get into an incline (30°-60°) push-up position using a high flat bench, a Smith machine, or an Olympic bar in a weight rack.
2. Resist the client's force by pushing down on their upper back as they extend their elbows to push up.
3. Instruct the client to engage the core, keep their chest up, and hold the position.

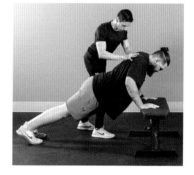

Training Tip

- This exercise can be used with a wider or closer stance to reduce or increase the intensity, respectively.

SHOULDERS

Standing Front Raise

Instructions

1. Have the client stand and hold their arms straight in front of their body at shoulder height.
2. The client lifts their arms up while you resist their force by pressing down on their forearms.
3. Instruct the client to engage the core, keep their chest up, and hold the position.

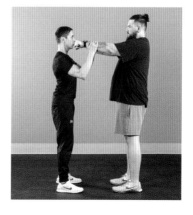

Standing Lateral Raise

Instructions

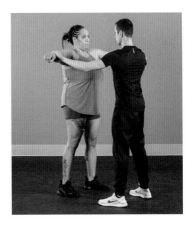

1. Have the client stand with their arms extended straight out to the sides at shoulder height.
2. The client lifts their arms up while you resist their force by pressing down on their forearms.
3. Instruct the client to engage the core, keep their chest up, and hold the position.

Seated Reverse Chest Fly

Instructions

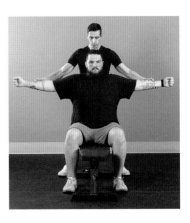

1. Have the client sit on a chair with the arms extended straight out to the sides at shoulder height.
2. The client pushes their arms backward while you resist their force by pressing forward on their forearms.
3. Instruct the client to engage the core, keep the chest up, and hold the position.

TRICEPS

Standing Triceps Extension

Instructions

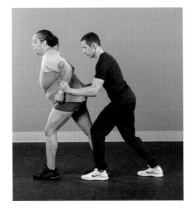

1. Have the client stand with a split stance and assume a triceps kickback position, with their upper arms held closely against the sides of the body.
2. The client presses their arms backward, keeping their elbows flexed in a 90° angle.
3. Resist the client's force by pressing forward on their forearms.
4. Instruct the client to engage the core, keep their chest up, and hold the position.

BICEPS

Standing Biceps Curl

Instructions

1. Have the client stand with their feet shoulder-width apart and their elbows flexed at 90°.

2. The client curls their arms upward while you resist their force by pressing backward on their forearms.

3. Instruct the client to engage the core, keep their chest up, and hold the position.

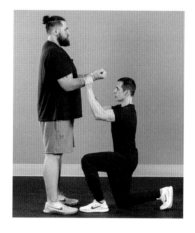

MODIFICATIONS AND PROGRESSIONS
LOWER BODY

SQUAT

Supported Bodyweight Squat

Instructions

1. Stand in front of a chair, feet shoulder-width apart, and place the hands on the chair for extra support (*a*).

2. Inhale, brace the core slightly, and squat as deeply as possible, keeping the heels flat and the knees out (*b*).

3. Exhale while returning to standing, or exchange air in the top position.

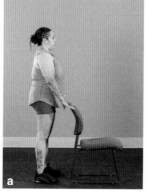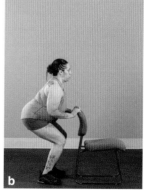

Squat on a Stability Ball (Inside Holder)

Instructions

1. Put a stability ball on a Pilates ring to make sure it is stable. Stand in front of the ball, facing away from it (*a*).
2. Inhale, brace the core slightly, and squat down on the stability ball, keeping the heels flat and the knees out (*b*).
3. Exhale while returning to standing, or exchange air in the top position.

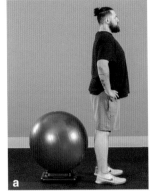
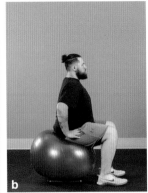

Chair Squat

Instructions

1. Stand just in front of a chair, facing away from it, and place the hands across the chest (*a*).
2. Keep the spine neutral and the chest up.
3. Inhale while sitting down on the chair with control, keeping the heels flat and the knees out (*b*).
4. Exhale and return to the starting position.

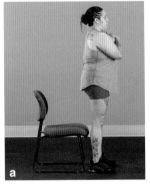
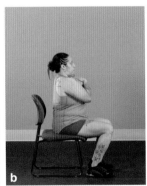

Stability Ball Wall Squat

Instructions

1. Stand with the feet shoulder-width apart, put a stability ball behind the back, and press up against a wall.
2. The feet should be slightly in front of the body and shoulder-width apart, and the arms should be held out for balance (*a*).
3. Inhale and squat down, keeping the heels flat and the knees out, and let the stability ball roll up the back (*b*).
4. Exhale and return to the starting position.

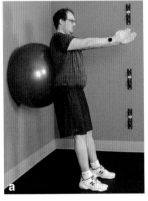
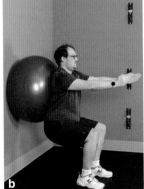

Bodyweight Squat

Instructions

1. Stand with the feet shoulder-width apart and place the hands across the chest (*a*).

2. Keep the spine neutral and the chest up.

3. Inhale, hinging at the hips to initiate the movement, then flex the knees to lower into a squat position until the thighs are almost parallel with the floor, keeping the heels flat and the knees out (*b*).

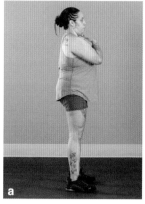
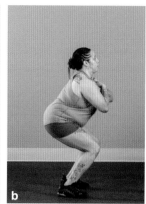

4. Exhale and return to the starting position.

Kettlebell Goblet Squat

Instructions

1. Stand with the feet shoulder-width apart and grab the bell of the weight such that the horns of the handle are pointed up and the bottom of the bell is pointed down (*a*).

2. Keep the spine neutral and the chest up, and hold the kettlebell 1 to 2 in. (3-5 cm) away from the chest throughout the movement.

3. Inhale and hinge at the hips to initiate the movement. Flex the knees to lower into a squat position until the thighs are almost parallel with the floor, keeping the heels flat and the knees out (*b*).

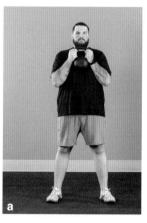
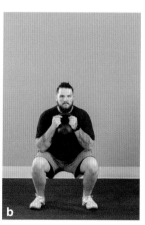

4. Exhale and return to the starting position.

HINGE

Wide Hip Hinging

Instructions

1. Stand with the feet shoulder-width apart and shift the body weight to the heels (*a*).
2. Keeping the chest open, back flat, and knees slightly flexed, push the hips back while hinging the torso forward while inhaling (*b*).
3. The movement comes from the hip joint. Pause once the torso is approximately at a 45° angle.

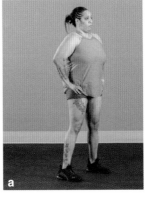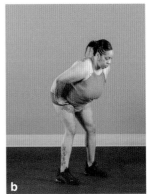

4. Exhale and reverse the movement by squeezing the glutes and pushing the hips forward and up to return to the standing position.

Sumo Deadlift Modified to Elevate Weight #1

Instructions

1. The kettlebell is positioned on a step aerobics platform with three blocks. Start with a wide foot stance and the toes pointing out, keeping the back straight and pulling the shoulders back and down.
2. Inhale, bend over from the hips, flex the knees, and grab the kettlebell with both hands (*a*).

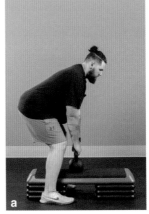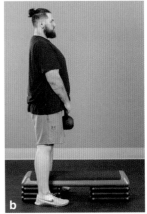

3. Shifting the body weight to the heels, extend the hips and knees to pull the weight off the step aerobics platform (*b*).
4. Slowly return to the starting position, let the kettlebell touch the platform, then drive back up again.

Sumo Deadlift Modified to Elevate Weight #2

Instructions

1. The kettlebell is positioned on a step aerobics platform with two blocks. Start with a wide foot stance and the toes pointing out, keeping the back straight and pulling the shoulders back and down.

2. Inhale, bend over from the hips, flex the knees, and grab the kettlebell with both hands (*a*).

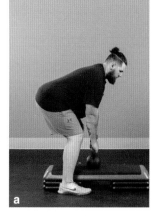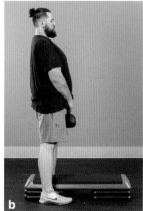

3. Shifting the body weight to the heels, extend the hips and knees to pull the weight off the step aerobics platform (*b*).

4. Slowly return to the starting position, let the kettlebell touch the platform, then drive back up again.

Sumo Deadlift Modified to Elevate Weight #3

Instructions

1. The kettlebell is positioned on a step aerobics platform with one block. Start with a wide foot stance and the toes pointing out, keeping the back straight and pulling the shoulders back and down.

2. Inhale, bend over from the hips, flex the knees, and grab the kettlebell with both hands (*a*).

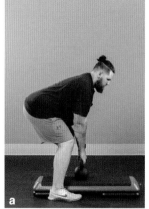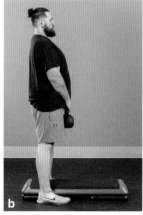

3. Shifting the body weight to the heels, extend the hips and knees to pull the weight off the step aerobics platform (*b*).

4. Slowly return to the starting position, let the kettlebell touch the platform, then drive back up again.

Sumo Deadlift Modified to Elevate Weight #4

Instructions

1. The kettlebell is positioned on a step aerobics platform without blocks. Start with a wide foot stance and the toes pointing out, keeping the back straight and pulling the shoulders back and down.

2. Inhale, bend over from the hips, flex the knees, and grab the kettlebell with both hands (*a*).

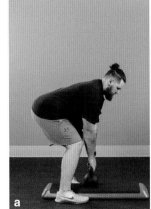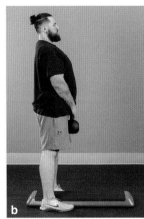

3. Shifting the body weight to the heels, extend the hips and knees to pull the weight off the step aerobics platform (*b*).

4. Slowly return to the starting position, let the kettlebell touch the platform, then drive back up again.

Sumo Deadlift

Instructions

1. Start with a wide foot stance and the toes pointing out, keeping the back straight and pulling the shoulders back and down.

2. Inhale, bend over from the hips, flex the knees, and grab the kettlebell with both hands (*a*).

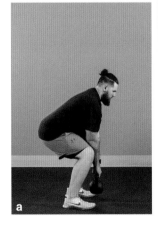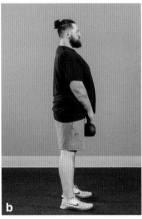

3. Shifting the body weight to the heels, extend the hips and knees to pull the weight off the floor (*b*).

4. Slowly return to the starting position, let the kettlebell touch the floor, then drive back up again.

<u>LUNGE</u>

Supported Static Lunge

Instructions

1. Stand in a split stance and hold on to a chair for balance.
2. Inhale and lunge as low as possible by flexing both knees to 90° and keeping the knees over the toes.
3. Exhale and stand back up with straight legs.
4. Repeat, then switch sides.

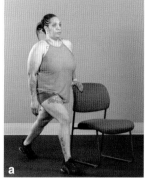
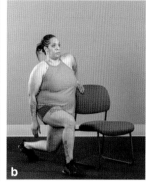

Static Lunge on a Balance Ball

Instructions

1. Stand in a split stance and place a balance ball under the rear knee (*a*).
2. Inhale and lunge by flexing both knees to 90° and keeping the knees over the toes. Lower until the rear knee touches the balance ball (*b*).
3. Exhale and stand back up with straight legs.
4. Repeat, then switch sides.

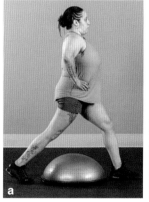
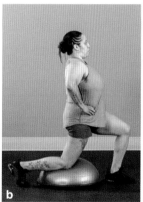

Static Lunge on a Balance Pad or Yoga Head Block

Instructions

1. Stand in a split stance and place a balance pad or yoga head block under the rear knee (*a*).
2. Inhale and lunge by flexing both knees to 90° and keeping the knees over the toes. Lower until the rear leg touches the pad or block (*b*).
3. Exhale and stand back up with straight legs.
4. Repeat, then switch sides.

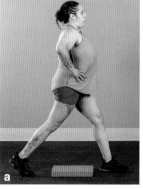
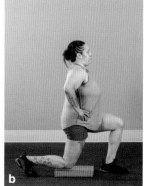

Bodyweight Static Lunge

Instructions

1. Stand in a split stance (*a*).
2. Inhale and lunge as low as possible by flexing both knees to 90° and keeping the knees over the toes (*b*).
3. Exhale and stand back up with straight legs.
4. Repeat, then switch sides.

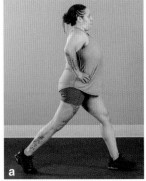
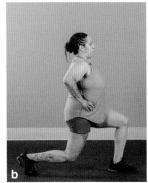

Bodyweight Dynamic Reverse Lunge

Instructions

1. Stand in a closed stance (*a*).
2. Inhale and take a big step backward with the left foot, landing on the ball of the foot.
3. Lower the body and flex the right knee until it forms a 90° angle (*b*).
4. Exhale and reverse the movement to return to the standing position.
5. Repeat on the other side.

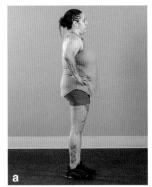
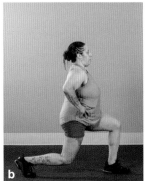

Bodyweight Dynamic Forward Lunge

Instructions

1. Stand in a closed stance (*a*).
2. Inhale and take a big step forward with the left foot, landing on the ball of the foot.
3. Lower the body and flex the right knee until it forms a 90° angle (*b*).
4. Exhale and reverse the movement to return to the standing position.
5. Repeat on the other side.

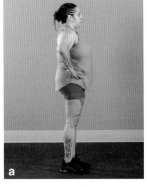
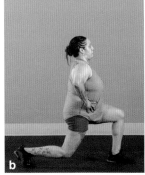

Kettlebell Goblet Reverse Lunge

Instructions

1. Stand in a closed stance and grab the bell of the weight such that the horns of the handle are pointed up while the bottom of the bell is pointed down (*a*).
2. Hold the kettlebell 2 to 3 in. (5-8 cm) away from the chest throughout the movement.
3. Inhale and take a big step backward with the right foot, landing on the ball of the foot.
4. Lower the body and flex the left knee until it forms a 90° angle (*b*).
5. Exhale and reverse the movement to return to the standing position.
6. Repeat on the other side.

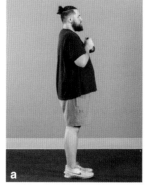
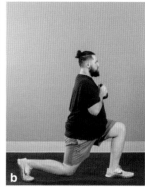

Kettlebell Goblet Forward Lunge

Instructions

1. Stand in a closed stance and grab the bell of the weight such that the horns of the handle are pointed up while the bottom of the bell is pointed down.
2. Hold the kettlebell 2 to 3 in. (5-8 cm) away from the chest throughout the movement.
3. Inhale and take a big step forward with the right foot, landing on the ball of the foot.
4. Lower the body and flex the left knee until it forms a 90° angle.
5. Exhale and reverse the movement to return to the standing position.
6. Repeat on the other side.

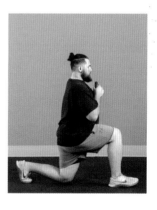

Kettlebell Goblet Forward and Reverse Lunge

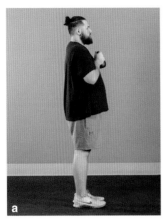 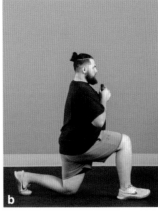 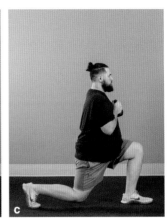

Instructions

1. Stand in a closed stance and grab the bell of the weight such that the horns of the handle are pointed up while the bottom of the bell is pointed down (*a*).
2. Hold the kettlebell 2 to 3 in. (5-8 cm) away from the chest throughout the movement.
3. Inhale and take a big step forward with the right foot, landing on the ball of the foot.
4. Lower the body and flex the left knee until it forms a 90° angle (*b*).
5. Exhale and reverse the movement to take a big step backward with the right foot, landing on the ball of the foot.
6. Lower the body and flex the left knee until it forms a 90° angle (*c*).
7. Exhale and reverse the movement to return to the standing position.
8. Repeat on the other side.

UPPER BODY

PUSH

Kneeling Push-Up

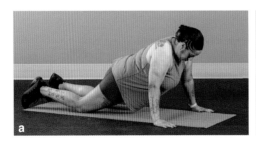 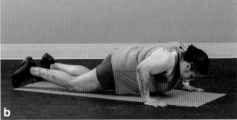

Instructions

1. Take a kneeling position.
2. Extend the arms and place the hands on the floor, slightly wider than shoulder-width apart (*a*).
3. Inhale, brace the core while flexing the arms, and lower the torso until the chest grazes the floor (*b*).
4. Exhale and push the torso back up by straightening the arms.

Modified Push-Up (Elevation: 60°)

Instructions

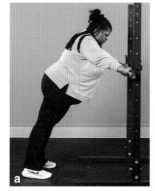
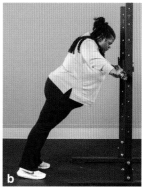

1. Stand facing a Smith machine or an Olympic bar in a weight rack.
2. Start with the bar set to about chest height and set up the stance and grip.
3. Extend the arms and legs, and position the hands on the bar slightly more than shoulder-width apart. Create a straight line from the head to the toes, making a 60° angle between the body and the floor (*a*).
4. Inhale, brace the core while flexing the arms, and lower the torso until the chest grazes the bar (*b*).
5. Exhale and push the torso back up by straightening the arms.

Modified Push-Up (Elevation: 45°)

Instructions

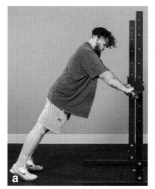
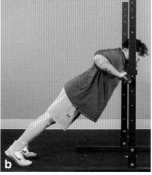

1. Stand facing a Smith machine or an Olympic bar in a weight rack.
2. Start with the bar set to about chest height and set up the stance and grip.
3. Extend the arms and legs, and position the hands on the bar slightly more than shoulder-width apart. Create a straight line from the head to the toes, making a 45° angle between the body and the floor (*a*).
4. Inhale, brace the core while flexing the arms, and lower the torso until the chest grazes the bar (*b*).
5. Exhale and push the torso back up by straightening the arms.

Kettlebell Overhead Press

Instructions

1. Stand with the feet shoulder-width apart and grab the bell of the weight such that the horns of the handle are pointed up while the bottom of the bell is pointed down (*a*).

2. Hold the kettlebell with both hands 1 to 2 in. (3-5 cm) away from the chest throughout the movement.

3. Press the kettlebell up until the arms are completely extended (*b*).

4. Reverse the movement and return to the starting position.

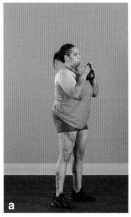
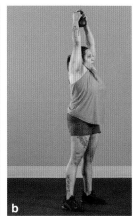

PULL

Inverted Row (Elevation: 60°)

Instructions

1. Use a Smith machine or an Olympic bar in a weight rack.

2. Start with the bar set high enough that when it is grabbed with both hands and the arms and legs are extended, the body is aligned without touching the floor.

3. Lie underneath the bar so that it is aligned with the chest. Grab the bar with the hands slightly more than shoulder-width apart and extend the arms and legs to the front, making a 60° angle between the body and the floor (*a*).

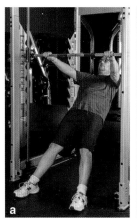
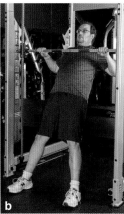

4. Create a straight line from the head to the toes. Exhale, and pull with the arms while squeezing the shoulder blades together to row the chest to the bar. Hold this position for 1 s (*b*).

5. Inhale and slowly lower the body back down, extending the arms with control and maintaining body posture at the bottom.

Inverted Row (Elevation: 45°)

Instructions

1. Use a Smith machine or an Olympic bar in a weight rack.

2. Start with the bar set high enough that when it is grabbed with both hands and the arms and legs are extended, the body is aligned without touching the floor.

3. Lie underneath the bar so that it is aligned with the chest. Grab the bar with the hands slightly more than shoulder-width apart and extend the arms and legs to the front, making a 45° angle between the body and the floor (*a*).

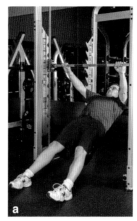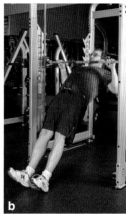

4. Create a straight line from the head to the toes. Exhale, and pull with the arms while squeezing the shoulder blades together to row the chest to the bar. Hold this position for 1 s (*b*).

5. Inhale and slowly lower the body back down, extending the arms with control and maintaining body posture at the bottom.

Modified Pull-Up

Instructions

1. Sit with the butt on the floor beneath a Smith machine or an Olympic bar in a weight rack, keeping the knees flexed and the feet flat (*a*).

2. Start with the bar set high enough to grab it with extended arms.

3. Grab the bar with the hands slightly wider than shoulder-width apart, using a pronated grip (palms facing downward). Keep the upper body at about a 90° angle with floor.

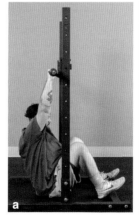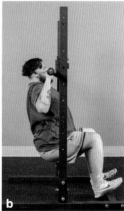

4. Exhale and pull with the arms, squeezing the shoulder blades together, until the eyes are positioned above the bar (*b*). Hold this position for 1 s.

5. Inhale and slowly lower the body back down, extending the arms with control and maintaining body posture at the bottom.

Kettlebell Upright Row

Instructions

1. Approach the bell on the floor. Hinge forward at the hips, grab the bell with both hands, and straighten the back to a standing position (*a*).

2. Engage the core, exhale, and drive the bell up, leading with the elbows, until the hands are just below the face (*b*).

3. Inhale and lower the bell with control.

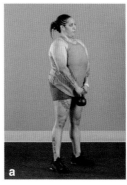
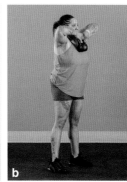

CORE

ANTIFLEXION OR EXTENSION

Vertical Force–Resisting Abdominal Bracing

Instructions

1. Have the client sit on a chair or bench without back support, keeping the arms straight in front of the body at shoulder height.

2. While the client lifts their arms up or down, resist their force by pressing down or up on their palms or forearms, respectively.

3. Instruct the client to brace the core, keep their chest up, and breathe normally.

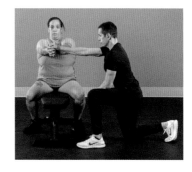

Variation

- To progress, this exercise can be performed on a stability ball or in a standing position.

Training Tip

- This exercise could also be performed in a supine lying, standing, or semi-kneeling position.

Kneeling Plank

Instructions

1. Take a kneeling position on a mat. Place the forearms flat on the floor, keeping the upper arms directly below the shoulders and the knees on the mat. The body should make a straight line at an angle to the floor.

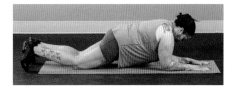

2. Brace the core, keep the spine straight, and hold for the desired amount of time while breathing normally.
3. Slowly release by pushing the hips back until they are over the heels.

Variations

- To progress, this exercise can be performed with straight arms and only the hands on the floor or with the forearms flat on a balance ball or foam roller.
- A half-kneeling version, with one leg extended and the foot resting on the floor, could be considered another progression.

Wall Plank

Instructions

1. Stand up straight facing a wall, with the feet shoulder-width apart. Flex the elbows, lean forward, and place the forearms against the wall.
2. The elbows should be at shoulder height, and the forearms should point vertically up the wall.
3. Brace the core, keep the spine straight, and hold for the desired amount of time while breathing normally.
4. Keep the body in line with the legs and pull the shoulder blades down and back.

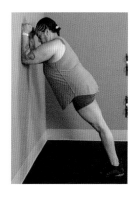

Variation

- To progress, this exercise can be performed with the feet hip-width apart.

Incline Plank

Instructions

1. Place the forearms firmly on a high bench with the feet shoulder-width apart and the elbows directly below the shoulders.
2. Extend the legs behind the body, resting the balls of the feet on the floor.
3. Brace the core, keep the spine straight, and hold for the desired amount of time while breathing normally.
4. Keep the body in line with the legs and pull the shoulder blades down and back.

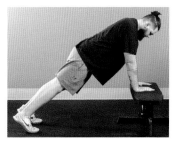

Variation

- To progress, this exercise can be performed with the feet hip-width apart or using a low bench.

Assisted Plank

Instructions

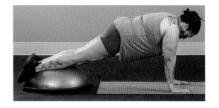

1. Lie face down on the floor with the elbows directly under the shoulders, the forearms extended to the front, and the palms against the floor.

2. Extend the legs behind the body, with a balance ball placed under the shins.

3. Brace the core, keep the spine straight, and hold for the desired amount of time while breathing normally.

4. Keep your body in line with the legs and pull the shoulder blades down and back.

Variation

- To progress, this exercise can be performed with straight arms, pressing the palms against the floor. Note that this progression may be challenging for clients with excess weight due to pressure in the wrists.

Bear Crawl Isometric Hold

Instructions

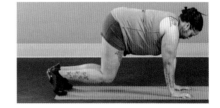

1. Take a quadruped position and keep the spine neutral. Ensure the knees are flexed, the hands are under the shoulders, and the knees are under the hips.

2. Lift the hips so the knees are hovering just above the floor.

3. Brace the core and hold for the desired amount of time while breathing normally.

4. Keep the arms straight and maintain the fixed position throughout the hold.

Variation

- To progress, walk forward or backward with control. Note that this progression may be challenging for clients with excess weight due to pressure in the wrists.

Training Tip

- The recommended durations are 10, 20, and 30 s for beginner, intermediate, and advanced clients, respectively.

Elevated Glute Bridge

Instructions

1. Lie on the back with the knees flexed and the feet flat on a low step platform.
2. Brace the core, squeeze the glutes, and lift the hips off the ground (*a*).
3. With control, lower the hips back to the ground.

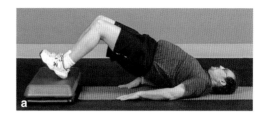

Variation

• To progress, this exercise can be performed using a balance ball or foam roller rather than a step platform to provide instability and greater core activation (*b*).

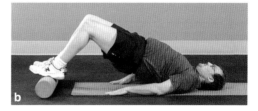

ANTI–LATERAL FLEXION

Asymmetric Loaded Carry

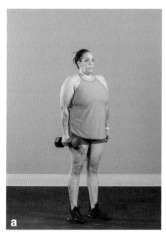 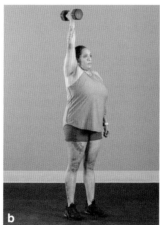 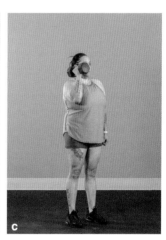

Instructions

1. Grab a weight (a dumbbell or kettlebell) in one hand only, as if holding a heavy suitcase (*a*).
2. Walk, aiming to keep the body balanced and upright (*b*).
3. During the movement, keep the shoulders back and the chin neutral, look straight ahead, and counterbalance with the free hand.

Variation

• To progress, carry the weight in a different position (e.g., rack, shoulder, or overhead) (*c*).

Training Tip

• A feasible distance for beginner, intermediate, and advanced clients with excess weight would be 10 to 15 yd (9-14 m), 20 to 25 yd (18-23 m), and 30 to 40 yd (27-37 m), respectively.

Modified Side Plank

Instructions

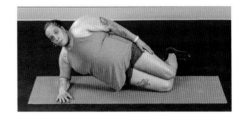

1. Lie on the right side of the body with the right elbow resting on the floor directly beneath the right shoulder.
2. Extend both legs out to left side and stack the knees. Flex both knees at a 90° angle so the lower legs are resting on the floor behind the body.
3. Engage the core and lift the hips off the floor, maintaining a straight line from the head to the knees.
4. Hold this position for the desired amount of time while breathing normally, then return to the starting position and switch sides.

Variation

- To progress the modified side plank, perform it with hip abduction (the top leg is extended straight and the bottom leg is flexed at the knee, with the knee remaining on the floor).

Abdominal Bracing to Resist Lateral Force

Instructions

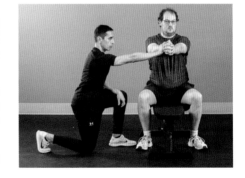

1. Have the client sit on a chair or bench without back support, with straightened arms extended in front of the body at shoulder height.
2. As the client pushes their arms to one side, resist their force by pressing in the opposite direction against their palms or forearms.
3. Instruct the client to brace the core, keep the chest up, and breathe normally.
4. Have the client switch sides.

Variation

- To progress, this exercise can be performed on a stability ball or in a standing position.

Training Tip

- This exercise can also be performed in a supine lying position; however, if such a position is uncomfortable for clients with excess weight, it should be avoided and substituted with a sitting or standing position.

Banded Half-Kneeling Pallof Press

Instructions

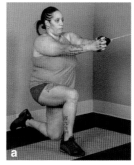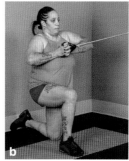

1. Anchor a band at chest height, grab the opposite end of the band in both hands, and step away from the anchor.

2. Take a half-kneeling position on the floor sideways to the anchor. Slowly extend the arms straight out in front of the body (*a*), hold for one count, then bring the hands back to the chest (*b*).

3. Engage the core and breathe normally. Do not let the torso twist toward the anchor.

4. Repeat for the desired number of repetitions, then switch sides.

Variation

- This exercise can be performed either in a contralateral (opposite arm and leg) or ipsilateral (same arm and leg) position. To progress this exercise, perform it in a kneeling or standing position.

Bird Dog

Instructions

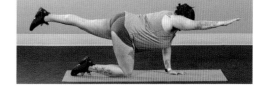

1. Take a quadruped position, find a neutral spine, and engage the core.

2. Raise one arm and the opposite leg during an exhale, and pause for one count at the top.

3. Inhale and return to the starting position.

4. Repeat on the other side.

Landmine Antirotation

Instructions

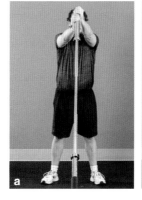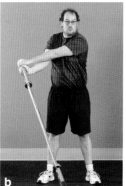

1. Grab a landmine with both hands and extend the arms in front of the body at shoulder height (*a*).

2. Stand with the feet slightly wider than shoulder-width apart, keep the chest up, and engage the core.

3. Pressing the landmine out, swipe it left and right while keeping the arms extended throughout the movement (*b*).

4. Resist the landmine wanting to pull the arms down, and breathe normally.

Landmine Twist

Instructions

1. Grab a landmine with both hands and extend the arms in front of the body at shoulder height (*a*).
2. Stand with the feet slightly wider than shoulder-width apart, keep the chest up, and engage the core.
3. Rotate the trunk and hips while swinging the weight all the way down to one side, keeping the arms extended throughout the movement (*b*).

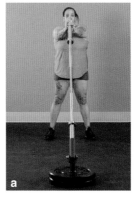
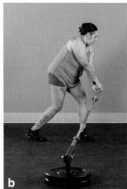

4. Return to the starting position and reverse the movement to swing the weight all the way to the opposite side while breathing normally.

Medicine Ball Rotational Swing

Instructions

1. Stand with the feet shoulder-width apart, holding a medicine ball with both hands at chest height (*a*).
2. Rotate the torso to one side, pivoting on the back foot, and then explosively rotate to the other side (*b*).
3. Engage the core and breathe normally throughout the movement.

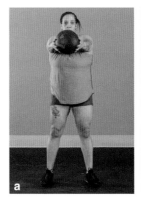
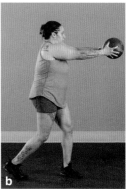

Rotational Chop

Instructions

1. Anchor a band high up. Grab the opposite end of the band in both hands, step away from the anchor, and stand sideways to the band's anchor point (*a*).
2. Make a sweeping, chopping-like movement diagonally downward with straight arms (*b*).
3. With control, return to the starting position.

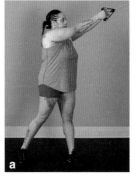
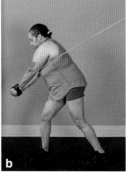

Variation

- The rotational chop can also be performed from low to high, anchoring the band to a stable object at roughly knee height.

CHAPTER SUMMARY

This chapter focused on muscular fitness and the psychophysiological adaptations to resistance training. It discussed in detail common myths and misconceptions linked to resistance training and described how to execute a large variety of training exercises using gym equipment, body weight, and partner-assisted manual resistance. The positive role of progressions was explored, along with modifications of fundamental movement patterns in muscular fitness activities within various exercise settings. In addition, the chapter emphasized that every weight management program should include muscle-strengthening activities on a regular basis.

KEY POINTS

- Resistance training should be a foundational piece of a multifaceted exercise training puzzle for individuals with overweight or obesity.
- Muscular fitness improvements play a vital role in various hormonal, biochemical, physiological, and psychological indicators linked to metabolic dysregulation.
- Muscle-strengthening activities are critically important for clients with overweight or obesity, helping this population manage common musculoskeletal health disorders and physical limitations.
- Any form of resistance training can be an injury-free, feasible, and effective exercise option; however, traditional strength training may be not always be an engaging strategy for every client.
- Partner-assisted manual resistance can be a nontraditional, joint-friendly, and pleasant muscle-strengthening mode for engaging clients with overweight or obesity in regular muscular fitness activities within various exercise settings.

CHAPTER QUIZ

Quiz answers can be found in the appendix.

1. One of the most promising chronic physiological adaptations to resistance training with respect to metabolic dysregulation is
   a. reduced cortisol
   b. reduced insulin resistance
   c. increased testosterone
   d. increased catecholamines

2. Which is the adaptation most commonly associated with resistance training?
   a. increased muscle fiber size
   b. increased muscle fiber number
   c. reduced fat cell size
   d. reduced fat cell number

3. One of the most promising acute psychological responses to resistance training is
   a. an improvement in self-confidence, self-esteem, and self-efficacy
   b. an increase in memory and concentration
   c. a reduction in the risk of Alzheimer's disease and dementia
   d. an increase in levels of endogenous opiates

4. Resistance training can chronically reduce
   a. behavioral regulation associated with exercise
   b. depression, anxiety, and other mental health disorders
   c. energy levels and mood
   d. focus and cognitive function

5. Resistance training may be more psychologically enjoyable than aerobic exercise for individuals with obesity, resulting in
   a. a more positive affective response
   b. a more negative affective response
   c. an equal affective response
   d. a more positive affective response, but only among young adults

6. Which of the following is NOT a negative psychological factor linked to resistance training that minimizes the positive effects?
   a. weight stigma
   b. lower levels of mental health
   c. internal motivation
   d. higher prevalence of diagnosable mental illness

7. Which of the following statements linked to resistance training for individuals with overweight or obesity is INCORRECT?
   a. Aerobic exercise is safer than resistance training.
   b. Both aerobic and resistance training should be regularly applied.
   c. Resistance machines and free weights are equally safe.
   d. Resistance training can be a pain-free and enjoyable exercise experience.

8. Which of the following statements linked to resistance training for individuals with overweight or obesity is correct?
   a. High volume (high repetitions) is better than high intensity (low repetitions).
   b. Muscle failure is the absolute way to success.
   c. Delayed-onset muscle soreness determines progress.
   d. Any type of resistance training equipment can be effective.

9. Are partner-assisted manual resistance exercises for a physically inactive adult with overweight or obesity beneficial during a muscle-strengthening session?
   a. yes—but only if there is no access to free weights or stationary resistance machines
   b. no—it is a boring approach with no sense for a client who just wants to lose weight
   c. yes—it is a feasible and pleasant exercise approach that promotes engagement in structured and supervised resistance exercise
   d. no—it is only a good option for novice clients without overweight or obesity

10. Which of the following exercises is recommended for previously inactive clients with overweight or obesity to activate core muscles?
    a. reverse crunches
    b. elevated plank
    c. Russian twists
    d. supine leg raises

CASE STUDY

Case study answers can be found in the appendix.

John is aiming to lose weight and improve his health, fitness, and well-being, but he has only had negative resistance training experiences in the past when he worked with other exercise professionals in various exercise settings. Particularly, over the past two years, he has implemented traditional strength training using stationary weight machines in a gym setting, where the prescribed exercises have not been body size–friendly. In addition, no interaction has occurred between John and the gym's hired exercise professionals who regularly supervise, instruct, and design his muscle-strengthening sessions. Importantly, John is struggling with chronic low-back pain, limited hip and shoulder mobility, and poor functional capacity. He is not an active person and regularly spends a lot of hours sitting. John is interested in improving his muscular fitness levels and functionality through engaging muscle-strengthening options in a fitness studio or at home. He is concerned about traditional strength training programs since a similar exercise strategy has not been a pleasant exercise experience for him in the past. He is hoping to try something different with respect to resistance training for 2 to 3 days per week because he is convinced that resistance training should not be avoided based on his current physical fitness status and health goals. Specifically, John's goals are to improve his muscular fitness while also experiencing a pain-free, feasible, and enjoyable form of resistance training in a supervised setting.

1. What mode of resistance training should John perform for his muscular fitness program to meet his goals from both a physiological and psychological perspective?
2. How would you program the muscle-strengthening routine in terms of the number of exercises, volume, intensity, and rest intervals?
3. What type of physiological responses might John expect when performing this exercise routine?
4. When will John begin to see results from his new workout routine, and what physiological adaptations can he expect with regard to his health and fitness profile?
5. Besides biological benefits, what other psychological and mental benefits might John experience from his new resistance training routine?

CHAPTER 9

Neuromotor Fitness

Alexios Batrakoulis, PhD, Leslie A. Stenger, EdD, and Elizabeth Kovar, MA

> After completing this chapter, you will be able to
> - describe the physiological adaptations to neuromotor and functional training,
> - list the benefits of adapted agility, balance, and coordination training,
> - apply adjunct modalities for improving motor fitness, and
> - explain the role of mind–body fitness activities as a feasible neuromotor fitness modality.

The role of exercise in preventing obesity and maintaining weight loss is complicated and has led to a vast amount of research. The focus of this section is to review the role neuromotor fitness plays within the process. The term *neuromotor* pertains to both nerves and muscles. Both are necessary for the neuromuscular system to produce movement. According to the American College of Sports Medicine (ACSM), neuromotor fitness is often referred to as *functional training* and involves skills such as balance, agility, speed, coordination, proprioception, endurance, strength, and flexibility (Garber et al. 2011). Research indicates that the terms *functional training* and *neuromotor fitness* are interchangeable when describing multiplanar, integrated movements that include acceleration, deceleration, stabilization, and destabilization and lead to improvements in neuromuscular efficiency (Da Silva-Gligoretto 2019; Stenger, 2018). However, the definition of *functional training* has not yet been well established, because inconsistent concepts in the current literature regarding this task-specific training modality create substantial confusion in the exercise community (Ide et al. 2022; La Scala Teixeira et al. 2017). Generally, functional training aims to improve the functional aspects of the neuromuscular system, and therefore, the desired objective is to restore neuromuscular function (Fleck and Kraemer 2014). Thus, the term *functional training* was initially used by sports medicine and rehabilitation professionals when working with older adults or athletes after injuries in a clinical setting (Stenger 2018).

That said, the term *functional training* no longer describes a specific physical training program. Instead, any exercise concept can be defined as functional training because it aims to increase performance for a specific functional task (Ide et al. 2022). People with obesity, in particular, need to improve their functional capacity for activities of daily living. With this in mind, any physical training program incorporating muscular strength, power, flexibility, and endurance exercises into the same session or within a periodized training regimen may efficiently improve the functional aspects of the neuromuscular system among individuals with excess body weight or adiposity. Importantly, movement-based exercise programs have been reported as a critical factor for inducing beneficial alterations in physical function and motor skills related to daily life among inactive populations affected by obesity or other common, lifestyle-related chronic diseases (King and Stanforth 2015). The broad definitions of *functional training* and *neuromotor fitness* enable fitness professionals to define the type of muscular fitness most appropriate for the desired population. There are common characteristics that emerge when defining neuromotor or functional training (Stenger 2018). This type of training

- is purpose-driven,
- is intentional,
- is multiplanar and multijoint,
- consists of activities from daily life,
- is specific,
- is task-driven,
- contributes to injury prevention, and
- creates a kinetic chain reaction.

Exercise professionals aiming to promote functional capacity among previously inactive people with overweight or obesity should consider these characteristics when designing client-centered muscular fitness programs in any exercise setting.

Physiological Adaptations With Neuromotor Fitness

Think of human movement as an orchestra. The conductor is the nervous system, which eloquently coordinates the muscular and skeletal systems to create gross and fine motor skills and produce endless movement patterns. As defined by the ACSM, *exercise volume* is "the summation of the total number of repetitions performed during a single training session multiplied by the resistance used and is reflective of the duration of which muscles are being stressed" (ACSM 2009, 690).

As mentioned in chapter 8, adaptations are based on manipulating the acute variables of exercise (muscle actions, volume, intensity and load, order of exercises, rest periods, and speed and tempo of movement) (Bird et al. 2005). Chronic adaptations related to neuromotor training include greater force production due to enhanced neuromuscular mechanisms. Neurological adaptations include greater recruitment of muscle fibers and enhanced rate of signal discharge to the muscle fibers. Muscular adaptations include an increase in the cross-sectional area of muscle tissue and changes in muscle architecture (ACSM 2009). Neuromotor exercise also seems to be effective in improving body composition in untrained populations (de Oliveira et al. 2019).

Training Adapted for Agility, Balance, and Coordination

Exercises incorporating balance and agility can be effective for improving motor control, proprioception, and overall quality of life (Garber et al. 2011). Agility and balance training may also reduce the risk of falling and fear of falling (Rodrigues et al. 2023). It has been noted in the research that individuals with abdominal obesity are more likely to experience falls than those with more equal distribution of fat weight throughout the body (Neri et al. 2020). Individuals with excess body weight are also more likely to have degenerative joint disease, thereby exhibiting a lower ability for stabilization and balance (Máximo et al. 2019).

Balance and strength training are important both physically and psychologically. Balance training can increase one's ability to control many of the destabilizing forces that occur during exercise, such as gravity, varying surface conditions, and the effects of some medications. These factors can influence a person's proprioception, or perception of their body's position and movement, but performing balance training can improve coordination due to a new understanding of how the body moves and how to control the movement (Brooks 2002). Being able to move one's body through space safely and efficiently is critical for the activities of daily living and for changing body position from standing to sitting and vice versa. Equally important is safely moving from the ground to a seated or standing position. These tasks can be much more difficult for individuals with excess body weight due to impaired proprioception.

To challenge the body, it is recommended to exercise in what is often described as a proprioceptively enriched environment. This may consist of an unstable yet controlled environment in which appropriate progressions are applied to allow the participant to adapt to the changing surroundings. Certain exercises using an unstable surface, such as a balance ball, stability ball, or foam roller, aim to reeducate the nerves and muscle tissues to work together in order to control a particular movement that engages different body parts at the same time. In other words, training in an unstable yet controlled environment increases the body's stability, balance, and coordination during a variety of movements (Romero-Franco et al. 2013). However, unstable surfaces result in limited muscular strength and power gains, because the increased difficulty reduces overloading compared to traditional resistance training. The transfer of gains from exercise performed on unstable surfaces to movement on stable surfaces (everyday life) is not optimal, and the potential risks of such adaptations do not appear to outweigh the potential benefits (Behm et al. 2015). In simple terms, heavy or explosive resistance training on unstable surfaces appears to be a useless and dangerous exercise concept for clients with excess weight.

Stabilization has been defined as the body's ability to provide optimal dynamic joint support and maintain correct posture during all movements. Balance training is a critical component of neuromotor exercise that requires an individual's mechanoreceptors to convert a neural message into a mechanical movement outcome. This type of training involves either maintaining a static position, controlling the body within a dynamic environment, or both. Proprioception involves multiple pathways within the body that deliver messages to and from the muscles via specialized neural receptors, referred to as mechanoreceptors, within the connective tissue. A mechanoreceptor is a sensory receptor that responds to mechanical pressure, converting the pressure into electrical signals sent to the central nervous system. A mechanoreceptor has the ability to detect and respond to certain kinds of stimuli in its environment, such as touch and changes in pressure or posture. Proprioception reflects the body's ability to adapt to the ever-changing environment that alters specific forces, tension, and, ultimately, body position (Aman et al. 2014), and mechanoreceptors detect signals both internally and externally from the environment and external forces on the body—such as gravity, varying surfaces, external weight, or body weight—that alter the center of mass.

The two mechanoreceptors that are on primary alert during balance, agility, stability, and coordination training are the Golgi tendons and muscle spindles. Golgi tendon organs are receptors in the musculotendinous junction, and they are sensitive to the amount of tension within a muscle and the rate at which that tension changes. The muscle fibers within the muscle spindles are intrafusal muscle fibers, which are parallel to the extrafusal fibers that make up the majority of the muscle tissue. Intrafusal muscle fibers are sensitive to changes in the length of muscle and the rate at which the length changes. Working in a proprioceptively enriched environment will place the body in conditions appropriate for activating the mechanoreceptors and refining the response to various stimuli (Zampieri and de Nooij 2021). These advancements play a significant role in maintaining good posture during exercise by enabling the body to make continuous, small adjustments that maintain the center of gravity over the base of support, which is a key to postural control.

Individuals with excess body weight, especially with an android shape (concentrated fat distribution in the abdominal and chest area—also termed *central obesity*, *abdominal obesity*, or *visceral obesity*), typically shift their base of support anteriorly when standing, which often leads to balance issues. To regain balance, the pelvis tends to shift anteriorly, creating lumbar lordosis (an extreme curve in the lumbar spine) and an additional external load on the lumbar area (Máximo et al. 2019). When the neurological and muscular systems are working at the highest efficiency, the agonists, antagonists, synergists, neutralizers, mobilizers, and stabilizers work together to provide effective movement through all three planes. Thus, implementing fitness games as an extension of a dynamic warm-up session (see chapter 7), along with some targeted neuromotor exercises during the main session, may be an optimal way to yield beneficial alterations in motor skills and body functionality among populations with overweight or obesity.

Using Adjunct Modalities to Enhance Training

Adjunct modalities, such as suspension exercise devices, balance balls, speed ladders, and battle ropes, may be useful training tools. Also known as training toys, such non-traditional equipment may be attractive and user-friendly to people with overweight or obesity who seek to improve their functionality through physical movement in a supervised, authentic fitness setting (Stanforth et al. 2015). One purpose of these modalities is to incorporate whole-body, multijoint movements that require the integration of various muscle groups. This type of training teaches clients how to control their body weight and assists in reestablishing a center of gravity, balance, and stability under a variety of conditions. This synergistic approach promotes maximum energy expenditure in the minimum time frame to promote reduction in body mass through efficient and safe movements.

Proprioceptive training involves both body awareness and stability and should teach the individual how to maintain or establish body alignment, stability, and awareness of their center of gravity during integrated movements on a variety of surfaces. The term *integrated or compound movement* implies that movements are closed-chain in nature and either the hands or feet are involved in supporting the weight of the body (i.e., squat, deadlift, hip thrust, push-up, pull-up, and dip), whereas open-chain movements are often considered isolated movements (i.e., knee extension, knee curl, hip extension, chest press, chest fly, pull-down, row, shoulder press, biceps curl, and triceps extension). Once individuals have established increased body awareness and the ability to maintain overall body stability, they are ready to participate in a wide range of activities that will challenge them both physically and psychologically using suspension training devices, battle ropes, balance and stability balls, and speed ladders, all while allowing for easy progressions that are not solely based on increasing weight but rather proprioceptive options. All four modalities address the fundamental principles of neuromotor training, which include being able to provide integrated movements involving multiple joints in multiple planes.

Suspension Device Training

Suspension exercise training seems to be one of the most feasible and promising modalities focusing on neuromotor fitness benefits among clients with excess weight, providing a variety of muscle-strengthening exercises activating the whole body in a safe, enjoyable, and efficient way (Campa et al. 2021). This nontraditional muscle-strengthening modality can induce beneficial changes in musculoskeletal, cardiometabolic, and mental health indices among older adults with metabolic dysregulation (Engel et al. 2019; Jiménez-García et al. 2019; Pierle et al. 2022; Samadpour Masouleh et al. 2021). Specifically, this form of exercise uses secured straps to place the individual in an unstable yet controlled environment by using the handles as a single anchor point for the hands or feet while the opposite end of the body (feet or hands, respectively) remains in contact with the ground. In essence, the body becomes the machine, and the method of altering the work is to change the leverage of the body to use body weight as the stimulus.

Because the body weight is the stimulus and the exercise professional selects the movements, suspension device training can focus on multiple neuromotor components, such as mobility, stability, balance, and coordination, as well as the traditional components of strength, endurance, and power (Dawes 2022). This can be an efficient training modality for clients with obesity, given that this population is typically characterized by poor functional capacity (Pataky et al. 2014). Beginners can use the system to add stability to movements by simply using the straps to control their body weight throughout a movement. Intermediate and advanced clients can change the position of the straps to increase the leverage, creating a mechanical disadvantage during the various exercises and thereby increasing the intensity of the movement. Movements can be created to mimic the same movement patterns used in everyday life, a sport, or a favorite leisure activity (Dawes 2022). This can be very motivating to individuals with excess body weight who find the traditional resistance training exercises on weight machines or with free weights to be boring or overly challenging (Burgess et al. 2017).

Suspension training depends on controlling the center of gravity as it moves through space to generate neuromuscular responses that change the mechanical advantage. Consider the following example: if a person were hanging from a pull-up bar, their center of gravity would be located within the body closer to the chest area. If that person released one hand, the body would rotate, and the center of gravity would move downward and possibly outside the body, depending on the body's position (Dawes 2022). Suspension training is a good option when the goal is to increase energy expenditure, because one exercise can allow the client to use large muscles through a full range of motion in an integrated fashion, moving through more than one plane of movement (Dudgeon et al. 2015; Smith et al. 2016).

Battle Ropes

Battle ropes, also known as heavy or functional ropes, have become a popular adjunct training modality in the fitness industry. They are an alternative type of equipment that enhances overall fitness and promotes muscular strength and endurance, power, coordination, and aerobic capacity, depending on the training program parameters. Battle ropes allow clients with excess weight to execute integrated movements at different speeds through various ranges of motion and planes. Although battle ropes primarily activate the upper body musculature, they appear to be an effective training tool for inducing general conditioning improvements (Fountaine and Schmidt 2015). Before prescribing battle rope training to clients with overweight or obesity, exercise professionals should consider some critical equipment-related variables affecting the intensity of the exercise, such as the length, diameter, and weight of the rope (Fountaine and Schmidt 2015). An advantage of battle ropes is the ability to promote coordination training regardless of the intensity of the prescribed exercise. This is critically important for clients with poor functionality and impaired motor skills (Pataky et al. 2014). On the other hand, the large space requirement and the limited range of motion when performing high-speed movements are disadvantages of battle rope training.

Balance and Stability Balls

Balance and stability balls are instability devices that permit multijoint or single-joint movements in an unstable environment. In theory, increasing the planes of motion or decreasing the number of contact points with the floor requires the client to exert greater effort to maintain balance and stability, thereby facilitating the completion of the desired movement. Consequently, numerous exercises using an instability device enhance core strength and muscular endurance, in addition to improving balance and stability at the specific joint or throughout the entire body.

Speed Ladder

Speed ladder exercises are a useful and enjoyable way for previously inactive clients with excess body weight or adiposity to enhance agility, which is a factor affecting physical fitness levels. Agility exercises for clients with overweight or obesity support their ability to move and change directions safely and efficiently. In addition, agility ladder drills are an effective tool for increasing aerobic capacity because they elevate the client's heart rate to a level that is beneficial for maintaining optimal cardiovascular health, resulting in the expenditure of a considerable quantity of calories. Thus, this particular equipment tool has been widely used in hybrid-type, multicomponent interval training programs tailored for people with overweight or obesity (Batrakoulis and Fatouros 2022; Batrakoulis et al. 2023; Batrakoulis et al. 2021). It also has the benefit of maintaining mental agility. The necessity to concentrate and focus on the task at hand, as well as the physical coordination required, ensures that the brain and body are engaged simultaneously. This type of exercise has been shown to improve overall coordination, which in turn has been linked to a reduction in the effects of aging on the mind.

Special Considerations for Adjunct Modalities in Training

In general, adjunct equipment appears to be an effective training tool for improving muscular fitness, static and dynamic balance, kinesthesis, proprioception, agility, and coordination. The use of an unstable surface, especially, triggers the core musculature to engage in an integrated movement, aiming to maintain the kinetic chain in a proper position. Thus, instability devices challenge individuals with obesity to enhance muscular strength and balance simultaneously while improving body composition (Campa et al. 2021).

Importantly, beginner clients with obesity should have solid balance skills on the ground before using an instability device. When incorporating balance exercises into a training session tailored to people with excess weight, exercise professionals should consider the following four variables to regress, progress, or modify an adjunct modality:

1. Movement
2. Eye gaze

3. External stimulus (e.g., equipment, trainer's touch, and wall)

4. Contact points (e.g., toes, hands, feet, and knees)

These four variables are of critical importance to exercise professionals when designing and supervising neuromotor fitness programs that are tailored to the needs, priorities, and goals of clients with excess weight. Such a training strategy may facilitate positive exercise experiences through injury-free, effective, pleasant, and inclusive workouts in any exercise setting.

In summary, exercise professionals should carefully consider using this alternative category of equipment with clients who have overweight or obesity, due to the higher skill level required to use these particular adjunct modalities compared to more traditional muscle-strengthening equipment. This is important when working with clients who have excess weight since these individuals may have poor functional capacity, limited stability and mobility in various joints, and impaired balance (Pataky et al. 2014). However, the integration of basic neuromotor exercises into an adapted exercise session for clients with excess weight could be implemented by using an easy drill at first. Afterward, progressions and modifications could be used to make clients feel more comfortable with adjunct modalities. Such a strategy would help clients establish the foundation they need to be able to pursue more challenging exercises.

EXERCISE TECHNIQUES

Each of the following neuromotor exercises should be performed for 15 to 30 s (8-12 reps) with a work-to-rest ratio of 1:1, aiming to ensure proper motor control without sacrificing movement quality.

COORDINATION EXERCISES

SUSPENSION DEVICE

Suspended Squat

Instructions

1. Face the anchor point of the straps.

2. Hold both handles in front of the waist, with the elbows flexed by the sides of the body (*a*).

3. Lower into a squat, extending the arms in front of the body at eye level (*b*).

4. Push back up to the starting position.

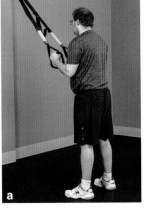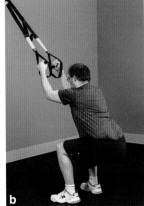

Variation

• Perform the same exercise using a wider stance.

Suspended Alternating Reverse Lunges

Instructions

1. Face toward the anchor point of the straps.
2. Hold both handles in a position where the straps are tight, with the elbows flexed at 90° (*a*).
3. Execute a backward lunge, allowing the arms to straighten (*b*).
4. Once the knees are flexed to 90° in the lunge, return to the top.
5. Switch sides, and continue alternating sides for the desired number of reps.

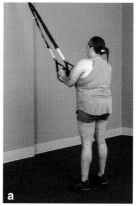 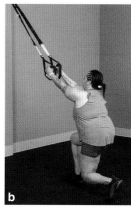

Variation

• Perform all repetitions on a single side consecutively, then switch to the opposite side.

Neutral-Grip Suspended Row

Instructions

1. Face toward the anchor point of the straps with the feet hip-width apart.
2. Hold the handles with a neutral grip (palms facing each other), with the elbows close to the waist.
3. Keep the body at a suitable incline (45°-60°) for the strength level (*a*).
4. Keep the chest up, engage the core, pull the torso up to meet the handles, and slowly reverse (*b*).

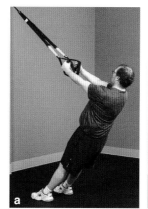 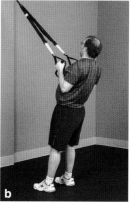

Variation

• Perform the same exercise with a pronated (palms facing downward at shoulder width), supinated (palms facing upward at shoulder width), or wide (palms facing downward with arms abducted closer to 90° from the torso) grip.

Suspended Staggered Chest Press

Instructions

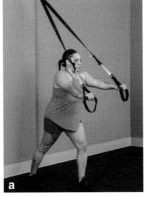
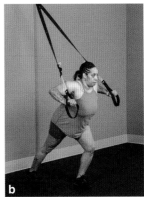

1. Face away from the anchor point of the straps with a staggered stance (feet slightly offset front to back).
2. The arms should be straight out in front of the body, barely wider than the torso at chest height (*a*).
3. Keeping a strong plank position in the torso, flex the elbows to lower the body toward the hands (*b*).
4. Straighten the elbows to press back up to the start position.

Variation

- Perform the same exercise, but alter the stance and base of support (e.g., feet shoulder-width apart, hip-width apart, or together).

Suspended Staggered T-Rows

Instructions

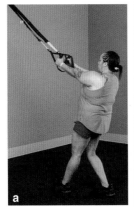
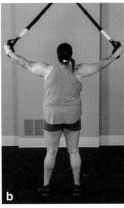
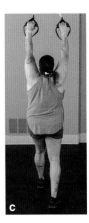

1. Face toward the anchor point of the straps, and stagger the stance (one foot should be slightly ahead of the other).
2. Hold the handles with a neutral grip (palms facing each other), with the arms extended in front of the chest.
3. Keep the body at a suitable incline (60°) for the strength level (*a*).
4. Keep the chest up, engage the core, pull the torso up to meet the handles, and slowly reverse (*b*).
5. Pull against the straps, shifting weight to one foot while opening the arms into a *T* position.
6. Return to the starting position.

Variation

- Perform the same exercise, but alter the stance and base of support (e.g., feet shoulder-width apart, hip-width apart, or together) or open the arms into a *Y* or *I* position (*c*).

BATTLE ROPE

Bilateral Wave

Instructions

1. Hold the ropes with a neutral grip, slightly flex the knees to lower into a shallow squat, and drive the hips back while engaging the core (*a*).

2. Raise both ropes to just below shoulder height at the same time quickly, then bring them down again (*b*).

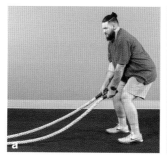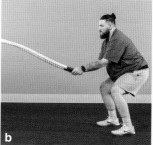

3. Hinge back, keeping the chest up and the shoulders down and back throughout the execution.

4. Repeat the up-and-down motion, creating simultaneous waves with the ropes.

Alternating Wave

Instructions

1. Hold a rope in each hand with a neutral grip, slightly flex the knees to lower into a shallow squat, and drive the hips back while engaging the core (*a*).

2. Raise one rope quickly to just below shoulder height, then bring that rope back to the start position while raising the other rope at the same time (*b*).

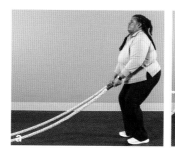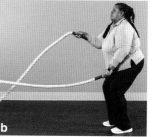

3. Repeat the up-and-down motion with the ropes moving in opposite directions, creating alternating waves.

Tsunami Wave

Instructions

1. Hold a rope in both hands, slightly flex the knees to lower into a shallow squat, and drive the hips back while engaging the core (a).

2. Be sure there is a little slack in the rope; it may be necessary to step forward.

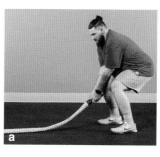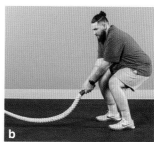

3. Raise and lower the arms to create quick, small waves with the rope (*b*).

Side-to-Side Wave

Instructions

1. Hold the ropes with a neutral grip, slightly flex the knees to lower into a shallow squat, and drive the hips back while engaging the core (a).

2. Be sure there is a little slack in the rope; it may be necessary to step forward.

3. With the arms extended, slam the ropes to the floor on one side (b). Then, forcefully slam the ropes on the other side.

4. Continue slamming the ropes quickly side to side.

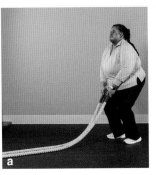
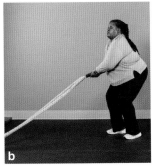

In-and-Out Wave

Instructions

1. Hold the ropes with a neutral grip, slightly flex the knees to lower into a shallow squat, and drive the hips back while engaging the core (a).

2. Be sure there is a little slack in the rope; it may be necessary to step forward.

3. Simultaneously slam the ropes to the floor apart from each other (outside), then quickly slam them to the floor close together (inside) (b).

4. Continue slamming the ropes quickly out and in.

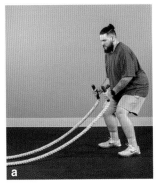
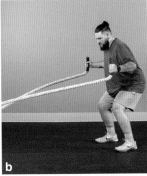

Rainbow

Instructions

1. Hold both ropes near the left knee with a neutral grip (a).

2. Be sure there is a little slack in the rope; it may be necessary to step forward.

3. In one fluid motion, extend the hips, knees, and back to swing the ropes up and overhead like a rainbow before squatting down to slam them to the ground near the right knee (b).

4. Quickly repeat the motion to the left side, and continue alternating side to side.

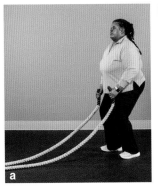
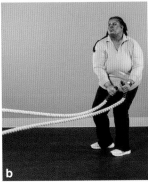

Slam

Instructions

1. Hold the ropes with a neutral grip, slightly flex the knees to lower into a shallow squat, and drive the hips back while engaging the core (*a*).
2. Be sure there is a little slack in the rope; it may be necessary to step forward.
3. Raise both ropes until the arms are level with the head. Slam the ropes down to the floor as hard as possible, then quickly repeat (*b*).

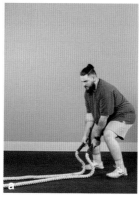 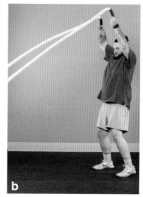

BALANCE EXERCISES

Single-Leg Balance

Instructions

1. Stand with the feet shoulder-width apart (*a*).
2. Extend the arms out to the sides and slowly lift the right foot off the floor (*b*).
3. Hold that position for 1 to 2 s, then relax.
4. Repeat on the other leg.

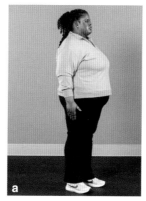 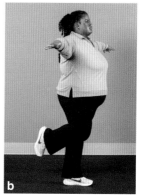

Modified Tree Pose

Instructions

1. Stand with the feet shoulder-width apart, holding the right hand to the chest and placing the left hand on a chair (*a*).
2. Raise the right leg straight up while turning the foot inward. Rest the sole of the right foot against the inside of the left thigh or calf (*b*).
3. Hold this position for 20 to 30 s.
4. Repeat on the other leg.

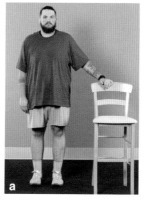 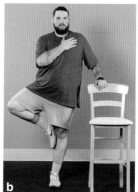

Tightrope Walk

Instructions

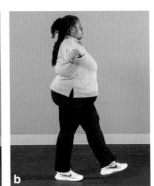

1. Stand on a line on the floor or next to a long rope. Place one foot in front of the other, heel to toe (*a*).

2. Like walking a tightrope, extend the arms out to the sides and start walking slowly, being careful to keep the feet on the line at all times (*b*).

3. Stop for at least 3 s before each step.

4. Take 10 steps forward, then turn around and repeat the exercise to return to the start position.

Flamingo Stand

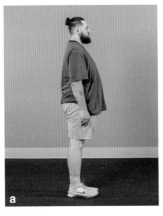
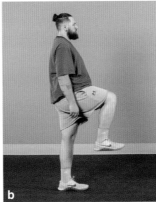
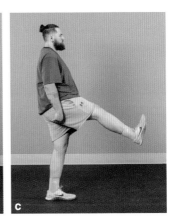

Instructions

1. Stand with the feet shoulder-width apart (*a*).

2. Raise the right knee up to hip height as though marching (*b*), then straighten the leg (*c*).

3. Reverse the movement, lower the leg, and repeat on the left side.

4. Repeat on both sides for 8 to 12 repetitions.

BALANCE BALL

Shin Balances

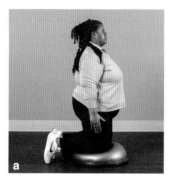
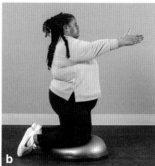
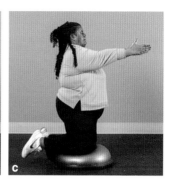

Instructions

1. Place the shins on top of a balance ball, keeping a neutral spine (*a*).
2. Place the toes on the ground, keep the hands in front of the shoulders, and hold this position (*b*).
3. To progress the exercise, lift the toes off the ground, close the eyes (*c*), or catch a ball thrown by the trainer.

Static Awareness Balance

Instructions

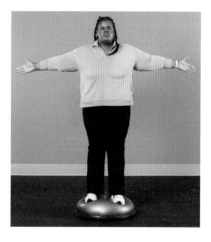

1. Stand upright on a balance dome with the feet hip-width apart.
2. Lift the arms out to the sides with the palms facing forward.
3. Focus on a focal point on the floor or wall directly ahead. Hold the position.
4. To progress the exercise, close one or both eyes.

Squat With Hand Tracking

Instructions

1. Stand upright on a balance dome with the feet hip-width apart.
2. Flex the knees and hips to lower the body into a squat. Place the arms in front of the body, with the elbows flexed and the palms facing forward (*a*).
3. Staying in the squat position, begin to move the hands up and down, while ensuring that the torso and head maintain stability throughout the movement (*b*).
4. To progress the exercise, keep the torso and head still while only moving the eyes to track the hands.

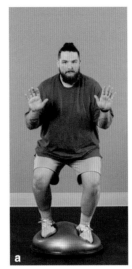
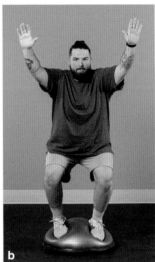

Standing Abduction Toe Taps

Instructions

1. Stand upright on the balance dome with the feet hip-width apart.
2. Place the arms in an athletic position in front of the body, with a 90° flex at the elbows (*a*).
3. Lift the left foot off the dome and tap the foot on the side of the dome (*b*). Return to the center and repeat with the right leg.
4. To progress the exercise, place the foot on the floor next to the dome and lower the body into a shallow squat position.

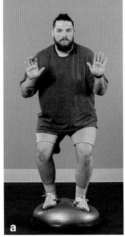
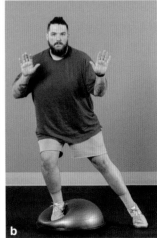

Static Lunge

Instructions

1. Stand with the right foot in the center of the balancing dome.
2. Keep the hands on the hips or in front of the body with the elbows flexed (*a*).
3. Lift the heel of the left foot and lower the left knee into a lunge position (*b*).
4. Return to the start position, then repeat.
5. Complete a set on the left leg, then switch to the right.

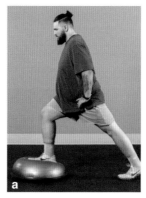
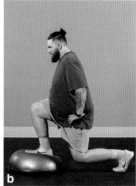

Walk-Ups

Instructions

1. Stand with a balance dome in front of the feet.
2. Place one foot on top of the dome (*a*), then the other foot (*b*), and then return both feet to the floor as if walking up and down on the dome.
3. Either lead with one foot for half the repetitions and then switch, or alternate the leading foot.
4. Use a body bar or wall to assist with balance if needed.

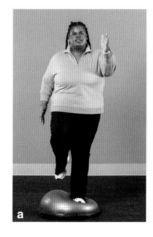
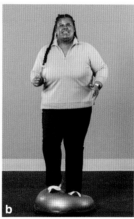

Variation

- To progress the exercise, perform step-ups, where only one foot at a time is placed on the dome instead of two.

Lateral Walk-Overs

Instructions

1. Stand with the outside of the right foot next to the balance dome.
2. Place the right foot on top of the dome (*a*), then the left, then bring the right foot to the floor on the other side of the dome (*b*), followed by the left. Imagine walking over the dome to the side.
3. Repeat in reverse to return to the start position: the left foot first on top of the dome, then the right, then the left foot to the floor, followed by the right.

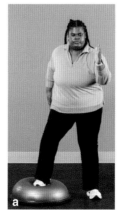
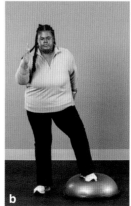

AGILITY EXERCISES

SPEED LADDER

Low-Knee Marching

Instructions

1. Begin at one end of the ladder, facing the rungs.
2. Walk with low knees into the first square with one foot and then into the next square with the other foot.
3. Repeat this process until the other end of the agility ladder is reached.
4. Turn around and repeat the exercise to return to the start position.

Variation

• Perform the same exercise laterally (lateral low-knee marching) to engage the frontal plane of motion.

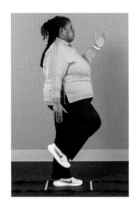

High-Knee Marching

Instructions

1. Begin at one end of the ladder, facing the rungs.
2. Walk with high knees into the first square with one foot and then into the next square with the other foot.
3. Repeat this process until the other end of the agility ladder is reached.
4. Turn around and repeat the exercise to return to the start position.

Variation

• Perform the same exercise laterally (lateral high-knee marching) to engage the frontal plane of motion.

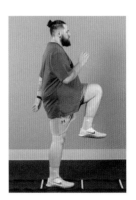

In-and-Out Steps

Instructions

1. Begin at one end of the ladder, facing the rungs.
2. Step the right foot to the outside (right) of the ladder, then step the left foot to the outside (left) of the ladder (a).
3. Step the right foot into the first box, followed by the left foot (b).
4. Continue this pattern to the end of the ladder.
5. Turn around and repeat the exercise to return to the start position, this time leading with the left foot.

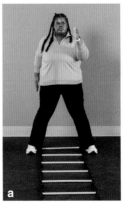 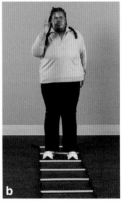

Variation

- Perform the same exercise standing on the side of the ladder, facing the first box (lateral in-and-out steps).

Side-to-Sides

Instructions

1. Stand with the ladder's first box on the left side of the body while facing the other end of the ladder.

2. Step into the first box with the left foot (leg closest to the ladder) (*a*), followed by the right foot.

3. Continue moving in the same direction (toward the leading leg) by stepping out of the box with the left foot (*b*), followed by the right foot.

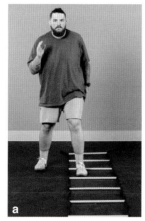 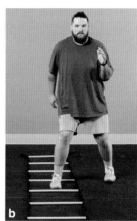

4. Continue this pattern through the remainder of the ladder.

5. Begin at the other end of the ladder, with the left side facing forward.

6. Place the left foot in the first box to start.

7. Bring the right foot into the same box, then step laterally into the next box with the left foot.

8. Move left and right in each box as quickly as possible.

9. Repeat the process, the next time beginning with the right foot.

Adaptations for Mind–Body Fitness

In the 21st century, the concept of mind–body fitness has grown in popularity and is one of the most sought-after types of exercise programming. During exercise, the mind signals the body to complete a movement or command, which connects the physical and mental aspects of the body. Technically, exercise in general involves mind–body fitness. However, the fitness industry recognizes mind–body fitness as a physical exercise approach executed with a profoundly inwardly directed focus (Shirley 2008). In the 1990s, the IDEA Health & Fitness Association narrowed down the five common characteristics of mind–body exercise as follows (Shirley 2008):

1. Inner mental focus

2. Concentration on muscular movements

3. Synchronization of movements with breathing patterns

4. Attention to form and alignment

5. A belief in the life energy, such as prana or chi, that is part of ancient Eastern disciplines

The Importance of Understanding the Nervous System When Working With People Who Have Obesity

Many fitness professionals know that mind–body exercise is beneficial, but they may not understand why. The missing link is usually a lack of understanding of the nervous system. Exercise mainly focuses on one of the branches of the peripheral nervous system: the autonomic nervous system (ANS). The ANS connects the brain to the internal organs. The three branches of the ANS include the sympathetic nervous system (SNS, responsible for fight-or-flight responses), the parasympathetic nervous system (PNS, with a rest-and-digest role), and the enteric nervous system (ENS, referred to as the gut brain) (Kiernan and Rajakumar 2013). The SNS and PNS work together like a seesaw; when one increases (activates), the other decreases (deactivates). When the SNS is activated, approximately 85% of the blood flow leaves the visceral organs and moves to the limbs and the working muscles to enable the body to flee danger. Within seconds after a (perceived) stressor, catecholamines such as epinephrine and norepinephrine (associated with the fight-or-flight response) are produced in the sympathetic nervous system and the adrenal medulla. They increase the heart rate and stroke volume and cause vasoconstriction of blood vessels in the skin and the gut (Kiernan and Rajakumar 2013).

With this knowledge, fitness professionals can recognize how often the human body operates in the SNS. The body activates the SNS during such stimulation, or stressors, as regular exercise, stressful moments, external distractions, and noise pollution, which is most of our daily existence.

Unfortunately, the brain does not know if one is fleeing a dangerous situation or stressed from a work email; it only knows how to respond to stress. As a result, the common habit of eating on the go (especially while feeling stressed) is not ideal. Consuming food while the SNS is responding to stress disrupts the natural flow of digestion and assimilation of nutrients, because the blood is flowing to the limbs to flee a perceived danger.

Conversely, the parasympathetic nervous system is the rest-and-digest part of the nervous system. Eating while in a PNS state is ideal because the blood flows to the visceral organs of the body to aid digestion. The PNS is also activated while one is at rest or asleep to help the body recover and heal. Individuals with sleeping issues or chronic diseases are at a disadvantage and may already have issues with the autonomic nervous system. According to the research, common conditions such as unmanaged type 2 diabetes, autoimmune and inflammatory conditions, benign and cancerous tumors, heavy metal toxicity, physical injury or trauma, and congenital conditions can disrupt or lead to dysfunction or disease of the ANS (Kiernan and Rajakumar 2013).

This knowledge is important, because modern living supports a fight-or-flight lifestyle. Mind–body exercise can be the key to healing and getting healthy. Mind–body exercise not only promotes better mental and physical health but also cares for the nervous system.

Today, mind–body exercise includes a mix of modern hybrid classes and traditional or ancient mind–body–spirit practices, with yoga, Pilates, and tai chi being the most popular. Mind–body exercise is like a meditation in motion. During mind–body exercise, there is a union between the physical state (movement), the mental body (awareness), and the spirit (breath). The word *spirit* derives from the Latin word *spiritus*, which means *breath*. Because of the heightened awareness in movement coupled with deeper breathing, individuals may reach a state known as flow during these forms of exercise. Being in flow is referred to as being in the zone. In simple terms, it is the union between action and consciousness. As a result, mind–body fitness can have profound mental, emotional, spiritual, and physical effects on individuals with obesity (Batrakoulis 2022a). In general, mind–body fitness seems to be an injury-free, enjoyable, and effective exercise option for people with obesity, given that such meditative training modalities induce beneficial changes in physical fitness, cardiovascular risk factors, and mental health among individuals with excess weight (Batrakoulis 2022b; Batrakoulis 2022c).

Mental, Emotional, and Physical Benefits of Mind–Body Exercise

Chronic stress or constant triggers from trauma responses such as posttraumatic stress disorder (PTSD) induce imbalances and functional impairments within the brain, resulting in ANS dysregulation. One benefit of mind–body exercise is that it stabilizes the ANS and can bring individuals back to a psychological baseline more quickly (i.e., it restores optimal homeostasis). Its emphasis on awareness of one's thoughts, breathing, and movements in the present time consciously retrains the mind to think instead of subconsciously reacting when in a stressful situation. Neurons that fire together wire together. In simple terms, mind–body exercise retrains a person with an autopilot lifestyle to live with more awareness and healthy behavior patterns. For example, if a person reacts moments after a stressful situation by eating candy to seek comfort, increased mind–body awareness would train the individual to recognize their reactive behavioral pattern. With practice, the person will be better able to recognize the trigger in the moment. Such mindfulness then allows them to initiate ways to mitigate stress in a healthy way, such as taking deep breaths instead of eating candy.

Many of the traditional and slower forms of yoga, such as restorative yoga and yoga therapy, along with practices such as qigong and tai chi, breathing exercises, and meditation, regulate the ANS by moving a person out of the SNS and activating the PNS. When the body is mindfully moving, the heart rate slows, awareness increases, and breathing is regulated, which stimulates a calming atmosphere. If a mind–body class includes soothing, ambient, or low-beats-per-minute music, the brain will also respond to the slower beat. Dr. Emma Gray of the British CBT and Counseling Service for Spotify has found through her research of music and the brain that humans are more relaxed when listening to music with 50 to 80 beats per minute, which puts the brain in the alpha wave state (Gray 2013). Gray indicates in her findings that it is not the genre of music but the tempo that has the most to do with creating a flow state.

Mental and Emotional Benefits

Body and breath awareness is key in all forms of mind–body exercise. Many people lack body awareness, and most are shallow chest breathers unless trained in deep, diaphragmatic breathing. A study investigating the role of 10 sessions of yoga in adult women with chronic PTSD indicated positive alterations in body awareness (Rhodes et al. 2016). In particular, yoga "can serve as a useful adjunctive component of trauma-focused treatment to build skills in tolerating and modulating physiologic and affective states that have become dysregulated by trauma exposure" (Rhodes et al. 2016, 1). Interestingly, women exerted important reductions in PTSD symptom severity during yoga and had a greater likelihood of overcoming a PTSD diagnosis. Also, female participants exhibited a meaningful reduction in using activities such as unhealthy eating to reduce negative tension and depressive symptoms compared to women who participated in consultation without any involvement in yoga practice (Rhodes et al. 2016).

Regular yoga practice helps the ANS become more flexible and adaptive, while mindfulness meditation, a key element of yoga, supports positive neural function changes (Hölzel et al. 2011; Streeter et al. 2012). The physical movements in yoga also release endorphins into the bloodstream, hormones that produce calmness and can remain in the body hours after practicing yoga. A study that evaluated the effects of hatha yoga and Omkar meditation on men demonstrated that yoga practice can help elevate the secretion of melatonin, resulting in an improved sense of well-being (Harinath et al. 2004). This is an important finding, given that melatonin is the hormone that regulates the sleep–wake cycle. After more frequent PNS activation, the mind and body positively transform. The mind becomes clearer and more aware, with the ability to make better decisions. Often, people naturally let things go or release deep-seated emotions from past wounds. This is all a process and is best experienced from a long-term practice coupled with lifestyle changes.

Physical Benefits

Many studies suggest that mind–body exercise contributes to weight loss; however, there is a need for additional studies and evidence. Studying clients with obesity who do not take medications would be ideal, because weight gain is a side effect of many medications that might present confounding factors. The caloric deficit incurred through mind–body exercise and the rating of perceived exertion are not as high as in other forms of exercise. Nevertheless, mind–body exercise has powerful effects on a person's stress level and requires constant core engagement, which may be why it contributes to weight management.

A well-rounded fitness regimen would include a mix of mind–body, cardiovascular, and resistance training. A 2021 study examining the therapeutic effects of 3 months of tai chi and conventional training on the management of abdominal adiposity in middle-aged and older adults with visceral obesity concluded that both interventions could prevent the progression of abdominal obesity (Siu et al. 2021). Considering that this population tends to experience a high risk of obesity-related illness, such outcomes enhance the important role of mind–body fitness modalities in cardiometabolic health among individuals with central obesity. Likewise, a meta-analysis evaluating the scientific evidence for the efficacy of Pilates in improving anthropometric characteristics and body composition indicators in adults with excess weight revealed that Pilates can induce a substantial reduction in body mass, body mass index, and body fat percentage in adults with overweight or obesity (Wang et al. 2021).

What Type of Mind–Body Fitness Class Is Best for Obesity?

Age and current fitness level affect where the client will begin. For older adults and sedentary individuals, it is best to start with the basics, learn the fundamentals, and progress over time. Individuals who are sedentary or have unresolved trauma can benefit from therapeutic or restorative mind–body exercise classes. As fitness endurance, skills, and coordination develop over time, progressing to intermediate classes is achievable without a higher risk of injury.

Many ancient forms of movement, such as yoga, have been modernized and incorporated into hybrid classes, such as a PiYo class. PiYo has emerged as a favorite class for individuals who seek to integrate the core-building of yoga, the strength-training of Pilates, and the nonstop action of an aerobic-based program into a single session. These classes are higher paced and use more modernized music (with a higher number of beats per minute) to keep the body moving. This may be more appropriate for an individual who has a current baseline of fitness, such as being able to walk or exercise for 30 to 60 minutes comfortably without taking frequent breaks or gasping for air.

Fitness professionals should recognize the following exercise risk factors for individuals with obesity:

- Higher risk of falling because of poor balance
- Chronic joint pain
- Poor mobility and posture due to a sedentary lifestyle
- Potential inability to get up and down from the floor
- Restrictive range of motion because of android obesity, especially during exercises that include forward folds
- Risk of overheating or heat intolerance, especially if one has a chronic disease such as multiple sclerosis
- Side effects from medication

During exercise, the body either moves through gravity or against gravity. Being upright and moving is ideal for building strength and burning calories but can put continuous stress on the joints. For example, the weight of the person's leg can be a significant challenge when lifting it to target major muscles. Too many activities requiring one-legged balance can also put a lot of stress on the standing leg. In addition, lying on a mat and moving against gravity for long periods may be uncomfortable with the person's body mass loaded on the spine and joints. Individuals with excess weight, especially older adults, could instead benefit from chair variations of yoga, Pilates, or tai chi to build strength, range of motion, and muscular endurance before progressing to standing and mat classes. Chair classes or modifications reduce the mechanical stress placed on the lower body's joints. Too much mechanical stress with underdeveloped ligament and tendon strength can lead to pain while moving or to injury.

Every person with obesity is different, and class recommendations will vary for each individual. The goal is to recommend smart progressions as well as making each class a positive experience to promote retention. People with obesity can participate in all forms of mind–body exercise. Some clients may require modifications (which might be temporary) or assistance (such as using a chair or bar) at the beginning stages of exercise, or specialized classes for their ability may be suitable (such as chair yoga for older adults).

CHAPTER SUMMARY

Obesity is a global epidemic and crisis affecting the minds and bodies of millions of people across the planet. Mind–body exercise is an effective form of exercise that can help individuals with obesity increase physical well-being as well as improve emotional and mental health. Regardless of the factors underlying obesity, mind–body exercise regulates the autonomic nervous system to help individuals return to optimal homeostasis, reduce overall stress, and better manage psychological triggers. Individuals with obesity can participate in any form of mind–body exercise, but modifications or adaptations may be required to assist them during the strength-building process.

KEY POINTS

- With physical education on the decline in the United States, obesity affects all ages, and children are raised with unhealthy learning behaviors.
- Obesity can develop from behaviors learned during childhood, or a stressful or traumatic event can affect one's health negatively if food is used for comfort when dealing with emotions.
- Chronic states of stress affect physical and mental well-being and also influence food choices that may contribute to obesity.
- Mind–body exercise is differentiated from conventional exercise by a direct inward focus that increases body awareness.
- Mind–body exercise positively affects the mind, body, and spirit due to activation of the parasympathetic nervous system and the release of positive hormones.
- Mind–body exercise focuses on awareness and deep breathing, which help retrain a person with an autopilot lifestyle to develop healthier behavior patterns.
- Sedentary individuals with obesity have more risk factors for injury, and therefore, they may require exercise modifications.
- All mind–body exercises or classes can be adapted, such as by using a chair to decrease the load and stress on lower-body joints.

CHAPTER QUIZ

Quiz answers can be found in the appendix.

1. During mind–body exercise, there is a union between movement, awareness, and _____.
   a. lifestyle
   b. breath
   c. music
   d. cueing

2. Because of the heightened awareness of movement coupled with deeper breathing, it is not uncommon for individuals to reach a state of _____ during mind–body forms of exercise.
   a. being
   b. contentment
   c. joy
   d. flow

3. Mind–body fitness has significant _____ effects on individuals with obesity?
   a. mental and physical
   b. mental, emotional, spiritual, and physical
   c. mental, emotional, and physical
   d. mental, spiritual, and physical

4. Mind–body fitness appears to be _____ exercise option for individuals with excess body weight and adiposity.
   a. an injury-free, enjoyable, and effective
   b. a safe, pleasant, but not physiologically effective
   c. a pain-free, feasible, but not psychologically effective
   d. an aversive, painful, and challenging

5. Chronic stress, negative thinking, and constant notifications keep a person in which branch of the nervous system?
   a. parasympathetic
   b. sympathetic
   c. enteric
   d. peripheral

6. The _____ nervous system is known for the rest-and-digest functions.
   a. parasympathetic
   b. sympathetic
   c. enteric
   d. peripheral

7. Which of the following does NOT occur when moving mindfully?

    a. the heart rate slows

    b. awareness increases

    c. the breathing rate increases

    d. relaxation is stimulated

8. When guiding a client with obesity in a mind–body class or program, it is best to _____.

    a. choose a class based on time

    b. push the body for a challenge

    c. start with the basics and focus on the fundamentals

    d. join the modern hybrids

9. Which of the following is NOT a risk factor for sedentary clients with obesity?

    a. Higher risk of falling because of poor balance

    b. Chronic joint pain

    c. Poor mobility and posture due to a sedentary lifestyle

    d. Having an easy time getting up from the floor

10. Being _____ and _____ is ideal for building strength and burning calories without continuous stress on the joints.

    a. upright; moving

    b. seated; moving

    c. seated; still

    d. supine; moving

CASE STUDY

Case study answers can be found in the appendix.

Sharon once had a natural and healthy lifestyle, especially while her children were little. Then, in a single year, she went through a divorce and had to quit nursing school to care for her mother and raise a family. During that same year, she lost her mother to multiple strokes, and she developed Graves' disease, for which her medical team treated her thyroid with radiation therapy and then ultimately removed her thyroid. After this experience, Sharon, who is 5 ft 10 in. (178 cm) tall, went from weighing 150 lb (68 kg) to weighing more than 200 lb (91 kg) and became embarrassed about her body. Over time, she kept to herself, mainly watching television, and became addicted to social media. She is unable to afford a gym membership but also has no interest in one because of how she feels about her looks. She does not even want to walk outside because she is embarrassed to be seen. Sharon used to get a lot of attention because of her attractiveness, but after her weight gain, she notes that she is treated differently and seen as lazy because of her weight. After having obesity for many years, Sharon has developed pain in her knees. She is also convinced that because she has no thyroid gland, weight loss is hopeless, and she figures that she may as well eat anything she wants because she cannot lose weight regardless. Sharon continuously eats junk food but has been in denial about her choices. She also has a history of abuse; her father, ex-boyfriends, and ex-husbands were all physically abusive to her. Now, after 22 years of being an individual with obesity, Sharon has high cholesterol and very low motivation.

1. If you were Sharon's personal trainer, explain how you would guide her after discovering her story during her initial assessment.

2. Explain your role, or scope of practice, with regard to helping Sharon live a healthier life.

3. Explain how Sharon's lifestyle choices of television and junk food contribute to her negative health cycle, regardless of her thyroid situation.

4. Given Sharon's history, explain how mind–body exercise could benefit her.

5. If you were guiding Sharon, how would you convince her of the benefits of mind–body exercise to encourage her to try it? Share three examples.

CHAPTER 10

Cardiorespiratory Fitness

Tony Nuñez, PhD, Elizabeth Kovar, MA, and Alexios Batrakoulis, PhD

After completing this chapter, you will be able to

- list psychophysiological adaptations to aerobic training,
- describe the benefits and limitations of continuous endurance training and high-intensity interval training,
- explain the similarities and differences between traditional and hybrid-type interval training, and
- explore the role of dance fitness activities as a feasible cardiorespiratory fitness modality.

Cardiorespiratory fitness (CRF), also referred to as *aerobic endurance*, is defined as the ability to perform large-muscle, dynamic, moderate- to vigorous-intensity exercise for prolonged periods (Liguori and ACSM 2021). Furthermore, CRF relies on the integration of three systems of the body: cardiovascular (heart and blood vessels), pulmonary (lungs) or respiratory (gas exchange and breathing), and musculoskeletal (muscles and bones). Improvements in CRF tend to be highly related to adaptations in the heart due to its role in pumping oxygenated blood to working muscle. Thus, the activities selected for aerobic exercise should require the heart to pump greater quantities of oxygenated blood to elicit an adaptation of the cardiovascular (CV) system that will lead to improvements in oxygen supply. This may explain why traditional aerobic activities, such as walking, jogging, and cycling, have been preferred over other modalities for improvements in CRF. Exercise involving more of the body's muscle mass (i.e., integrating both the lower and upper body) requires a greater amount of oxygenated blood to be sent from the heart. Ultimately, the need to pump blood to working muscles comes from the requirement of oxygen in muscles during aerobic exercise.

Maximal oxygen consumption ($\dot{V}O_2max$) is the standard measurement for CRF and is defined as the maximal amount of oxygen an individual can consume and use during exhaustive aerobic activity. Additionally, $\dot{V}O_2max$ has been viewed as the strongest predictor of mortality risk when compared to other established cardiovascular disease (CVD) risk factors (Ross et al. 2016). This value is especially important in individuals with obesity, who are at greater risk of CVD (NHLBI 1998). $\dot{V}O_2max$ can be expressed in a few different units: liters per minute, milliliters per minute, or milliliters per kilogram per minute. The third measurement (milliliters per kilogram per minute) is referred to as relative $\dot{V}O_2$max and is directly affected by the body mass of an individual, meaning that individuals with similar absolute $\dot{V}O_2$max values (liters per minute and milliliters per minute) may have different relative $\dot{V}O_2$max values if there is a wide discrepancy in body weight. Additionally, the classification of CRF based on relative $\dot{V}O_2$max may be improved simply by a reduction in body weight. Improvements in $\dot{V}O_2$max might lead to an extended life span, or at the very least, to improved quality of life at an equivalent life span (Aoike et al. 2018).

Adaptations in the previously mentioned physiological systems (pulmonary, cardiovascular, and musculoskeletal) depend on the type of exercise training performed. Researchers who have examined the effects of aerobic exercise training have noted that there may be differences between continuous endurance training (CET), high-intensity interval training (HIIT), and combined training (a combination of aerobic and resistance exercise) when it comes to physiological and psychological adaptations as well as weight loss and cardioprotective health (Batrakoulis et al. 2022; Swain 2000; Tabata et al. 1996). This chapter will discuss CET and HIIT (traditional and hybrid) as techniques for improving CRF, along with recommendations, special considerations, and limitations of each technique.

CET

Traditionally, when individuals are asked about aerobic exercise, they think of CET. This is the performance of one continuous aerobic exercise bout at low to moderate intensity without rest intervals to elicit an aerobic response—for example, performing exercise on a treadmill at a constant speed and grade equivalent to 45% to 70% of the $\dot{V}O_2$max for 30 to 60 minutes. Programming CET in this fashion has traditionally been considered the most beneficial format for the prevention of CVD (Boutcher and Dunn 2009; Swain 2000). Furthermore, performing CET allows for a ramp-up period of the physiological systems to meet the oxygen requirements of the activity. Once the body can meet the oxygen demands, a steady state can be maintained for a prolonged period, providing an aerobic response. To reach and maintain a steady state, the exercise intensity must be low to moderate. As mentioned previously, research suggests that moderate-intensity continuous training (MICT) is a strong enough stimulus to improve CRF over time, assuming that the participant meets the recommended duration (not including the warm-up and cool-down).

Acute Physiological Responses to CET

When an individual performs CET, their cardiovascular system will immediately begin to adjust. Specifically, the person will experience an increase in **heart rate** (HR), which is the number of heart beats per minute, and **stroke volume** (the volume of blood pumped per heartbeat). This ultimately leads to an increase in **cardiac output** (Q), or the volume of blood the heart pumps per minute. The rise in Q will lead to an increase in the oxygenated blood being sent to working muscles while limiting blood flow to nonworking tissue. Also related to the CV system is **blood pressure**; exercise will lead to an increase in systolic blood pressure (SBP), with little to no change in diastolic blood pressure (DBP). For reasons that will be mentioned later, the responses of the CV system to CET are due to an increase in **sympathetic nervous system** (SNS) drive, as well as withdrawal of **parasympathetic nervous system** (PNS) stimulation.

Pulmonary responses to CET are an increase in **ventilation** (the flow of air into and out of the alveoli in the lungs) due to an increase in respiratory rate (breaths per minute) and **tidal volume** (amount of air per breath), with the latter increasing to a greater extent. Increased ventilation allows for an increase in the rate of oxygen consumption ($\dot{V}O_2$) to match changes in Q. Alterations in ventilation can be observed during exercise through a method known as the **talk test**, which refers to a participant's ability to talk comfortably during exercise at a given exercise intensity. An intensity indicative of a negative talk test (an inability to talk comfortably during exercise) is related to increased ventilation demands that are not sustainable for prolonged exercise. Research has demonstrated that the talk test is a useful tool for managing exercise intensity, especially for keeping exercise intensity in the moderate range for CET (Reed and Pipe 2014).

A secondary marker of $\dot{V}O_2$ is energy expenditure, which also increases during CET compared to rest. Research examining $\dot{V}O_2$ and energy expenditure during exercise has unequivocally determined that they are largely affected by exercise intensity (Swain 2000); as exercise intensity increases, $\dot{V}O_2$ and energy expenditure will also increase linearly, mostly because of the energy demands of muscle tissue. Thus, the musculoskeletal system will require greater blood flow during CET, due to an increase in oxygen and nutrient demand. The requirement for more nutrients during CET is directly related to increased energy demands in muscles (Kenney et al. 2021). Energy metabolism is a complicated topic, but in brief, changes in enzyme activity and hormone concentrations promote conversion of blood glucose and fat into energy during exercise.

Regardless of a person's body size (i.e., healthy, overweight, or obese), responses to aerobic exercise appear to be similar. However, more recent research suggests that these responses might be altered in individuals with obesity. According to a review by Boutcher and Dunn (2009), reductions in SNS activity might limit energy expenditure during and after exercise. Furthermore, the review discusses alterations in hormones related to fat oxidation and storage, which also might lead to lower oxidation of fat during MICT. Oxidative enzymes also appear to be altered in individuals with obesity who are insulin resistant, leading to lower enzyme activity that contributes to a reduction in fat burned during and after exercise (Ortega et al. 2016).

Chronic Physiological Adaptations to CET

For chronic adaptations to CET to take place, an individual must complete a workout a minimum of 3 to 5 days per week for several weeks (typically >8-12 wk) (Batrakoulis et al. 2022). If this level is achieved, an individual will likely begin to see improvements in physiological variables, both at rest and during exercise. Adults with overweight or obesity tend to have many other comorbidities, especially if they are sedentary (Ortega et al. 2016). Examples of these comorbidities are type 2 diabetes, **hypertension** (high blood pressure), and dyslipidemia (a poor blood lipid profile). Adaptations to CET improve many, if not all, of these comorbidities related to CRF, glucose uptake, fat oxidation, and arterial blood pressure (Batrakoulis et al. 2022).

When following a CET program, adults with overweight or obesity will typically experience improvements in CRF, specifically increases in $\dot{V}O_2$max (Su et al. 2019). Research in this area has determined that major improvements in $\dot{V}O_2$max are related to increases in Q and stroke volume following training, which will also allow for a lower exercising HR at similar exercise intensities before training (Wilmore et al. 2001). Although $\dot{V}O_2$ remains relatively constant at an absolute exercise intensity, attainment of a greater $\dot{V}O_2$max will allow an individual to achieve greater exercise intensities.

Furthermore, improvements in CRF will lead to lower ratings of perceived exertion at similar submaximal exercise intensities. Adults with overweight or obesity also experience a reduction in SBP during exercise following CET (Batrakoulis et al. 2022), which may lead to lower arterial pressure, a major determinant of blood flow during exercise.

At rest, the HR experiences a downward trend following CET (Batrakoulis et al. 2022) in adults with overweight or obesity. Although mechanisms explaining the decrease in resting HR are not completely understood, they may be related to improvements in peripheral resistance in the CV system, allowing for a greater stroke volume or improvements in PNS stimulation at rest. Changes in blood pressure appear to be greatest in individuals with obesity or overweight who have been diagnosed with hypertension or prehypertension (Arboleda-Serna et al. 2019). A decrease in SBP will lead to a decrease in arterial blood pressure and ultimately reduce peripheral resistance in the CV system (Kenney et al. 2021).

Ventilation is not typically a limitation to CET; however, adaptations to ventilation do occur following aerobic training. During submaximal exercise, ventilation may be decreased by as much as 20% to 30% following CET, which signifies an improvement in system efficiency. Talk test results (i.e., positive versus negative) improve following CET, allowing individuals to reach higher exercise intensities before having a negative talk test during CET (Reed and Pipe 2014). Lastly, tidal volume during exercise appears to increase following aerobic training, allowing for reductions in respiratory rate at similar relative exercise intensities (Chen et al. 2017), which may explain improvements in talk test results. At rest, there appear to be minimal, if any, changes in ventilation following CET in adults with overweight or obesity.

Body composition changes also occur following CET and can be related to both fat mass and fat-free mass. While there is some debate over the effectiveness of CET on body composition, research in this area has demonstrated that CET can improve body composition through a reduction in fat mass or an increase in fat-free mass (Donnelly et al. 2000). According to Chen and colleagues (2017), 8 weeks of CET led to an increase in muscle mass in elderly adults with sarcopenic obesity performing aerobic training 2 days per week. Donnelly and colleagues (2000) found that continuous participation in CET led to significant weight loss following an 18-month program. The weight loss experienced by these participants (approximately 2.1% of the baseline body weight) represents a noteworthy decrease in CVD risk. However, according to a meta-analysis of randomized controlled trials by Thorogood and colleagues (2011), isolated MICT provided only modest weight loss in adults with overweight or obesity and was not an effective weight loss therapy.

Acute Psychological Responses and Chronic Adaptations to Exercise

Obesity, inactivity, and poor psychological health, often referred to as *the triangle*, are intertwined among adults with overweight or obesity (Batrakoulis and Fatouros 2022). Exercise alone does not appear to influence changes in mental health in individuals with serious mental illness, but it can be beneficial as part of a greater, multifaceted treatment (Carraça et al. 2021). Data suggest that physical inactivity is correlated with depression and obesity and that it would be beneficial to use CET to combat symptoms related to both disorders (Batrakoulis and Fatouros 2022). To keep within the scope of this textbook, the psychological outcomes that will be discussed are related to adherence, exercise enjoyment, affect valence, depression, and anxiety following the implementation of exercise among adults with overweight or obesity.

Adherence

Adherence to an exercise program has been highly researched, especially when comparing the effects of different exercise intensities. Limiting findings to CET at a moderate intensity, research suggests that this type of exercise may be highly suitable for adherence among adults with overweight or obesity (Batrakoulis and Fatouros 2022). Because intensity appears to have a major effect on exercise adherence in this population, low- to moderate-intensity exercise could prove favorable in individuals starting an exercise program (Martinez et al. 2015). Counter to exercise intensity is the inverse relationship between exercise duration and adherence. For CET to be effective, there is a minimum time commitment of 30 minutes per session and 3 to 5 days per week, with greater frequency being best for weight loss (Liguori and ACSM 2021). Research suggests that a lack of time is the greatest deterrent to starting and adhering to an exercise program (Salmon et al. 2003) and that adults with overweight or obesity are less likely to adhere to an exercise program with a greater time commitment (Batrakoulis and Fatouros 2022). In response to the time conundrum, the American College of Sports Medicine (ACSM) has suggested breaking up 30-minute exercise sessions into multiple bouts of 10 minutes to match the total volume for the day and week (Liguori and ACSM 2021).

Exercise Enjoyment

Salmon and associates (2003) surveyed more than 1,300 people and found that enjoyment and preference were major barriers to physical activity. Other research on this topic has found similar results. The findings suggest that exercise programs for adults with overweight or obesity should allow them to choose activities they prefer and enjoy to achieve superior adherence. Given that the research is equivocal as to whether CET or other modalities are more favored in this population, if CET is the preferred and more enjoyable form of exercise, it is certainly a viable option for improving CRF, assuming adherence to the time recommendations.

Affect Valence

Affect is an instinctive mood response that does not require considerable thought and is associated with pleasure or displeasure and tension or calmness (Batrakoulis and Fatouros 2022). Research on the affective response to CET among adults with overweight or obesity has determined that intensity during this form of exercise is a strong influence. The affective response is much higher during and following MICT compared with high-intensity (HI) continuous training in this population (Batrakoulis and Fatouros 2022; Martinez et al. 2015).

Anxiety and Depression

Anxiety and depression disorders are complicated and multifaceted but may have a relationship with the presence of overweight or obesity. According to research, obesity in adults may lead to an increased incidence of anxiety due to weight-related discrimination and psychological discrimination (Batrakoulis and Fatouros 2022). Depression also appears to have a greater presence in sedentary adults with obesity compared to their physically active counterparts. Research investigating exercise-related improvements in symptoms of depression and anxiety is limited; nevertheless, exercise may be a helpful tool for lowering anxiety levels in adults with obesity (Carraça et al. 2021). The effects of exercise on depression in adults with overweight or obesity appear to be limited, but exercise does improve symptoms related to depression in populations with mood barriers (Batrakoulis and Fatouros 2022).

Special Considerations for CET

According to the ACSM's guidelines for exercise prescription, low- to moderate-intensity exercise is recommended for most adults (Liguori and ACSM 2021). Individuals not currently meeting minimum physical activity guidelines (3 days per week, 30 minutes per day for at least 3 months) may immediately begin taking part in a low-intensity program but should seek medical clearance for higher exercise intensities. The risk of experiencing a fatal cardiac event during low- to moderate-intensity exercise is extremely minimal, even in individuals with previously diagnosed CV, metabolic, or renal disease (Liguori and ACSM 2021). Nonetheless, carefully monitoring exercise intensity using HR, the talk test, or the rating of perceived exertion to ensure a low to moderate intensity is imperative for maintaining the safety of a program.

Recommended Modalities for CET

When performing CET, the recommended modes of exercise provide some form of rhythmic, continuous movement and include a comprehensive list of activities. A few examples are walking, jogging, cycling, rowing, and swimming. The advantages of each modality will be outlined, but it is important to highlight that the best mode for a person is the one that leads to the greatest exercise adherence (Liguori and ACSM 2021). According to a review by Baillot and colleagues (2021), pain or physical discomfort during exercise is a primary barrier to physical activity, and based on a small number of studies, walking was the preferred mode of physical activity in people with obesity. Cycling, rowing, and swimming were also mentioned as preferred modes of physical activity for people with obesity.

Walking

Walking is a simple form of exercise that can be accomplished in many different settings but may be limited based on the environment (weather, accessibility of neighborhoods or parks, etc.). Using techniques for judging exercise intensity during walking will help ensure the individual meets recommended guidelines. Walking is a low-impact activity that does not overly stress the joints but does provide some weight-bearing activity that will aid in the maintenance of bone mineral density in adults with overweight or obesity who may be susceptible to osteoporosis. Jogging has similar benefits as walking but does place greater stress on joints due to greater ground-reaction force during the activity, which may not be suitable for adults with overweight or obesity.

Stair Climbing

Stair climbing is a great alternative to jogging because it has lower impact, but it also increases physical demand compared to simply walking. Stair climbing requires the individual to balance and push on a single leg as they advance vertically from step to step. If stair climbing is performed outdoors, adults with overweight or obesity should be cautious of overloading when descending stairs, due to the high level of eccentric contraction (lengthening of the muscle under tension). This form of contraction might lead to greater levels of postexercise soreness and pain.

Cycling and Rowing

Stationary cycling and rowing are low-impact activities that minimize stress on joints. Unlike walking, both cycling and rowing are non-weight-bearing activities; thus, they have limited benefit for bone mineral density. Nevertheless, they are great alternatives for individuals who want to increase exercise intensity without the added stress on joints that jogging requires.

Upright cycling and recumbent cycling are great options for CET. Each has advantages. Upright cycling requires more activation of midtorso muscles to maintain an upright posture. Recumbent cycling is performed in a position where the upper torso is supported, and it may be more comfortable for adults with obesity who have poor mobility.

Another modality, the rowing machine, offers three primary advantages: (1) it provides a comprehensive, full-body workout that engages all major muscle groups; (2) it causes minimal to no impact, offering a joint-friendly exercise experience; and (3) it is a versatile piece of equipment that can be used for a multitude of training goals. Rowing ergometers introduce the upper body into the activity, which may lead to greater energy expenditure compared to cycling. There is slightly more skill required in rowing than in cycling, but both are great options, especially for individuals who may be experiencing knee or ankle issues during walking or jogging.

HIIT

Seen as a favorable alternative to CET, HIIT has grown in popularity since research by Tabata and colleagues in 1996. It is important to define traditional HIIT programming and how it compares to CET. First, HIIT uses repeated HI bouts of activity dispersed between low-intensity (LI) bouts of recovery. Research investigating HIIT focuses on the use of HI bouts at a duration of anywhere from 30 seconds to 4 minutes and LI bouts of equal duration or half the duration of the HI bout. While the duration of HI bouts can be highly variable, reviews of research on HIIT programming have determined that a period of 30 seconds to 4 minutes provides the optimal results for CRF (Liguori and ACSM 2021). Exercise intensity for the HI bouts can range from 65% to 100% of the $\dot{V}O_2$max, whereas the LI intervals are performed at a lighter intensity (about 50% of the maximum HR) to allow for recovery between HI bouts. A key aspect of performing HIIT, and a major contributor to its popularity, is its efficiency. It can be performed in less time while achieving similar results as CET, even among adults with overweight or obesity (Ramos et al. 2016). This is especially true when performing HIIT at a low volume, or for less than 15 minutes—the cutoff for high-volume versus low-volume HIIT (Williams et al. 2019).

Acute Physiological Responses to HIIT

Physiological responses to HIIT and CET are similar, but in HIIT, the magnitude of change is greater during HI intervals and relatively equal or lower during LI bouts. This can sometimes lead to relatively similar or even lower average physiological responses over a training session during HIIT compared to CET (Taylor et al. 2019). Specifically, compared to CET, the percentage of the maximum HR may be higher during the HI interval but will likely be lower during recovery. Depending on the duration of the HI and LI intervals, this can ultimately lead to a lower percentage of the maximum HR for the overall training session, especially compared to MICT. Pertaining to the CV system, SBP will increase during the HIIT session, with a linear relationship to the exercise intensity. In other words, SBP will increase to a greater extent during HIIT compared to CET and MICT (Batrakoulis et al. 2022).

Pulmonary responses to HIIT are like those in response to CET, with the caveat that ventilation will need to match the increased exercise intensity. Increases in ventilation allow for an increase in $\dot{V}O_2$ to match the increase in Q. The talk test is useful for monitoring exercise intensity during CET, but it might not be as useful during HIIT. As described by Reed and Pipe (2014), limitations in the usefulness of the talk test during HIIT are due to intervals of HI exercise that do not allow for optimal time for the ventilatory response. Conversely, HI bouts of longer duration (3-4 min) with longer LI bouts in between may provide adequate time for the talk test to be useful, but to our knowledge, there is currently no research on this topic.

Using $\dot{V}O_2$ to estimate energy expenditure is only valid during steady-state aerobic exercise. Thus, to estimate energy expenditure during HIIT, researchers must use other methods of estimating the anaerobic contribution during the HI bout (Panissa et al. 2018). Research has found that overall energy contribution to HI exercise is greater than for moderate-intensity exercise (Swain 2000). Gerosa-Neto and colleagues (2019) observed that when energy expenditure between MICT and HIIT sessions was matched, the HIIT session required approximately 15 minutes less time to achieve the same expenditure.

Skeletal muscle response during HIIT is also similar to that during CET but with nuances related to aerobic and anaerobic metabolism. Because HIIT requires a higher exercise intensity compared to CET, there is more involvement of fast-twitch (anaerobic) muscle fibers, along with continued involvement of slow-twitch (aerobic) fibers. This necessitates the use of both anaerobic and aerobic metabolism during HIIT. Enzymes related to both types of metabolism will increase during HIIT, and therefore, the concentration of hormones related to breakdown of substrates (the molecules on which enzymes can act) tends to be higher following HIIT compared to CET (Peake et al. 2014).

Chronic Physiological Adaptations to HIIT

When comparing physiological adaptations to HIIT versus MICT in adults with overweight or obesity, similarities and differences between research findings depend on the programming. For instance, according to a study by Arboleda-Serna and colleagues (2019), there was no difference in CRF as measured by $\dot{V}O_2$max following 8 weeks of MICT versus HIIT in adults with healthy weight versus overweight. However, according to a review by Batrakoulis and colleagues (2022), HIIT appeared to lead to a clinically significant (≥ 3.5 mL $\cdot$ kg^{-1} $\cdot$ min^{-1}) increase in $\dot{V}O_2$max in adults with overweight or obesity, whereas CET did not. Differences in results comparing HIIT and MICT may be due to discrepancies in the duration of HI intervals, with HI intervals lasting 2 minutes or longer leading to the greatest CRF improvements (Su et al. 2019).

Most of the research comparing adaptations between MICT and HIIT has found that HIIT leads to adaptations sooner in a program but eventually results in a similar $\dot{V}O_2$max as MICT at the end of programs lasting between 8 and 12 weeks. Su and colleagues (2019) concluded that adults with overweight or obesity participating in HIIT compared with MICT spent 9.7 fewer minutes per session, on average, to achieve similar improvements in CRF, body composition, and total cholesterol. Greater improvements in CRF also are observed following HIIT compared to MICT when energy expenditure is equal between the two formats.

In addition, HIIT may lead to improvements in resting-state CV variables such as SBP, DBP, and HR, but these findings are mixed, and the improvements may be inferior compared to those achieved with CET (Batrakoulis et al. 2022). According to Batrakoulis and colleagues (2022), a combination of resistance training and CET, known as combined training, may be best for improving SBP and DBP. Hybrid training, a form of training that uses any intermittent multicomponent exercise mode engaging both the CV and the musculoskeletal systems throughout a single session, may be best for improvements in resting HR.

Adaptations to respiratory and musculoskeletal physiology following HIIT appear to be superior to those following CET, especially related to improvements in anaerobic, lipid, and glucose metabolism. During HI bouts, activation of fast-twitch muscle fibers will lead to greater glucose uptake and energy demands during exercise, which might be a precursor to improvements in insulin resistance following HIIT. While these results are clearer in adults with type 2 diabetes, longer interventions (20 weeks or more) appear to produce meaningful improvements in women with overweight or obesity (Donnelly et al. 2000). Improvements in lipid metabolism appear to favor combined training and hybrid training compared to other modalities. However, HIIT contributes to the greatest reduction in triglycerides compared to other training formats. Both HIIT and CET may ultimately lead to improvements in fasting blood glucose levels in adults with overweight or obesity but with no clear advantage between modalities (Batrakoulis et al. 2022).

Similar to CET, HIIT may reduce body weight, fat mass, and waist circumference in adults with overweight or obesity. Despite the differences in muscle fiber involvement between HIIT and MICT, there are no meaningful differences in the improvements in fat-free mass between the two formats. Nonetheless, Su and colleagues (2019) suggest that HIIT is superior to MICT for weight loss in adults with overweight or obesity due to its ability to promote the secretion of hormones that promote fat breakdown during and after exercise. The discrepancy in results related to weight loss in most studies may be related to less time on task and energy expenditure during HIIT compared to MICT. Furthermore, energy intake during these types of programs may not be controlled and might offset any losses experienced during either program (Thorogood et al. 2011).

Acute Psychological Responses and Chronic Adaptations to HIIT

Although HIIT appears to be a similar, if not superior, strategy for improvements in whole-body physiology compared to MICT, there are concerns about the high demand for this format among adults with overweight or obesity. Greater demand may lead to lower levels of adherence, affect valence, and enjoyment. However, research on this matter is not straightforward. According to a review by Batrakoulis and Fatouros (2022), HIIT performed in both supervised and unsupervised settings achieved high adherence rates in men with overweight or obesity. Furthermore, HIIT led to significantly higher adherence compared to MICT during a 4-week intervention among individuals with abdominal obesity.

Affect Valence

Affect valence appears to be mixed following HIIT and MICT. The lower volumes of exercise required to meet similar adaptations following HIIT compared to MICT are associated with better feelings of pleasure, but the inherent intense nature of HIIT has revealed variations in affective response (Batrakoulis and Fatouros 2022). Current evidence on affect response in adults with overweight or obesity suggests that a similar response is achieved during HIIT and MICT but that workouts of higher intensity continuously lead to inferior affect response, likely due to the combination of increased intensity and time.

Mood Disorders

Traditional HIIT does not appear to lead to high levels of enjoyment or feelings of pleasure among inactive adults with overweight or obesity. Greater enjoyment is experienced among adults with overweight or obesity when HI intervals are shorter ($\leq$30 s) compared to longer (60-120 s). Thus, it may be recommended that HIIT programs initially use shorter HI bouts to promote greater exercise enjoyment and potentially improve adherence among adults with overweight or obesity. In summary, HIIT and MICT appear to be similarly effective at improving exercise enjoyment and adherence.

Special Considerations for HIIT

ACSM guidelines for exercise participation strongly recommend that any individual seeking to partake in vigorous or high-intensity exercise seek medical clearance prior to beginning a program (Liguori and ACSM 2021). While some HIIT programs have integrated moderate-intensity intervals in place of the HI bout, most entail greater intensity than what is recommended for inactive adults. This is especially the case in adults with overweight or obesity who have been diagnosed with a CV, metabolic, or renal disease. Furthermore, overweight and obesity may increase the likelihood of injury during HIIT. Therefore, it is recommended that these individuals participate in preparatory training to reduce the risk of injury. HIIT requires careful monitoring of exercise intensity during the HI and LI bouts to ensure proper programming. Preparing an appropriately periodized program of HIIT will help to limit the likelihood of injury and an adverse event.

Traditional HIIT Versus Hybrid Training

Traditional HIIT uses cardio equipment, as previously described in this chapter. Both the HI and the recovery bouts are performed on the same piece of equipment during the workout. Conversely, hybrid training is a multicomponent exercise routine that integrates CV and musculoskeletal systems simultaneously at various intensities in a single session. These sessions typically last from 30 to 45 minutes but result in responses and adaptations in both CV fitness and muscular strength, which will decrease the time requirements for meeting recommendations for both fitness areas. The ACSM recommends aerobic training on 3 to 5 days and muscular fitness training on 2 or more days per week, which will likely require about 300 to 400 total minutes. According to Batrakoulis and colleagues (2022), the average time commitment for hybrid training is approximately 130 minutes per week, whereas combining both HIIT and resistance training will require approximately 215 minutes per week. Therefore, hybrid training would be the second-best option, just behind a combination of CET and resistance training (about 230 min/wk), for inducing overall improvements in cardiometabolic health among adults with overweight or obesity.

Recommended Modalities for Interval Training

As with CET, in the context of interval training, there is an extensive list of recommended modes of exercise that provide the client with rhythmic and continuous movement. Examples of such activities include walking, jogging, stair climbing, cycling, rowing, swimming, bodyweight exercises, and adjunct modalities such as resistance-training accessories (Stanforth et al. 2015). Each modality has advantages and disadvantages; however, the optimal mode for an individual with overweight or obesity is the one that fosters the greatest adherence to exercise (Liguori and ACSM 2021). Given that pain is a significant impediment to exercise among previously inactive individuals with excess body weight or adiposity, it is preferable to implement interval training protocols in a manner that avoids causing discomfort.

Traditional

Traditional HIIT necessitates the use of cardio equipment or modes of CET without equipment, such as walking, jogging, or cycling. When using devices such as a treadmill, elliptical trainer, or stationary bike, the individual has the choice of adjusting speed, stride frequency, and revolutions per minute (RPM) as well as the grade (incline), resistance, and power. For adults with overweight or obesity, it may be more suitable to set the same walking speed on a treadmill for both the HI and LI bouts and increase the grade (percentage of incline) for the HI bouts. On devices such as elliptical trainers and stationary bikes, stride frequency and RPM eventually reach a peak, and only the resistance can be adjusted to increase intensity. Thus, it is recommended that adults with overweight or obesity find a comfortable stride frequency (typically about 150 steps per minute) on an elliptical trainer or RPM (typically about 80) on a stationary bike for the LI bout and increase the resistance while maintaining that stride frequency or RPM for the HI bout. Unique to elliptical trainers is the use of the upper body during exercise, which may allow for recruitment of more muscle tissue.

Hybrid

Integration of many modalities at various intensities into a single session (hybrid training) has boomed in popularity (Newsome et al. 2024), and it appears to be effective for adults with overweight or obesity (Batrakoulis et al. 2022). Recommendations for hybrid training include the performance of about 10 to 12 exercises in a circuit fashion for a prescribed duration of time (such as 20-40 s) followed by an equivalent recovery period to elicit both CV and muscular responses and adaptations. These exercises can include bodyweight calisthenics or traditional resistance training movements, depending on equipment availability and the participant's fitness level. In particular, adjunct modalities, also known as training toys (Stanforth et al. 2015), are widely used in these exercise regimens and include equipment such as kettlebells, suspension exercise devices, medicine balls, stability balls, balance balls, battle ropes, and foam rollers. It is recommended that recovery periods be longer than work efforts in the initial stages of these programs, progressing toward longer work efforts and shorter recovery periods once fitness improves (Batrakoulis et al. 2018). If programmed properly, hybrid training appears to be an effective strategy for improvements in CRF, muscular fitness, body composition, and metabolic health in adults with overweight or obesity (Batrakoulis, Jamurtas, et al. 2021; Batrakoulis et al. 2023; Batrakoulis, Tsimeas, et al. 2021). This nontraditional exercise concept also seems to be effective for psychological alterations in critical indicators such as subjective vitality, distress, and regulation of exercise behavior among people with excess weight (Batrakoulis et al. 2020).

Dance Fitness

Dance fitness, an aerobic form of exercise, is among the earliest forms of human communication and expression and is regarded as one of the most coordinated activities carried out by the body (Hincapié-Sánchez et al. 2021). Dance fitness has evolved over the past 100 years. It started with self-improv in the 1920s; progressed to Ballet Burn in the 1950s, Hustle Muscle in the 1970s, and Jazzercise and Step Aerobics in the 1980s and 1990s; then transformed into popular Zumba and Hip-Hop dance classes in the new millennium. Dance fitness can range from nonconventional aerobic exercises to choreographed sequences and cultural dances. *Dance* is broadly defined as moving one's body rhythmically to music, usually as a form of artistic or emotional expression (Fong Yan et al. 2018). Dancing can be a general form of exercise or used as a modality of physical or emotional healing and self-expression (known as dance therapy).

Dance Therapy

Dance therapy, or *dance movement therapy*, is defined by the American Dance Therapy Association (ADTA) as the psychotherapeutic use of movement to promote emotional, social, cognitive, and physical integration of the individual as a way to improve health and well-being (ADTA 2023). Dance movement therapy is a holistic healing approach rooted in the evidence-based belief that the mind, body, and spirit are interconnected and inseparable, with changes in one influencing the other (ADTA 2023).

The ADTA (2023) states that dance movement therapy relies on the following concepts:

- Movement is a language, our first language. Nonverbal and movement communication begins in utero and continues throughout the life span.
- Mind, body, and spirit are interconnected.
- Movement can be functional, communicative, developmental, and expressive.
- Movement is both an assessment tool and a primary mode of intervention.

Fitness professionals may have clients who love dance fitness without a clear understanding of why they like it. While observing a dance class, many people smile, unaware of their expression. With the mind, body, and spirit interconnected, dance can be an empowering form of exercise.

The Body, the Breath, and the Beat

There is a union or synchronization of body, breath, and beat during dance fitness that can lead to moments of joy, defined by *The Merriam-Webster Dictionary* as an experience of great pleasure or delight. In dance, the movement of the body flows with the rhythm of the musical beat along with a connection to the breath and an increase of oxygen flow. The type of music and style of dance go hand in hand to either generate an energizing workout or create a healing environment. For example, ballet can evoke deep emotions while moving the body to classical music, almost to the point where it can bring people to tears. The number of musical beats per minute (bpm) affects the brain and how the body will respond to movement. Based on the apparent relationship between the bpm (tempo) of music and the desire to move (for example, tapping the feet) induced while listening to that music, it is hypothesized that musical tempo may evoke movement-related activity in the brain (Daly et al. 2014). Tempo is also an important musical element that affects human emotional processes when listening to music (Liu et al. 2018).

Music is claimed to be one of humanity's most expressive and oldest forms of language. In most music, the tempo ranges from 40 to 300 bpm; music with a walking speed ranges between 76 and 108 bpm. The body responds with quicker movements to a more rapid beat, such as electronic music with 120 to 150 bpm. Such music energizes a workout, mentally pushes people, and gets participants' adrenaline flowing. Slower music, including classical, chill, or ambient music, ranges between 40 to 80 bpm and is used in some forms of creative dance or ballet. Musical tempo can cause a flow state that leads to joy. An energetic dance program can be subconsciously therapeutic, such as by building confidence, even if it is not moving with intentional healing purposes, as in guided dance therapy.

Dance Fitness and Exercise Adherence

Individuals with obesity may struggle with confidence and motivation for exercise. It also is not uncommon for people to express that going to the gym or lifting weights feels like a chore. Why do people feel this way? It is possible that working out on a machine or lifting weights seems mechanical, similar to daily tasks that include high amounts of repetition, such as vacuuming or chopping vegetables. As science continues studying the effects of dance and music on the brain, creative expression, or free-flowing movement, may create joy that increases exercise adherence. In simple terms, dance fitness is just fun. Humans were meant to be upright and moving, and free movement in dancing is consistent with human design.

Several researchers have noticed higher rates of exercise adherence in dance fitness studies. Various clinical trials using dance as an intervention strategy found a minimal dropout rate when compared with traditional physical exercise interventions, for which decreased interest in participating in clinical studies or continuing with the rehabilitation process was identified (Hincapié-Sánchez et al. 2021). Studies implementing dance protocols to identify health effects found that participants described dance as a pleasant, innovative, and safe method of achieving the expected results, generating an increase in attendance to scheduled sessions (Hincapié-Sánchez et al. 2021).

Dance Fitness Benefits for the Brain and Body

Dance is an innovative intervention strategy for patients with comorbidities or underlying pathologies as well as for those in good health (Hincapié-Sánchez et al. 2021). It is noteworthy that clinicians can suggest dance as a safe and effective alternative exercise for persons with obesity, who are at higher risk for disease, aiming to decrease fat mass, lower triglycerides, enhance cardiovascular fitness, improve flexibility, and support daily functional abilities (Fong Yan et al. 2018). Research indicates that Zumba improves peak $\dot{V}O_2$ and provides many health benefits, including parameters related to quality of life (such as physical self-perception and psychological well-being), anthropometrics, body composition, blood pressure, and physical fitness (Chavarrias et al. 2021).

Dance practice also benefits the brain, promoting neuroplasticity, which is the nervous system's capacity to adapt its activity in response to internal or external stimuli by reorganizing its structure, functions, or connections following injuries like strokes or traumatic brain injuries (Puderbaugh et al. 2023). The study noted positive structural and functional changes after dance practice. Functional changes included alterations in cognitive function, such as significant improvement in memory, attention, body balance, psychosocial parameters, and altered peripheral neurotrophic factor (Teixeira-Machado et al. 2018). Psychologically, dance influences mood while promoting fluid movement, posture, and body control, making it a supportive therapy for managing stiffness, bradykinesia, and postural instability (Hincapié-Sánchez et al. 2021). There is enough evidence to suggest that dance fitness is a beneficial form of exercise for people with obesity.

Special Considerations

Uncoordinated and sedentary people will need to ease into dance fitness just as they would other forms of exercise. Fitness professionals should consider the following:

- Chair dance programs may be appropriate for clients with morbid obesity and those rehabilitating after injury to build stamina and coordination.
- For novice dancers, the moves should be kept basic and the sequences easy to follow to increase confidence and movement skills. Using music with a tempo at walking speed can help participants keep up with the sequence.
- Movements should be kept simple and fun, and progressing to complex moves should be done over time. This reduces embarrassment for those who cannot keep up.
- Dance fitness is balance in motion. Elderly and highly immobile participants may require more stationary sequences with limited lateral or front-to-back movement (for example, grapevines).

- Fitness professionals should learn how to progress or regress movements, such as designating upper- or lower-body movement as level 1 and full-body movement as level 2.

CHAPTER SUMMARY

This chapter focused on cardiorespiratory fitness and the acute responses and chronic adaptations of physiological systems, such as musculoskeletal, cardiovascular, and pulmonary. It discussed in detail the benefits and limitations of CET and HIIT. It also described hybrid training for cardiorespiratory fitness and its potential benefits for adults with overweight or obesity. Finally, the chapter explored dance fitness as an adjunct form of exercise and its positive role in physical fitness, exercise adherence, mood, and neuroplasticity among clients with excess weight.

KEY POINTS

- Improvements in cardiorespiratory fitness rely on the integration of the following systems: cardiovascular, respiratory, and musculoskeletal.
- Maximal oxygen consumption is the standard measurement for cardiorespiratory fitness and is considered the strongest predictor of mortality risk.
- Continuous endurance training (CET) is the traditional form of aerobic training but may have limitations for adults with overweight or obesity in the areas of energy expenditure and fat oxidation.
- High-intensity interval training (HIIT) is a suitable format for improving cardiorespiratory fitness in adults with overweight or obesity when proper programming and precautions are used.
- Psychological benefits from CET and HIIT appear to be relatively similar, with some findings gravitating more toward the latter training format.
- Hybrid training appears to be the best strategy for improving cardiorespiratory fitness in adults with overweight or obesity who have time limitations.
- Dance fitness can range from a variety of nonconventional aerobic exercises to choreographed sequences that revolve around a specific theme or cultural dance.
- Dance is an innovative intervention strategy for individuals who have excess weight, with or without obesity-related comorbidities.
- Clinicians can recommend dance as a safe alternative form of physical activity or exercise to reduce physical function and cardiometabolic health.
- Everyone can dance. However, as with any other form of exercise, sedentary individuals will need to ease into dance fitness or can use a chair for modification, especially if rehabilitating after an injury.

CHAPTER QUIZ

Quiz answers can be found in the appendix.

1. According to exercise adherence factors, why might continuous endurance training be a suitable aerobic activity in adults with overweight or obesity?

   a. exercise intensity
   b. exercise time per session
   c. total exercise time per week
   d. mental effort

2. Which exercise modality is the most suitable progression for adults with overweight or obesity currently participating in walking?
   a. jogging
   b. cycling
   c. stair climbing
   d. rowing

3. To improve feelings of enjoyment during a HIIT program in adults with overweight or obesity, what should trainers shorten?
   a. duration of high-intensity intervals
   b. duration of low-intensity intervals
   c. number of high-intensity intervals
   d. total exercise time

4. Which of the following training formats best integrates both cardiovascular and muscular-strength responses?
   a. CET
   b. HIIT
   c. hybrid training
   d. resistance training

5. Which of the following statements is true about recommendations for the progression of hybrid training for cardiovascular fitness?
   a. Participants should maintain recovery durations and increase work efforts.
   b. Participants should shorten recovery durations and increase work efforts.
   c. Participants should increase recovery durations and maintain work efforts.

6. The American Dance Therapy Association notes that dance movement therapy "is a holistic approach to healing, based on the empirically supported assertion that mind, body, and spirit are _____ and _____."
   a. inseparable; disconnected
   b. separable; interconnected
   c. inseparable; interconnected
   d. inseparable; connected

7. Dance is one of the most _____ forms of human communication and expression.
   a. important
   b. primitive
   c. effective
   d. nonverbal

8. _____ is defined as "as the ability of the nervous system to change its activity in response to intrinsic or extrinsic stimuli by reorganizing its structure, functions, or connections after injuries, such as a stroke or traumatic brain injury."
   a. Neuroplasticity
   b. Neurology
   c. Neuroscience
   d. Neuropathy

9. Which of the following is NOT a special consideration regarding dance fitness among people with obesity?
   a. Keep sequences simple and fun, and progress to more complex movements over time.
   b. For elderly individuals with severe obesity, use a chair if necessary to help build stamina.
   c. Use music with a tempo at walking speed for novice dancers and exercisers.
   d. Include many lateral and front-and-back movements.

10. It is possible that dance fitness is effective because it is _____ and does not feel _____.
    a. funny; silly
    b. fun; mechanical
    c. fun; painful
    d. trendy; mechanical

CASE STUDY—CARDIORESPIRATORY FITNESS

Case study answers can be found in the appendix.

Aubrey is not a fan of the idea of improving her aerobic fitness with traditional, long-duration cardiorespiratory exercise. Over the past 5 years, she has transitioned from a very active job to a very sedentary one, so she knows she needs to do something to stress her heart, lungs, and muscles. However, she experienced a severe foot injury a couple of years ago, and jogging or running can lead to serious foot pain during and after exercise. She owns a hybrid commuter bicycle and recently purchased a stationary bike for her home gym. Aubrey also has the following equipment in her home gym: resistance bands, light dumbbells (2.5 lb [1.1 kg] to 15 lb [7 kg], in 2.5 lb [1.1 kg] increments), a foam roller, and a suspension trainer. She is hoping to put together a routine she can perform 3 days per week but wants a lot of variety. She was told that performing traditional HIIT 2 days per week and hybrid HIIT 1 day per week could be a good start. Her goal is to improve her cardiorespiratory fitness while also achieving a muscular response.

1. What mode of exercise should Aubrey perform for her HIIT program, and how should she set up her initial intervals?
2. How would you program the hybrid-type interval training in terms of the number of exercises, sequence, and rest intervals?
3. What type of physiological responses might Aubrey expect when performing these exercise routines?
4. When will Aubrey begin to see results from her new routine, and what physiological adaptations can she expect?
5. Besides physical benefits, what other psychological and mental benefits might Aubrey gain from her new routine?

CASE STUDY—DANCE FITNESS

Case study answers can be found in the appendix.

Nicole has never been a traditional exerciser. Working long hours at a veterinary clinic, pet sitting on the side, and taking care of her own pets, her schedule is very busy. As she has gotten older, she has gained weight and has noticed things have changed in her body. She knows she needs to exercise, but in the past, when she tried going to the gym or boot camp classes, they left her so sore she was unable to walk much for days. She never continued with those programs or a membership after her trial period; in general, she does not like to exercise. Single and looking for new friends, she loves music and felt that dance fitness could be a fun way to meet new people as well as get her body moving. With her work schedule varying in both hours and days, she is not always consistent with attending dance fitness but has found it enjoyable. She claims dancing doesn't feel like her other exercising attempts in the past. She has noticed that once she began dance fitness, her sleep improved.

1. For someone like Nicole, what are three reasons dance fitness may be beneficial for her health and exercise adherence?
2. As an exercise professional, what would you say to Nicole for encouragement to attend dance fitness sessions, even if her attendance is irregular?
3. Nicole's past experiences of attending fitness classes have left her sore and unable to walk much for days. As an exercise professional, what recommendations do you have for her to ease into dance fitness so she does not experience the same results?
4. Based on the theory you learned above, why is dance fitness so much more appealing for many people than traditional exercise?
5. Besides physical benefits, what other emotional or mental benefits can Nicole gain from dance fitness?

CHAPTER 11

Flexibility Training and Cool-Down Techniques

Elizabeth Kovar, MA, and Alexios Batrakoulis, PhD

After completing this chapter, you will be able to

- list the benefits of participating in an effective flexibility training program,
- describe the components of the cool-down phase,
- explain the value of cooling down following a workout,
- design engaging cool-down routines for clients with excess weight, and
- supervise client-centered, multicomponent flexibility training programs and cool-down routines.

Flexibility is the range of motion of a joint and the ability of the joint to move freely through its normal, full range of motion (Haff and Triplett 2015). In the fitness world, it is not very common for exercise professionals to spend a whole session on teaching mobility and flexibility training. Ideally, separate sessions are recommended for optimal benefits in both mobility and flexibility. Thus, providing mobility and flexibility training in multiple sessions is a common strategy for individuals of all ages and levels with no limitations in weekly time commitment and exercise programming (Garber et al. 2011).

Considering that client-centered exercise sessions for persons with excess weight are characterized by a multicomponent training approach, mobility training is primarily included in the warm-up, while flexibility training is primarily included in the cool-down (Garber et al. 2011). However, the cool-down phase offers excellent timing for performing both mobility and flexibility exercises, especially for individuals with excess weight, because this particular population tends to have poor functional capacity (Pataky et al. 2014), limited range of motion in all joints (Jeong et al. 2018), a high risk of orthopedic injuries (Sabharwal and Root 2012), and insufficient musculoskeletal fitness levels (Wearing et al. 2006).

The Benefits of Flexibility Training and Cool-Down Techniques

The cool-down phase decreases postexercise hypotension, allows better dissipation of body heat, removes lactic acid, mitigates the increase in stress-response hormones called catecholamines that can potentially cause cardiac arrhythmia, and possibly reduces the risk of cardiac events during the recovery period (McQueen 2009). Given that an increase in the joints' range of motion is important at the beginning of a session for clients seeking to have that range of motion while they train and keep that new range of motion throughout the session, dynamic stretching fits better into the warm-up than the cool-down phase (Garber et al. 2011). A stretching routine following the cool-down period has been shown to improve flexibility and reduce the potential for muscle soreness; however, this evidence has been reported as ambiguous (Andersen 2005).

Instead, static stretching better suits the cool-down as a way to promote relaxation and stress relief. Low-intensity movements are beneficial for an optimal postexercise recovery process to help alleviate any discomfort the day after a difficult workout. Mobility exercises of low to moderate intensity may also help attenuate muscle tightness and soreness and enhance blood flow in sedentary individuals with excess weight (Funk et al. 2003). Such an exercise strategy may help individuals with overweight or obesity and poor functional capacity not only increase their body functionality but also achieve a complete recovery following an exercise session, with the aim of entering a repair mode through a positive exercise experience.

Components of the Cool-Down Phase

In a 60-minute session, the cool-down should last approximately 10 to 15 minutes. This phase should include activities of low to moderate intensity, such as walking, stretching, breathing, and relaxation techniques for physical and mental stress relief. The goal is to incorporate lighter movement that allows the heart rate and breathing rate to recover from exercising and move toward homeostasis. Some dynamic movements used in the warm-up may also be applicable in the cool-down, aiming to enhance mobility among people with excess weight and poor body functionality. This cool-down phase is directed at preventing the tendency for blood to pool in the lower extremities, which may occur when exercise ends.

Movements and exercises performed during the cool-down can improve flexibility, muscle recovery, and movement efficiency in addition to inhibiting overactive muscles and reducing pain (Hopper et al. 2019). The cool-down phase may include the following techniques:

1. *Mobility exercises.* Performing multiplanar movements at a variety of rhythmic speeds can elevate body temperature, allowing layers of fascia and muscle to slide over one another (Samson et al. 2012). Mobility exercises focus on the range of motion of a specific joint or area of the body. Examples include shoulder circles, cat–cow, and hip swings.

2. *Self-myofascial release (SMR).* SMR techniques involve small, continuous back-and-forth movements on a foam roller or with a massage device (e.g., a massage ball), covering an area of 2 to 6 in. (1-2 cm) over a tender region for 30 to 60 seconds. An exercise professional can assist with myofascial release if a client is unable to perform SMR in specific positions or for certain muscle groups (Cheatham et al. 2015).

3. *Proprioceptive neuromuscular facilitation (PNF) stretching.* PNF is when a client performs a hold–relax stretch, holding the isometric contraction of the agonist muscle for a minimum of 6 seconds, followed by a 10- to 30-second assisted or passive stretch (Hindle et al. 2012). For individuals with excess weight, PNF stretches should be assisted to make them feasible and safe.

4. *Static stretching.* Static stretching requires the client to lengthen a muscle as far as possible without feeling any extreme pain or discomfort, then hold that position for 15 to 60 seconds (Page 2012).

5. *Diaphragmatic breathing.* Diaphragmatic breathing helps clients to ease out of the sympathetic nervous system state, flood the brain with oxygen, and feel better. This change in state will give them greater range of motion in all joints (Reid and McNair 2004), because a reduction in muscle tightness and pain allows a person to relax both physically and mentally.

Stretching for Clients With Excess Weight

Exercise professionals will get a better idea of a client's abilities, needs, and priorities after a postural and functional movements assessment. Stretching can be beneficial for clients with excess weight, but there are some considerations concerning flexibility training for this population. Individuals with obesity need mobility but do not need to focus on becoming extremely flexible. Flexibility training alleviates discomfort, but the ability to touch one's toes is not an important goal when exercise adherence and behavior changes are the priorities.

Generally, the human body adapts to the stimuli to which it is exposed. Davis's Law states that soft tissue adapts along lines of stress (Frost 2003). The principle posits that the configuration and orientation of soft tissues, including fasciae, tendons, ligaments, and cartilage, undergo a process of adaptation over time in response to the physical stresses exerted on them. Gravity affects posture, which may worsen over time with technology use and a sedentary lifestyle. Typing on a computer or texting can put the shoulders in a position of internal rotation. Gravity also pulls the spine down, potentially developing a forward curve in the upper back that also internally rotates the shoulders when the head is tilted forward. In addition, abdominal obesity causes an imbalance in the muscles around the pelvis, triggering hip joint contracture, anterior pelvic tilt, and excessive activity of the hip joint flexors to compensate for weakened abdominal muscles; this results in lordosis (an excessive inward curve in the lower back) and, therefore, low-back pain (Park and Seo 2014).

With this in mind, stretches should focus on the major muscles of the body that improve posture and alleviate spinal pain. Hip and thoracic spine mobility should be a priority for clients with excess weight, because these two regions are the most mobile areas of the body that affect low-back and knee health. Sedentary people with excess weight are likely to have a high risk of injury and of musculoskeletal health disorders (e.g., osteoarthritis) in the knees and lower back due to physical limitations, postural deviations, and muscular imbalances (Shumnalieva et al. 2023). Hence, chest openers, hip flexor stretches, and forward folds to stretch the posterior chain of the body can be beneficial.

Stretching should be eased into and progressed over time. Stretching can cause delayed-onset muscle soreness for beginners due to microtears in muscles, especially if clients push beyond their limits (Stecco et al. 2020). Sessions should progress through intelligent stretching sequences that are appropriate for the person's current fitness level and ability. Physically active individuals with overweight or obesity may be able to perform a wider variety of stretches and cool-down exercises compared to sedentary clients with severe obesity, who may require modifications or alternative programming. Although stretching and SMR are beneficial to everybody, there are special considerations and contraindications for clients with overweight or obesity.

Special Considerations for Flexibility Training

Due to various physical limitations and postural deviations, individuals with excess body weight or adiposity may experience several difficulties when performing flexibility exercises such as vertical and horizontal stretches and SMR techniques. Specifically, in a workout tailored to the psychophysiological profile of a client with excess weight (i.e., aiming to avoid pain, uncomfortable positions, and embarrassment), the following five factors may impede the use of flexibility exercises (Jeong et al. 2018; Pataky et al. 2014; Sabharwal and Root 2012; Schvey et al. 2017; Wearing et al. 2006):

1. Effects of different positions against gravity on the client's body and adipose tissue
2. Inability to get down to or up from the floor
3. Inability to stand up from a seated position
4. Lack of a full range of motion to bend over
5. Limited range of motion in the shoulder and hip joints

Special Considerations for SMR Techniques

1. Massage balls or sticks are ideal tools to use in seated and vertical positions before progressing to foam rolling. For active individuals with overweight or obesity who can foam roll, use a softer foam roller and focus on the larger muscle groups before moving to more sensitive areas. The goal is to build tolerance for rolling out the major muscles, creating a positive experience rather than one associated with pain. Avoid rolling with dense objects, such as golf balls, baseballs, baseball bats, metal poles, or metal water bottles. These harder surfaces may cause damage and pain.

2. Foam rollers are not ideal for beginners with obesity. Sitting or lying on a foam roll places the person's body weight on an unstable surface. Balance and coordination to stay on top of the roller may be difficult for the client. In addition, loading the body's weight onto a small, dense surface may cause pain or bruising. Foam rolling also requires enough upper-body and wrist strength and shoulder-blade stability to lift and move the body in supine and prone positions.

3. There are several contraindications to foam rolling. Individuals with inflammatory diseases, neuropathy, nerve damage, extreme hypertension, or diabetes or who have peripheral neuropathy should avoid foam rolling or modify it with other SMR techniques. Also, individuals with inflammation from recent injuries should avoid foam rolling and follow a protocol from their doctor or physical therapist. Foam rolling also increases inflammation and blood pressure to trigger the healing response, which can cause issues for those with certain preexisting conditions.

4. Foam rolling is too challenging for many individuals to do independently, which presents an opportunity for the exercise professional to foam roll the client in a lying-down position. This involves placing the soft roller on top of rather than underneath the person. This option may be feasible for a client with overweight,

but it may be aversive for individuals with obesity, especially for those with abdominal obesity and a large waist.

Special Considerations for Stretching

1. Previously sedentary individuals with overweight or obesity may have muscles that are sensitive to touch and to general stretching. Vertical and seated chair stretching may be more advantageous for beginning and deconditioned clients before progressing to floor stretching.

2. People of any age with severe obesity may not be able to get down to and up from the floor for stretching or SMR. Individuals with excess weight may require a massage table or a bed for stretches done while lying down to make it easier to get into a seated or lying position. If such a surface is not available, the client should perform vertical and seated stretching.

3. Floor stretching may be restricted by excess weight. Some individuals may feel uncomfortable on the ground or be unable to move into a stretch because of body size. In addition, when a client with overweight or obesity is lying down, gravity pulls the abdominal adipose tissue (and breast tissue) onto the organs and spine, which may restrict the range of motion.

4. Seated stretching on the floor, specifically in forward-fold and spinal-twist positions, may also be difficult for those with higher levels of abdominal obesity. Elevating the hips helps people with inflexibility to achieve seated stretches more easily than sitting on the ground. Elevated surfaces could include a step bench, weight bench, plyo box, or balance ball. Note that stable surfaces are recommended before using unstable surfaces, such as a balance ball, because adequate core strength is required to stay on the ball without the risk of falling off.

Tips for an Inclusive Cool-Down Phase

The cool-down phase is an excellent opportunity not only to promote relaxation and restoration but also to offer a positive exercise experience through client-centered exercises. Such an approach will provide beneficial psychophysiological adaptations to clients with excess weight while offering a pain-free and engaging fitness journey in various exercise settings.

1. A low-impact cardiorespiratory fitness activity, such as easy walking with deep breathing, is a priority to transition the body to final stretching. A cool-down can also include some dynamic movement exercises, similar to a warm-up.

2. Excessive foam rolling should be avoided, and the client should use a soft foam roll or something such as a massage ball or a stick. Individuals who cannot place their body on top of a device can be rolled out by the exercise professional to aid in the release of adhesions and muscle tension.

3. Static stretching should not be overused. The focus should be on the stretches that will benefit the client most, such as posterior chain or chest stretches to aid better posture.

4. Prescriptions of SMR, PNF, and static stretching for clients with abdominal obesity should avoid lying positions (prone and supine), because these positions may cause awkwardness and discomfort that are not worth the effort. Standing, seated, and quadruped positions are recommended instead.

5. Stretches should be demonstrated at the client's ability level. When clients see the exercise professional going to a maximum range of motion, they can get discouraged because their own range of motion may be less.

6. The exercise experience should be positive. The goal is to make the cool-down phase enjoyable and help clients feel empowered, confident, and comfortable by avoiding painful techniques. Such a strategy provides exercise professionals with the possibility to increase clients' adherence and get results.

7. The opportunity to connect emotionally with clients during the cool-down should not be missed. This is perfect timing for an honest conversation and productive consultation, aiming to empower clients with excess weight who may have mental health challenges.

COOL-DOWN MOBILITY EXERCISES

Dynamic Knee Pull

Primary Muscles Stretched
- Glutes
- Hamstrings

Instructions
1. Stand tall and maintain a neutral spine (*a*).
2. Lift the right leg, placing the hands around the front of the knee or behind the hamstrings (*b*).
3. Hold for 1 s, then release.
4. Repeat with the left leg.
5. Continue to alternate between lifting the right and left leg for 15 to 30 s.

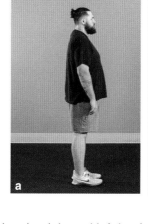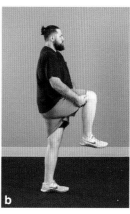

Variation
- Perform the exercise while seated in a chair.

Dynamic Spinal Twist

Primary Muscles Stretched
- Erector spinae
- Rhomboids
- Latissimus dorsi

Instructions
1. Find a seated position and bring the spine into neutral alignment.
2. Inhale while reaching the arms overhead (*a*).

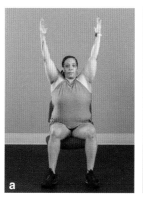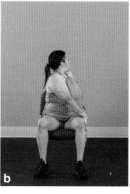

3. Exhale while twisting the spine toward the left. Place the left hand either on the seat or near the lower back (*b*).
4. Hold for 3 to 5 s.
5. Inhale while rotating to the center with the arms overhead.
6. Exhale while twisting the spine toward the right. Place the right hand either on the seat or near the lower back.
7. Continue this motion for 30 s.

Variation

- Perform this stretch while standing with the feet shoulder-width apart. Move the hands toward the hips and lower back.

MYOFASCIAL RELEASE TECHNIQUES ASSISTED BY AN EXERCISE PROFESSIONAL

Assisted Supine Myofascial Release

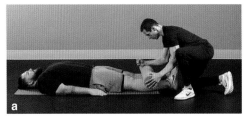 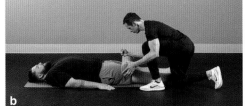

Note that a supine position may be feasible for a person with overweight but may not be comfortable or even possible for a person with obesity. Therefore, the following techniques may not be recommended for all clients, especially those with abdominal obesity or a large waist.

Primary Muscles Released

- Peroneal muscles
- Quadriceps

Instructions

1. Have the client lie face-up on a table or a mat. Support their head with pillows if necessary.
2. Initiate the rolling process with a soft foam roller or massage stick.
3. Use the forearm to push the roller up and down the peroneal muscles. Perform this for about 30 s, then move to the quadriceps (*a*).
4. Use the forearm to push the roller up and down the quadriceps for 30 s (*b*). Focus on the medial, lateral, and central areas of the quadriceps. Avoid rolling the knee and the hip joint.
5. Repeat the rolling process on the opposite leg.

Assisted Prone Myofascial Release

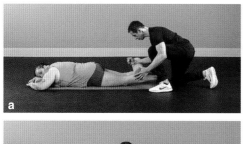
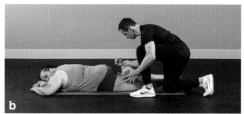
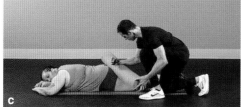
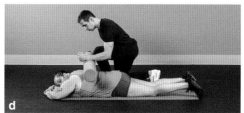

Note that a prone position may be feasible for a person with overweight but may not be comfortable or even possible for a person with obesity. Therefore, the following techniques may not be recommended for all clients, especially those with abdominal obesity or a large waist.

Primary Muscles Released

- Calves
- Hamstrings
- Gluteus maximus
- Thoracic spine muscles

Instructions

1. Have the client lie face-down on a table or a mat. Support their head with pillows if necessary.
2. With the client lying comfortably, initiate the rolling process with a soft foam roller or massage stick. Begin with the calf (*a*), then proceed to the hamstrings (*b*), glutes (*c*), and thoracic spine muscles (*d*).
3. Use the forearm to push the roller from the bottom to the top of the calf for 30 s, avoiding the ankle and the back of the knee.
4. Use the forearm to push the roller up and down the hamstrings for 30 s. Focus on the medial, lateral, and central areas of the hamstrings. Avoid rolling the back of the knee and the hip joint.
5. Use the forearm to push the roller up and down the glutes for 30 s.
6. Use the forearm to push the roller up and down the thoracic spine muscles for 30 s. Avoid rolling the neck.

PNF STRETCHING

Seated Pectoral PNF Stretch

Primary Muscles Stretched

- Pectorals
- Anterior deltoids

Instructions

1. Have the client sit in a chair with a neutral spine and their hands behind their head, with their elbows winging wide.
2. Place your hands on the inside of the client's lower arms, near the elbows.
3. Have the client push into your hands, holding for about 6 s.
4. After the contraction, have the client relax into the stretch. Apply light pressure to the client's arms to trigger a stretch through the pectoralis major. Hold for 10 to 30 s.
5. Complete 3 sets of this contract-and-relax cycle.

Supine Lying Hamstring Stretch

Primary Muscles Stretched

- Hamstrings
- Calves

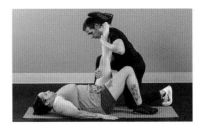

Instructions

1. Lie supine on the floor or on a massage table.
2. Lift one leg and place the calf on the fitness professional's shoulder, pressing the leg and calf into the shoulder for about 6 s.
3. After the contraction, relax into the stretch, applying light pressure to the leg to stretch the hamstrings.
4. Keep the foot flexed and hold for 10 to 30 s.
5. Complete three sets of this contract-and-relax cycle. Then perform this same sequence on the other leg.

Variation

- Perform this stretch with a yoga strap placed over the sole of the foot.

Supine Lying External Hip Rotation Stretch

Primary Muscles Stretched

- External rotators of the hip

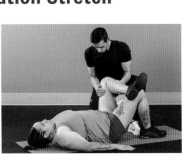

Instructions

1. Have the client lie supine on the floor or on a massage table, crossing the left ankle over the right thigh and keeping the right foot on the ground.
2. If the client is capable, have them lift the right leg and place their hands behind their right hamstring.

3. Place one hand on the lower part of the client's left inner thigh.

4. Have the client resist or push into the hand for about 6 s.

5. After the contraction, have the client relax the leg. Apply light pressure on the leg to externally rotate the hip.

6. Complete three sets of this contract-and-relax cycle, then perform the same cycle on the other leg.

Variations

- This can be performed with the client seated in a chair if the client is able to cross their ankle over the opposite thigh.

- A yoga strap can also be used to support the leg if the client is unable to cross the ankle over the thigh.

STATIC STRETCHING EXERCISES

Palm and Forearm Stretch

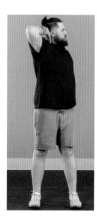

Primary Muscles Stretched

- Extrinsic and intrinsic muscles of the hand and forearm

Instructions

1. Sit or stand tall with a neutral spine.

2. Inhale while interlocking the fingers in front of the chest.

3. Exhale while extending the arms forward with the palms facing out.

4. If possible, exhale and press the arms overhead with the palms facing the ceiling.

5. Hold for 15 to 30 s.

Variation

- Add dynamic or static lateral flexion to lengthen the side of the body.

Seated or Standing Pectoral Spinal Twist

Primary Muscles Stretched

- Pectoral muscles
- Anterior deltoids

Instructions

1. Sit or stand tall with a neutral spine and the feet slightly more than shoulder-width apart. Standing will also stretch the obliques.

2. Inhale while interlocking the hands and placing them behind the head.

3. Exhale and rotate to the right into a spinal twist; hold for 30 s.

4. Inhale and return to center.

5. Exhale and rotate to the left; hold for 15 to 30 s.

Iliotibial Band Lateral Side Bend

Primary Muscles Stretched

- Lateral hip
- Iliotibial band area
- Obliques

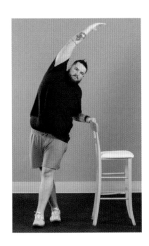

Instructions

1. Stand with the left hand holding on to a chair, wall, or windowsill.
2. Cross the right foot behind the left leg.
3. Inhale and lift the right arm overhead.
4. Exhale and shift the right hip to the right while laterally flexing the spine to the left.
5. Hold for 15 to 30 s, then switch to the other side.

Variation

- Stand with the feet together if unable to cross one foot behind the other, or place the hand behind the head if unable to hold the arm in the air.

Elevated Forward Fold

Primary Muscles Stretched

- Glutes
- Hamstrings
- Calves

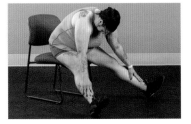

Instructions

1. Find an elevated surface, such as a chair, weight bench, or step bench. (A balance ball can also be used by individuals who are comfortable with unstable surfaces.)
2. Sit on the elevated surface and extend the legs out in front.
3. Place the heels on the ground, with the legs shoulder-width apart and the feet flexed.
4. Inhale and sweep the arms overhead, extending the spine.
5. Exhale and fold forward, lengthening from the naval center and placing the hands on the legs.
6. Hold for 15 to 30 s.

Variation

- If extending the legs is too intense, place the feet flat on the ground with the knees flexed.

Supported Hip Hinge

Primary Muscles Stretched

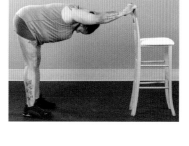

- Hamstrings
- Calves
- Glutes
- Erector spinae
- Pectorals

Instructions

1. Find a stable surface, such as a bar, doorknob, or countertop.
2. Face the stable surface and hold on to it while standing with the feet slightly more than shoulder-width apart.
3. Walk the feet away from the stable surface until the arms are straight.
4. Exhale and hinge forward at the hips until the hips are behind the feet and the spine is parallel to the ground. Imagine the torso melting toward the ground with gravity.
5. Keep breathing while holding the stretch for 15 to 30 s.

Variations

- Advanced clients can use a TRX suspension trainer as the unstable surface.
- Placing the hands flat on a tabletop is also effective.

High Lunge With Pectoral and Calf Stretch

Primary Muscles Stretched

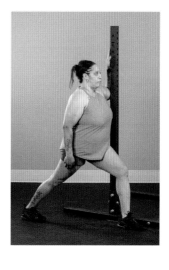

- Calves
- Hip flexors
- Pectorals

Instructions

1. Stand with the left side of the body near a wall or a doorway.
2. Place the left forearm against the wall or doorframe so that the left shoulder and elbow are at 90° angles.
3. Bring the left foot forward and flex the knee into a lunge position, moving the body forward until a stretch is felt in the chest.
4. Extend the right leg back and press the heel to the ground to stretch the calf.
5. Keep the pelvis in neutral alignment and tuck the pubic bone forward while keeping the ribs and hips facing forward to enhance the hip flexor stretch on the right leg.
6. Hold for 15 to 30 s, then perform the stretch on the other side.

Variation

- Each stretch can be performed separately if combining them is too complicated for hand and foot coordination.

Chest Stretch With Strap

Primary Muscles Stretched

- Pectoral muscles
- Anterior deltoids

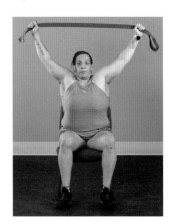

Instructions

1. Sit or stand tall with a neutral spine.
2. Hold a strap in both hands and exhale while lifting the arms overhead, making a *Y* shape with the arms.
3. Hold for 15 to 30 s.

Variation

- Perform lateral flexion, with the spine moving from right to left.

Seated Spinal Flexion With Twist

Primary Muscles Stretched

- Rhomboids
- Latissimus dorsi

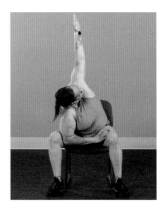

Instructions

1. Sit in a chair and hinge forward at the hips, placing the right forearm (or hand) on the thighs.
2. Exhale and lift the left arm upward while twisting the thoracic spine.
3. Hold for 15 to 30 s while breathing naturally, then repeat on the other side.

Seated Leg Stretch With Strap

Primary Muscles Stretched

- Calves
- Hamstrings

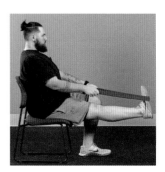

Instructions

1. Sit in a chair with a neutral spine and place a strap under the arch of the right foot.
2. Exhale, extending the right knee to lift the leg. Support the strap with both hands.
3. Hold the stretch for 15 to 30 s, then switch legs.

Quadriceps Stretch With Strap

Primary Muscles Stretched

- Quadriceps

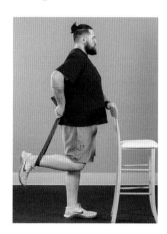

Instructions

1. Stand tall and bend the right knee so that the right foot is lifted behind the body. Place a strap around the top of the right foot or ankle, and hold the strap with the right hand.
2. Use the left hand for balance support if needed.
3. Use the strap to pull the lower right leg up to the point where a quadriceps stretch is felt.
4. Keep the inner thighs parallel and imagine pushing the right thigh bone backward.
5. Hold for 15 to 30 s, then repeat with the left leg.

Variation

- Perform with the hands rather than a strap if the client is capable of holding their foot.

DIAPHRAGMATIC BREATHING TECHNIQUES

Diaphragmatic Breathing— Matching Inhale With Exhale

Primary Muscles Stretched

- Diaphragm

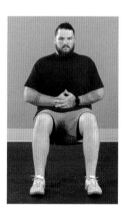

Instructions

1. Sit in a chair and maintain a neutral spine. Support the spine with pillows if needed.
2. Place the hands on the belly between the navel and the base of the ribcage.
3. Inhale for a count of five to balloon the diaphragm into the hands.
4. Hold the breath for 1 s.
5. Exhale for a count of five, feeling the diaphragm moving toward the spine.
6. Continue for 2 to 3 min while maintaining a tall posture and neutral spine.

Three-Part Breath

Primary Muscles Stretched
- Diaphragm

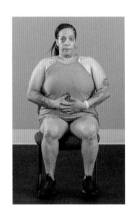

Instructions
1. Sit in a chair and maintain a neutral spine. Support the spine with pillows if needed.
2. Place the hands on the diaphragm.
3. Inhale three short breaths through the nostrils, feeling the diaphragm expand into the hands.
4. Exhale one long breath out of the mouth.
5. Repeat for five cycles.
6. Inhale one long breath through the nostrils, feeling the diaphragm expand into the hands.
7. Exhale three short breaths out of the mouth.
8. Repeat for five cycles.

Seated Cat–Cow With Chest Opener

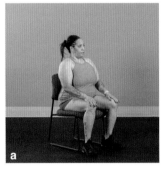 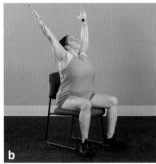 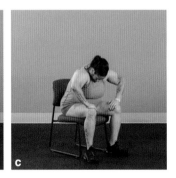

Primary Muscles Stretched
- Diaphragm
- Pectorals
- Rhomboids
- Trapezius

Instructions
1. Sit in a chair and maintain a neutral spine, resting the hands on the thighs.
2. Inhale to puff the ribs into thoracic extension, then sweep the arms open above the shoulders in a *Y* shape.
3. Exhale, rounding the thoracic spine and tucking the chin to the chest; bring hands to the thighs. Repeat for 5 to 10 cycles.

Variation
- Keep the hands on the thighs and move the spine only.

Quadruped Cat–Cow

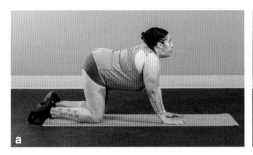 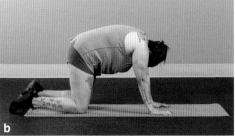

Primary Muscles Stretched
- Diaphragm
- Pectorals
- Rhomboids
- Trapezius

Instructions
1. Begin on the hands and knees in the table pose, with a neutral spine and the knees in line with the hips.
2. Inhale while lifting the sit bones upward. Press the chest forward and drop the belly while lifting the head and relaxing the shoulders away from the ears (*a*). Gaze straight ahead.
3. Exhale while rounding the spine outward, tucking in the tailbone, drawing the pubic bone forward, and relaxing the head toward the floor (*b*).
4. Repeat for 5 to 10 cycles.

CHAPTER SUMMARY

The cool-down phase of a fitness session is essential to transition the body from the workout back toward homeostasis. A cool-down includes a mix of low- to moderate-intensity movements and static stretches to release metabolic waste and decrease the chance of muscle tightness and soreness. A postexercise flexibility and cool-down strategy can include a mix of diaphragmatic breathing and selected SMR techniques as well as feasible PNF and static stretching. All of this is beneficial to clients with overweight or obesity, but modifications and special considerations may be necessary, depending on the fitness level and abilities of the client. However, considering that exercise professionals may only have 2 to 3 hours per week to check off a lot of parameters in each session, many common flexibility and mobility exercises are not completely necessary for people with overweight or obesity during a cool-down. As long as clients with excess weight are able to incorporate foundational, pain-free, muscle-strengthening exercises with a great range of motion into their workouts, this is sufficient given the limited time per week.

KEY POINTS

- The cool-down phase should be a fundamental component of a personal training session or group exercise class.
- The cool-down phase includes light- to moderate-intensity activities to decrease the heart rate, followed by diaphragmatic breathing techniques and selected SMR, PNF, and static stretching.
- People are under the influence of gravity at all hours, and a long-term sedentary lifestyle can affect posture through the development of a forward curve in the upper back, internally rotated shoulders, and an excessive inward curve in the lower back (lordosis).
- Clients with excess weight can benefit from SMR and stretching but may require modifications based on their physical fitness level, abilities, and body size.
- Clients do not need to make it a goal to become extremely flexible but should use stretching and SMR to alleviate pain and aid in developing better posture.
- Contraindications for foam rolling are important to understand, because foam rolling can be painful and may irritate inflammatory and nerve issues. It can also be awkward to balance on a foam roller.
- The goal for exercise professionals is to make stretching a positive fitness experience and avoid any painful techniques.

CHAPTER QUIZ

Quiz answers can be found in the appendix.

1. Which of the following is NOT one of the purposes of the cool-down phase?
   a. dissipate heat
   b. remove lactic acid
   c. reduce the risk of cardiovascular events
   d. increase heart rate

2. The duration of the cool-down should be _____ that of the warm-up.
   a. as intense as
   b. the same as
   c. shorter than
   d. longer than

3. Which of the following types of stretches should NOT be part of the cool-down phase?
   a. active isolated stretching
   b. static stretching
   c. SMR
   d. PNF stretching

4. _____ is a hold–relax stretch in which a client holds the isometric contraction of the agonist muscle for at least 6 seconds, followed by an assisted or passive stretch for 10 to 30 seconds.
   a. Ballistic stretching
   b. SMR
   c. PNF
   d. Active isolated stretching

5. Static stretches are held to the point of tension for _____ seconds.
   a. 30-90
   b. 30-60
   c. 15-60
   d. 15-45

6. When on the floor, _____ may help inflexible people get into stretches more easily and comfortably.
   a. pushing forward
   b. lifting the spine
   c. relaxing the legs
   d. elevating the hips

7. Which of the following pieces of equipment should be avoided for SMR?
   a. foam roller
   b. baseball
   c. massage ball
   d. massage stick

8. Which of the following is NOT a contraindication for foam rolling and SMR?
   a. stiff muscles
   b. neuropathy
   c. elevated blood pressure
   d. inflammation issues

9. Exercise professionals should focus on stretches that
   a. are performed while lying down
   b. can assist clients in being able to touch their toes
   c. improve posture and alleviate areas of tension or pain
   d. make clients as flexible as possible

10. Which of the following is NOT a special consideration for clients with overweight or obesity when stretching?
    a. how the body is affected by gravity
    b. SMR contraindications
    c. ability to get down to and up from the floor
    d. client age

CASE STUDY

Case study answers can be found in the appendix.

Aditya is a 28-year-old man with a body mass index of 37 kg/m^2 who works in the technology industry and has led a sedentary lifestyle for decades. He is a computer programmer who spends most of his day working as a software engineer and his spare time on technology or watching television. Because he is highly dedicated to his job, Aditya does not move much and has decided to hire a personal trainer to help him get into better shape. Due to sitting for long periods of time, he has some low-back pain, and while initiating the first couple of sessions, basic exercises and lateral movements have initiated hip pain. During the assessment, it is clear that Aditya has limited range of motion, especially on the floor; however, he can get down to and up from the floor easily. He has great coordination and tends to move quickly, but because he is unconditioned, just 15 minutes of basic continuous movements (e.g., lateral steps, toe taps on a bench, or standing from sitting in a chair) ignite pain in his lower-body joints. It seems that a 30-minute personal training session that primarily includes being upright and moving is too much for his body. Aditya clearly needs help with conditioning but also with building stability and mobility in his body. If he loses weight, much of the pain may be decreased, but at present, he cannot handle more than 15 minutes of continuous movement.

1. Do you think someone like Aditya is within your scope of practice?
2. Within your scope of practice, how would you structure Aditya's fitness program?
3. Knowing that Aditya's hip pain flares up with the specific exercises mentioned, what cool-down exercises would you incorporate into his program?
4. What stretches would you incorporate into Aditya's cool-down program?
5. What SMR techniques would you incorporate, knowing that Aditya should not sit on the foam roller?

PART IV

THE PROGRAMMING

CHAPTER 12

Program Design

Alexios Batrakoulis, PhD, and Anoop Balachandran, PhD

After completing this chapter, you will be able to
- describe the training principles for effective and safe exercise programming;
- explore the fundamental concepts in training and exercise prescription;
- use exercise engagement strategies;
- explain the components of a tailored exercise session;
- design progressive, multicomponent training programs; and
- incorporate special considerations and precautions when programming exercises for individuals with excess body weight and adiposity.

This chapter will present a number of evidence-based program design strategies and proven training concepts, with a goal of enabling practitioners to design client-centered exercise programs under authentic conditions. The interpretation of scientific principles and guidelines into practical applications represents a crucial step in the design of an effective and safe exercise program while also fostering exercise enjoyment and reducing negative beliefs, fears, and stress. This is of critical importance for exercise professionals working with clients who have excess weight; each client is unique and each case is distinct, influenced by a multitude of individual and environmental factors.

Training Principles

There are six key principles of exercise training: overload, reversibility, progression, individualization, periodization, and specificity (Garber et al. 2011; Piercy et el. 2018).

1. *Overload:* This principle refers to the need for an organ system or tissue to be exercised at a level beyond its accustomed state to achieve training adaptations. The exercise variables that constitute overload include intensity, duration, and frequency. For example, aerobic exercise places stress on the cardiorespiratory system and muscles, requiring the lungs and heart to transport more oxygen and deliver it to the working muscles. This increased demand enhances the efficiency and capacity of the lungs, heart, circulatory system, and exercising muscles.

2. *Reversibility:* The principle of reversibility indicates that fitness and performance gains achieved through training are quickly lost when training is stopped and the overload is removed. According to this principle, the body adapts to the cessation of a specific exercise program and inadequate training load, resulting in atrophy and reductions in fitness and performance.

3. *Progression:* The principle of progression refers to gradual and systematic increases in training stress to evoke continued training adaptation. Training parameters (e.g., frequency, intensity, and time) should be increased to provoke further adaptation. Importantly, such increases must take place gradually to avoid injury, burnout, and overtraining, although very slow progressions may result in delayed goal accomplishment. Once a person reaches a certain fitness level, they can progress to higher levels of physical activity through continued overload and adaptation. Gradually, progressive changes in overload help the body adapt to increased stress while minimizing the risk of injury. The recommended rate of progression in an exercise program depends on an individual's health status, physical fitness, training responses, and exercise program goals. For aerobic activities, progression may involve increasing any of the four components of the FITT principle (frequency, intensity, time, and type) that the individual can tolerate. In resistance training, progression can be achieved by (1) reaching muscular failure without changing the number of repetitions, (2) increasing the amount of weight lifted by 2.5% to 5% once the goal repetitions and sets can be achieved in at least two consecutive sessions, (3) increasing the number of sets per muscle group, or (4) modifying the rest interval between sets in accordance with the training goal. For instance, shorter rest intervals while performing high repetitions encourage greater adaptations in muscular endurance, while longer rest intervals while performing low repetitions stimulate greater gains in muscular strength. However, resistance training without reaching muscle failure may evoke similar or even more favorable muscular fitness improvements compared to training until muscle failure (Vieira et al. 2021).

4. *Individualization:* The principle of individualization involves the adjustment of training to consider a person's unique capacity and response to it. Each exercise program should be characterized by differences in a client's capacity for adaptation compared to that of other clients. Otherwise, adherence to a prescribed exercise program cannot be ensured, because numerous factors (e.g., physiologic, psychologic, environmental, and genetic) affect the person's capacity. This particular principle scientifically explains why a one-size-fits-all exercise approach should not be applied.

5. *Periodization:* This principle underlines the planned systematic and structural variation of a training program over time. Training parameters (e.g., frequency, intensity, time, and type) should be constantly cycled within an exercise program, aiming to ensure optimal training stimuli; manage changing goals and personal variability; and avoid injury, burnout, and overtraining.

6. *Specificity:* The principle of specificity emphasizes that exercise is specific to the muscles involved in the activity, the recruited fiber types, the engaged energy system, the velocity of contractions, and the type of muscle contractions. For instance, the physiological benefits of walking primarily target the lower body and cardiovascular system. On the other hand, engaging in strength training will primarily lead to adaptations in strength and muscle mass.

Fundamental Components of Exercise Prescription

In terms of exercise prescription, the four FITT principles (frequency, intensity, time, and type) are fundamental components of exercise prescription used to design and modify exercise programs (Donnelly et al. 2009; Garber et al. 2021). They guide how to structure workouts for optimal results and safety. The following are recommended guidelines for both aerobic and resistance training under each category.

F: Frequency (How Often)

Frequency refers to how many times per week a person should engage in their exercise routine. Generally, the frequency depends on fitness goals, schedule, and the type of exercise the person is doing. Aerobic exercise is recommended to be performed at least three days per week. For most adults, it is best to spread the exercise sessions across three to five days per week to reach the recommended amount of physical activity. Moderate- and vigorous-intensity exercise options can be combined weekly, which is suitable for most individuals.

Resistance training exercises that target all major muscle groups with at least one set of 8 to 12 repetitions in a session should be performed at least two days per week on nonconsecutive days.

I: Intensity (How Hard)

Intensity refers to how hard a person works during their exercise sessions. It can be measured in various ways, such as heart rate, weight lifted, or perceived effort. The minimum threshold of intensity for benefit seems to vary depending on an individual's current fitness level and other factors, such as age, health status, habitual physical activity, and social and psychological considerations.

Aerobic exercise can be performed in either moderate-intensity or vigorous-intensity activities or as a combination of both. Moderate to vigorous exercise (65%-85% of the maximum heart rate [HRmax]) is recommended for people with overweight or obesity. However, beginners, deconditioned individuals, and older adults need to start with lower intensities (55%-70% of the HRmax) and gradually progress to more vigorous intensities, as tolerated. The talk test is a simple and reliable approach to gauging intensity for aerobic exercises. As a rule of thumb, a person engaged in moderate-intensity aerobic activity should be able to talk but not sing during the activity. A person involved in vigorous-intensity activity should not be able to say more than a few words without pausing for a breath. In general, on a scale of difficulty from 1 to 10, progress from a 5 to an 8 throughout the workout is recommended.

In resistance training, intensity refers to the amount of weight lifted during exercises, typically expressed as a percentage of an individual's 1-repetition maximum (1-RM) for a given exercise, such as 80% of the 1-RM, or using different repetition maximums, such as the 5-repetition maximum (5-RM) or 10-repetition maximum (10-RM). For general muscular fitness goals, a load corresponding to 8 to 15 repetitions at 60% to 80% of the 1-RM is usually recommended. In general, on a scale of difficulty from 1 to 10, progressing from a 5 to a 7 throughout the workout is recommended. However, beginners, deconditioned individuals, and older adults with overweight or obesity and comorbidity should start with lower intensities (12-15 reps at 40%-60% of the 1-RM, with at least 2-3 reps in reserve).

T: Time (Duration)

The time principle relates to how long each exercise session should last. It is important to consider the duration of both the entire workout and the individual exercises or sets within the workout.

Light-intensity activity is defined as 1.1 to 2.9 metabolic equivalents (METs), moderate-intensity activity as 3.0 to 5.9 METs, and vigorous activity as more than 6 METs. There appears to be a dose–response relationship between the amount of time habitual physical activity is performed and weight loss. Typically, being physically active for 225 to 420 minutes per week or more results in a bodyweight reduction of approximately 2 lb (1 kg) (Donnelly et al. 2009). For aerobic exercise, most adults should aim to accumulate 30 to 60 minutes per day of moderate-intensity exercise, 20 to 60 minutes per day of vigorous-intensity exercise, or a combination of both to meet the recommended target of 150 to 300 minutes of exercise per week. A general rule of thumb is that 2 minutes of moderate-intensity activity are equivalent to 1 minute of vigorous-intensity activity. For instance, 30 minutes of moderate-intensity activity is roughly equal to 15 minutes of vigorous-intensity activity. It should be noted that additional health benefits can be obtained by engaging in physical activity beyond the equivalent of 300 minutes of moderate-intensity physical activity per week.

While there is no specific recommended duration for muscle strengthening, it is important to perform muscle-strengthening exercises to the point where completing another repetition would be challenging. When using resistance training to improve muscle strength, one set for each exercise is effective, although 2 to 3 sets may be more effective. In general, 2 to 4 sets per major muscle group are recommended, although the total sets per muscle group can be from one exercise or multiple exercises. Approximately 1-minute rest intervals should be applied between sets; however, this time frame may vary according to the muscle groups used and client recovery. Importantly, resistance training to failure is not recommended for beginners, deconditioned individuals, and older adults with overweight or obesity and comorbidity. Also, 1 to 2 sets per exercise is enough training volume for these particular populations.

T: Type (Mode)

The type principle involves choosing the type or mode of exercise that aligns with one's goals and preferences. Exercise modalities include running, swimming, cycling, weightlifting, yoga, and many more. Selecting the appropriate type ensures that an individual enjoys their workouts and that the workouts are catered to the person's specific fitness objectives.

Aerobic exercise, performed in either a continuous or intermittent manner and involving major muscle groups, is recommended for most adults. Fully or partially weight-bearing modalities are recommended, including walking, cycling, aquatic activities, and slow dancing. These require minimal skill or fitness to perform and engage major muscle groups.

A wide variety of resistance training equipment can effectively improve muscular fitness, including free weights (e.g., barbells and dumbbells), machines (e.g., weight-stack and plate-loaded), resistance bands or tubing, and one's own body weight. Resistance training regimens can consist of (1) multijoint exercises targeting multiple muscle groups (e.g., bench press, push-ups, pull-ups, squats, lunges, and deadlifts) and (2) single-joint exercises focusing on individual muscle groups (e.g., biceps curls, triceps extensions, leg extensions, and leg curls). Multijoint exercises are primarily recommended because they target multiple muscles in less time, enhance intermuscular coordination, and may promote greater functional gains and caloric expenditure compared to single-joint exercises (Paoli et al. 2017). However, equipment selection is based on the client's ability, experience, body size, comfort, and preference.

Exercise Recommendations

For weight loss and prevention of weight regain, exercise recommendations and prescriptions vary (Donnelly et al. 2009).

- To prevent weight regain, engaging in 150 to 250 minutes of physical activity per week can help prevent weight gain exceeding 3% in most adults.
- There is a dose–response relationship between exercise and weight loss: 150 minutes per week promotes minimal weight loss, while more than 150 minutes per week results in a modest weight loss of approximately 4 to 7 lb (2-3 kg) when following a consistent program of aerobic-based activities with no diet changes for 12 consecutive months. Engaging in 225 to 420 minutes per week can lead to weight loss of 11 to 17 lb (5-8 kg).
- Physical activity is essential for weight maintenance after weight loss. Some studies suggest that participating in at least 200 to 300 minutes of physical activity per week during weight maintenance can help reduce weight regain. However, direct evidence for the amount of physical activity required to prevent weight regain after weight loss is currently lacking.
- It is important to note that resistance training itself does not typically result in clinically significant weight loss. However, resistance exercise can enhance muscular strength and physical function in individuals with overweight or obesity. Furthermore, participating in resistance exercise may offer additional health benefits, including improvements in risk factors for cardiovascular disease, diabetes, and other chronic diseases.

Designing a Program

Before prescribing client-centered exercise programs, exercise professionals should carefully consider the health-related physical fitness assessment results of each individual (see chapter 6). Such a strategy will guide exercise programming safely and effectively, because the information collected from these field tests and the client's medical and exercise background provide the exercise professional with individual data about health and fitness status. In other words, program design will be easier and more effective if exercise professionals respect the assessment outcomes, aiming to create and customize personalized workout plans and set goals that are SMART—specific, measurable, attainable, realistic, and timely (see chapter 4) (Feito and Magal 2022; Liguori et al. 2022).

Special Safety and Training Considerations

Considering that people with overweight or obesity often have poor functional capacity and common musculoskeletal health disorders (Pataky et al. 2014), exercise professionals should be equipped to address several physical limitations in a gym setting. These physical limitations play a critical role in exercise programming because it may be challenging to prescribe pain-free and feasible cardiorespiratory and muscle-

Exercise and Bariatric Surgery

Despite a rise in bariatric surgeries being performed worldwide, no specific exercise prescription guidelines for people with overweight or obesity have been published (Petering and Webb 2009). Thus, further research is warranted. The scientific field needs more high-quality studies investigating the dose–response relationship between exercise and health-related effects in this population (Baena-Raya et al. 2024). Importantly, among individuals with severe obesity, bariatric surgery has been reported as an effective solution for improvements in body composition but not in physical function compared to a long-term, multicomponent exercise program (Gilyana et al. 2024).

Summary of Current Evidence

Considering recent evidence, the role of exercise in patients after bariatric surgery is summarized as follows (Bellicha et al. 2021; Coen et al. 2018):

- Exercise may be a feasible and clinically effective adjunct treatment option.
- Exercise may also be a critical factor for long-term weight loss maintenance.
- Exercise may help patients manage some of their existing comorbidities (e.g., insulin resistance, type 2 diabetes, raised blood pressure, and dyslipidemia).
- Exercise improves all physical fitness components, enhancing functional capacity and health-related quality of life.
- Exercise promotes small additional weight and fat loss.
- Exercise helps prevent weight regain and supports bone metabolism.

Special Considerations and Precautions

Exercise professionals working with patients after bariatric surgery in various exercise settings should be familiar with the following special considerations and precautions, aiming to supervise and instruct their clients accordingly. However, the recommended activity guidelines for this patient population have not yet been determined (Livhits et al. 2010; Ren et al. 2018).

Exercise During the First 2 to 8 Weeks

- Most patients can begin an exercise regimen between 2 and 6 weeks after surgery; however, it is critically important to be medically cleared by their bariatric surgeon before starting a moderate to vigorous exercise program.
- Patients can engage in regular muscle-strengthening activities no sooner than 6 to 8 weeks after bariatric surgery. This time frame would be longer (3-6 mo) for those who seek to perform trunk flexion or extension exercises.
- If patients had gastric bypass surgery as an open operation with one large incision, they need longer recovery and healing time before safely performing resistance training, including abdominal exercises.
- In the first 2 to 4 weeks after surgery, it is recommended to start with a small amount of movement, aiming to gradually increase physical activity levels, because these patients are likely to be sore and uncomfortable immediately after surgery. In particular, a simple walking program lasting 5 to 10 minutes

a few times a day appears to be a safe, tolerable, and effective approach that supports the patient's recovery.

- Swimming, water fitness activities, or biking can be used as suitable and effective exercise options for inducing gradual increases in physical activity through short aerobic activities lasting 15 to 30 minutes 3 to 5 days a week.

- Muscle-strengthening activities also can be added once or twice per week; however, heavy lifting (more than 10-15 lb [5-7 kg]) should be avoided for the first 6 to 8 weeks after surgery.

- Balance training and unilateral lower-body resistance exercises, such as single-leg squats, single-leg deadlifts, static and dynamic lunges, and single-leg step-ups, should be avoided in the first 6 months after surgery, because changes to the body's center of balance due to rapid weight loss may adversely affect the patient's stability.

Exercise After the First 3 to 6 Months Following Bariatric Surgery

- Overheating during exercise is common among clients who have undergone bariatric surgery; excess fat mass and a limited ability to consume fluids are critical factors. Therefore, exercising in a cool, climate-controlled environment appears to be the ideal initial scenario.

- After the first 3 to 6 months, patients can implement structured exercise programs in a gym setting. They may not be comfortable fitting into various aerobic and resistance stationary machines due to their large body size. Thus, free weights may be a better option. In terms of aerobic training modalities, recumbent bikes are often a good choice because of the large seats.

- In a supervised exercise setting, training programs with low volume and low intensity should be implemented no sooner than 3 to 6 months after bariatric surgery. This is important, because these patients typically present with low energy levels, rapid loss of lean body mass, reduced balance, and fatigue due to a very low-calorie diet.

- After the 6-month mark, patients are encouraged to gradually increase both exercise volume and intensity, aiming for 30 to 45 minutes of aerobic exercise at least 4 days a week and resistance training at least twice a week.

strengthening exercises. This is critically important and seems to be one of the greatest barriers exercise professionals working with these populations are called to overcome. In brief, the excess weight may affect the following (Jeong et al. 2018; Pataky et al. 2014; Sabharwal and Root 2012; Wearing et al. 2006):

- Joint range of motion
- Ability to fit into machines
- Ability to get up from the floor
- Ability to stand up from a seated position
- Full range of motion to bend over
- Ability to move around the gym quickly and easily

Training Limitations

More specifically, when designing workout routines for individuals with excess weight, the following limitations may exist and should be taken into account to ensure safety, comfort, and effectiveness. Exercise professionals should try not to make assumptions or stereotype what their clients may be able to do and not do for any exercise. The following are some specific exercise programming considerations for clients with overweight or obesity.

Aerobic Training Limitations

- *Joint stress:* Increased body weight can lead to greater stress on weight-bearing joints, such as the knees, hips, and ankles, which can cause pain or discomfort during high-impact activities (e.g., running or jumping). Thus, to reduce joint stress, opt for low-impact aerobic exercises, such as swimming, cycling, or using an elliptical machine.

- *Balance and stability:* A larger body mass can affect the center of gravity, making it more difficult to maintain balance during certain movements and increasing the risk of falls during activities that require coordination.

- *Endurance:* Individuals may have lower cardiovascular endurance, which can make sustained aerobic activity challenging. They may tire more quickly and require more frequent breaks.

- *Heat regulation:* Excess body fat may cause individuals to overheat quickly during exercise, leading to discomfort and potential risk of heat-related illnesses. Hence, the implementation of measures to manage overheating, such as exercising in a cool environment, using fans, and staying hydrated, is highly recommended.

- *Equipment size and fit:* Standard exercise equipment may not accommodate larger body sizes comfortably or safely, which can limit the types of aerobic exercise that can be performed.

Resistance Training Limitations

- *Machine accessibility:* Weight machines often are not designed for larger bodies. They may have restrictive seats and pads that can make it difficult for clients with overweight or obesity to perform exercises correctly or comfortably. In addition, gyms often put pieces of weight equipment close together, and clients with a larger body size may not be able to walk in between them. Thus, equipment alternatives should be used. Select cardio equipment designed for larger bodies or adapt exercises that do not rely on traditional gym equipment. Exercise professionals should also implement free weights, resistance bands, or bodyweight exercises that can be performed in a seated or standing position with support, and they should modify movements to accommodate a limited range of motion.

- *Range of motion:* Excess body fat, particularly around the abdomen, can restrict the range of motion. For instance, bending over for a deadlift or squat may be difficult, and abdominal fat can restrict deep breathing when bending forward.

- *Core strength:* Core muscles of clients with overweight or obesity may be weaker, which can affect their ability to perform exercises that require a strong core, such as certain weightlifting movements or compound exercises.

Flexibility and Mobility Training Limitations

- *Modifications*: Reduced flexibility affects the ability to perform exercises through a full range of motion. Modifications may be needed.

- *Posture and alignment:* Maintaining proper posture and spinal alignment during weight training can be more challenging for clients with excess weight, but it is essential for preventing injury and ensuring that the correct muscles are being engaged.

Obesity-related physical limitations make the program design process more difficult and can adversely affect health-related quality of life among people living with excess weight (Warburton et al. 2001). By understanding and addressing these specific limitations, exercise professionals can design programs tailored to meet the needs of individuals with overweight or obesity while promoting inclusivity and encouraging a positive exercise experience. Coaching and exercise programming are not only about physiological adaptations but also psychological ones. It can be very challenging for exercise professionals to create client success stories if they just translate science into application without considering the psychosocial component included in a multifaceted exercise approach for clients with overweight or obesity.

Exercise Engagement Strategies

According to a global obesity consensus statement (European Association for the Study of Obesity 2023), obesity is a complex, multifactorial, relapsing chronic disease that requires a highly comprehensive, individualized treatment approach. Thus, multifaceted obesity treatment, including the exercise component, is not just about weight loss. Obesity care is about health, not weight; therefore, positive exercise experiences promoting health at every size and spreading the word that there is no one-size-fits-all exercise solution for populations with excess weight should be high priorities for the health and fitness industry. Taking this into account, exercise professionals working with previously inactive clients who have overweight or obesity should consider applying the following three key strategies, aiming to respect the aforementioned physical limitations and enhance exercise engagement.

1. Apply a realistic process.
   - Start slowly, introducing basic and simple drills.
   - In the first days or even weeks, avoid exercises that may cause extreme soreness and exhaustion.
   - Build client confidence and self-efficacy and create a positive exercise experience from the beginning.
   - Do not focus on perfection. Just inspire your client to be more active on a daily basis.

2. Implement recreational sessions.
   - Avoid painful, boring, or exhausting exercise experiences, especially during the first days, weeks, or even months.
   - Apply fitness games and partner exercises while keeping the sessions varied and simple.

- Apply exercises based on activities of daily living, focusing on fundamental movement patterns.

3. Set priorities.

   - Use elevated or modified versions of foundational exercises.
   - Limit the use of static stretching, foam rolling, or balance drills.
   - Avoid uncomfortable abdominal and back exercises (i.e., crunches, reverse crunches, and back extensions).
   - Minimize traditional warm-up drills.
   - Avoid plyometrics, explosive exercises, and ballistic movements.
   - Design hybrid routines that combine cardiorespiratory and muscle-strengthening activities.
   - Choose cardio and weight machines that are comfortable for clients with respect to their body size.

Exercise Snacks

According to the World Health Organization and its current guidelines on physical activity and sedentary behavior, every step counts; therefore, any amount of physical movement daily has value compared to inactivity (Bull et al. 2020; Piercy et al. 2018). Thus, it is critically important for people with excess weight to understand the real value of any kind of physical activity. In 2007, Dr. Howard Hartley coined the term *exercise snacks*, which he defined as brief periods of vigorous-intensity bodily movement or exercise that typically last for no more than 2 minutes (Hartley 2007). This is a quick and easy way to get moving without requiring equipment or going to a gym and is something that your clients can and should do in their daily life.

In 2014, the first peer-reviewed study investigating the effect of short, intermittent bouts of vigorous walking on glucose metabolism among people with prediabetes was published (Francois et al. 2014). In particular, movement or exercise snacks appear to be a vital approach for cardiometabolic health improvements, even without weight loss (Islam et al. 2022). Also, such short activity breaks appear to be effective for enhancing various well-being indicators, such as vigor and fatigue, as well as cognitive function, especially when the exercise break is more extended (Albulescu et al. 2022). Evidence regarding benefits of short bouts of physical activity is valuable because such micro-breaks can help previously inactive clients with excess weight break up their sedentary behavior and engage in regular bodily movement through small daily doses at a self-determined pace and intensity (Moore et al. 2022).

Benefits of Exercise Snacks

Incorporating short bouts of movement throughout the day is a critical strategy commonly ignored by clients with excess weight and by exercise professionals when designing personalized exercise programs and behavior-change strategies. Considering that individuals with overweight or obesity likely have insufficient physical activity levels (Gray et al. 2018), movement or exercise snacks could be a clever and efficient concept for increasing physical activity levels in an efficient, user-friendly way. This is important because adults with overweight or obesity tend to have low adherence and high dropout rates when engaging in traditional cardiorespiratory fitness activities (Burgess et al. 2017). One of the biggest mistakes exercise professionals make when designing training programs for clients with excess weight is an exclusive focus on weight loss, which is a long-term goal, without considering the process. In other words, many exercise professionals emphasize the destination without paying attention to the journey to get there.

Taking this into account, exercise professionals should find ways to regularly engage clients who have excess weight in physical movement anywhere they spend time throughout the day, not only in a structured exercise program in a gym setting. Considering that only one in five of those who try to lose weight succeed in maintaining a 10% loss for at least a year (Wing and Phelan 2005), it is clear that the primary goal is not rapid weight loss. Instead, gradual weight loss and long-term weight loss maintenance seem to be the optimal goals for these clients since weight regain is common after losing weight, especially for individuals with low physical activity levels, regardless of their current body weight (Wing and Phelan 2005). Hence, increased physical activity appears to be a key factor in successful long-term weight loss (Soini et al. 2015). However, emerging evidence shows that although exercise snacks can improve cardiorespiratory fitness, they do not improve maximum fat oxidation in healthy, young, inactive adults with healthy body weight (Yin et al. 2024). This observation may indicate an adjunct role of exercise snacking in weight loss while underlining the need for further research in this area, with a focus on people with overweight or obesity.

When to Use Exercise Snacks

Emerging research shows that exercise snacks with greater intensity but that are still well-tolerated provide better results concerning cardiorespiratory fitness and neuromuscular performance in inactive adults. In general, this strategy involves 15 to 30 seconds of vigorous activity (rating of perceived exertion of 6-7 classified as a somewhat hard to hard effort on a scale of 1-10), such as from cycling or stair climbing, three times per day. However, these brief daily movement sessions are not meant to replace structured exercise sessions supervised by qualified exercise professionals. The primary role of exercise snacks is to complement client-centered exercise programming, aiming to engage clients with excess weight in efficient regular bodily movement. In other words, supervised exercise is about being physically active in various fitness settings to achieve health and fitness goals, whereas movement snacks are about opposing sedentarism and improving the client's health in daily settings, such as at home or at work (Islam et al. 2022).

Tips for Using Exercise Snacks

Given that any movement is better than no movement, exercise professionals should try to inspire their clients with excess weight to be more active every day. Clients can be advised to try the following options, each resulting in 10 to 15 total minutes of activity (Fountaine 2023):

- Set reminders on their smartphone to interrupt sedentary behavior and break up sitting time with 1 to 2 minutes of light- to moderate-intensity walking once every 20 to 30 minutes.
- Walk in place at a moderate pace during TV commercials. This is a clever strategy for breaking up prolonged sitting as an exercise snack at home.
- Store healthy snacks and their water bottle away from their desk (i.e., on a separate floor or in the farthest room on the same floor) so that they have to climb a flight of stairs or walk each time they want to eat or drink something.

- Spend a few minutes on a movement snack before their lunch break, using foundational bodyweight exercises such as chair squats, incline push-ups, chair dips, supported static lunges, an incline plank, or seated or standing marching.
- Plan short walks with a colleague outside the office before or after their work schedule.
- Use lightweight, portable muscle-strengthening equipment (e.g., a set of dumbbells, a medicine ball, or a stability ball) two or three times per day, if they have access to a home or office gym.
- Walk to a local coffee shop located at least one block away from the office or house each morning.

The Fitness Fun Concept

Weight loss and weight loss maintenance are complex endeavors influenced by a variety of factors, including diet, physical activity, and behavioral changes. Traditional exercise regimens may be effective, but research suggests that unique and enjoyable workouts can enhance adherence to and effectiveness of a weight management program (Blair 1993; Freedman et al. 2001). Incorporating unique and enjoyable workouts into weight management regimens has several science-backed benefits, ranging from enhanced adherence to optimized caloric expenditure and psychological well-being. These workouts can involve fitness games, friendly competition, partner exercises, and dance fitness activities that make the exercise experience more enjoyable and entertaining for clients with excess weight (see chapters 7, 8, and 10). Such a strategy promotes inclusion and body positivity while inducing meaningful improvements in overall well-being, both physically and mentally (Blair 1993; Foreyt and Goodrick 1993; Freedman et al. 2001).

Enhanced Adherence Rates

Adherence to a regular exercise regimen is a significant predictor of weight loss success (Blair 1993). Studies indicate that enjoying exercise increases adherence rates (Foreyt and Goodrick 1993; Freedman et al. 2001). Unique and fun workouts can transform exercise from an obligatory task into an enjoyable activity, thereby improving long-term adherence. The psychology behind this is rooted in the principle of positive reinforcement; when an activity is enjoyable, individuals are more likely to repeat it, thereby forming a habit (Foreyt and Goodrick 1993).

Optimized Caloric Expenditure

Engaging in a variety of physical activities can optimize caloric expenditure, crucial for creating a caloric deficit (Blair 1993; Freedman et al. 2001). This aligns with the fundamental principle behind weight loss: reducing caloric intake while increasing physical activity. Varied workouts can also prevent physiological adaptation, thereby maintaining a higher level of caloric burn over time (Blair 1993).

Psychological Well-Being

The psychological benefits of enjoyable physical activities extend beyond mere mood enhancement. Research shows that exercise can act as an adjunct treatment for conditions such as depression and anxiety, which are often barriers to weight loss. Also, the endorphins released during physical activity serve as a natural mood booster, further enhancing the likelihood of adherence (Foreyt and Goodrick 1993).

Multicomponent Workout Structure

Given that lack of time has been reported as the primary exercise barrier among adults (Salmon et al. 2003; Trost et al. 2002), clients with excess weight seeking either personal training services or a gym membership may be struggling to reserve time for separate aerobic or resistance training sessions each week with the aim of meeting exercise recommendations. Hence, multicomponent workouts that include aerobic, resistance, and neuromotor training in one session have value for people with overweight or obesity. It is critical to design multicomponent workouts for these populations, promoting all fitness parameters and integrating several modalities simultaneously into a session lasting no more than 60 minutes in various exercise settings (e.g., gym, studio, and home). The suggested basic workout structure in table 12.1 provides a general and applicable concept for designing a supervised session for clients with excess weight.

Table 12.1 Basic, Multicomponent Workout Structure

Phase	Modality	Time, min
Warm-up (chapter 7)	Cardiopulmonary load	3-5
	Mobility	2-3
	Dynamic stretching	2-3
	Movement preparation	3-5
	Neuromuscular activation	2-3
	Total time	**15-20**
Conditioning (chapters 8-10)	Muscular training	10-15
	Neuromotor exercise	5-10
	Cardiorespiratory training	10-15
	Total time	**25-35**
Cool-down (chapter 11)	Mobility	2-3
	Self- or assisted myofascial release	2-3
	Static stretching	2-3
	Diaphragmatic breathing	1-2
	Total time	**5-10**

The suggested structure in table 12.1 is not a mandatory workout plan for all clients with overweight or obesity, because each client is unique and has specific goals and priorities. Any training phases included in a multicomponent exercise session may need modifying according to the individual's needs and abilities as well as to the exercise setting. On the other hand, if clients with excess weight have limited free time during the week to devote to improving their overall health and fitness through two to three supervised exercise sessions, a multicomponent workout structure can be a feasible, effective, and engaging solution. In fact, combined aerobic and resistance training has been documented as the optimal exercise mode for cardiometabolic health improvements in populations with overweight or obesity and without comorbidities (Al-Mhanna, Leão, et al. 2024; Batrakoulis, Jamurtas, Metsios, et al. 2022; Sorace et al. 2024) as well as an effective training modality for people with excess weight and various health complications (Al-Mhanna, Wan Ghazali, et al. 2024).

The Mixed Exercise Approach

The mixed exercise approach—incorporating muscle-strengthening, cardiorespiratory, mobility, and recovery activities into a single session supervised by a qualified exercise professional two to three times per week—seems to be the best scenario for most clients with excess weight. Small-group training sessions designed for people with overweight or obesity also may be an excellent exercise solution that customizes the prescribed exercises, modifies the FITT principles, and creates an engaging environment among individuals with similar psychophysiological profiles. Such an approach aims to apply scientific guidelines to real-life practice, integrating various components of physical fitness into one workout routine in an efficient and pleasant fashion. This exercise solution also leaves space in clients' schedules for daily exercise snacks and for self-paced aerobic activities on other days of the week.

Exercise for weight loss in small-group training sessions has been reported as a popular trend in the health and fitness industry (Newsome et al. 2024). Small-group training can take place indoors (e.g., at a health club or fitness studio) or outdoors (e.g., in a park or field). It provides clients with the possibility of sharing the cost of an exercise session, making it a more affordable option compared to one-on-one training. Small-group training sessions are also attractive to exercise professionals, because they are reasonably profitable compared to personal training sessions. Additionally, small-group training sessions designed for clients with excess weight may be more engaging than private sessions because of the additional benefits of social connections and companionship. Working out with people who have similar needs, abilities, and goals for health and fitness provides powerful social benefits, which can be critically important for exercise engagement. Clients with overweight or obesity may feel more confident if they exercise with other people who have similar anthropometric characteristics, physical fitness levels, and performance goals (Wayment and McDonald 2017). It has also been reported that individuals feel more motivated to continue being physically active in various fitness settings when they have the opportunity to select what exercise modes they use during a workout and when they feel connected to others (Teixeira et al. 2012).

A mixed exercise approach can also be used in home-based workouts, using the client's body weight as resistance along with portable fitness equipment (e.g., light dumbbells, bands or tubing, medicine balls, suspension exercise devices, foam rollers, and weight sticks). This may be an attractive, simple, and effective solution for clients with overweight or obesity who work from home or do not have access to or time to attend a fitness club. Home exercise gyms were reported to be significantly popular during the COVID-19 pandemic (Kercher et al. 2022) and appear to be a flexible fitness scenario for individuals with excess weight who prefer their privacy.

The Cardioresistance Exercise Concept

A mixed exercise approach is a comprehensive, feasible, safe, effective, and pleasant training option for many clients who have excess weight, with or without obesity-related complications. Exercise professionals may also consider going one step further in terms of program design by using cardioresistance training, which also appears to be an effective exercise approach for this population. Cardioresistance training combines cardiorespiratory and musculoskeletal fitness stimuli into the same session, rotating aerobic and resistance-based exercises in a hybrid format without recovery periods in between. Such a session structure provides clients with both cardiovascular and neuromuscular improvements through an exercise experience that they may find to be more engaging than traditional combined (i.e., concurrent) aerobic and resistance training (American College of Sports Medicine 2009). A sample conditioning phase of a cardioresistance training program tailored for beginners with overweight or obesity is shown in table 12.2.

Table 12.2   Sample Beginner Cardioresistance Training Program

Exercise	Intensity	Time or volume
AEROBIC ACTIVITY		
Stationary cycling	55%-70% of HRmax (RPE of 11-14; light to moderate effort)	3-5 min
Treadmill walking	55%-70% of HRmax (RPE of 11-14; light to moderate effort)	3-5 min
Elliptical training	55%-70% of HRmax (RPE of 11-14; light to moderate effort)	3-5 min
RESISTANCE-BASED ACTIVITY		
2-3 lower-body exercises (e.g., knee-dominant, hip-dominant, and single-leg variations)	40%-60% of 1-RM with at least 2-3 reps in reserve	1 set of 12-15 reps per exercise; 1-min rest between sets
2-3 upper-body exercises (e.g., pushing and pulling variations)	40%-60% of 1-RM with at least 2-3 reps in reserve	1 set of 12-15 reps per exercise; 1-min rest between sets
2-3 core exercises (anteflexion or extension, anti–lateral flexion, and antirotation variations)	N/A	1 set of 12-15 reps per exercise; 1-min rest between sets

Note: 1-RM = 1-repetition maximum; HRmax = maximum heart rate; N/A = not applicable; RPE = rating of perceived exertion.

As the client progresses, the exercise volume and intensity of the cardioresistance training program should be increased to induce greater gains in cardiorespiratory and muscular fitness while avoiding a training plateau, boredom, and monotony, resulting in reduced psychophysiological adaptations (American College of Sports 2009).

The Pain-Free Concept

Pain has been documented as a major exercise barrier for sedentary individuals with overweight or obesity when engaging in structured fitness programs or trying to elevate their physical activity levels. In particular, exercise-induced hyperalgesia (increased sensitivity to pain) promotes inappropriate beliefs, fear, and avoidance, resulting in reduced exercise tolerance (Raja et al. 2020). Assisted and modified movements can help exercise professionals prescribe pain-free exercises in a gym setting, aiming to build self-confidence, create positive exercise experiences, teach appropriate posture, and enhance injury prevention.

Prescribing Pain-Free Exercises

Many exercise professionals believe that every client should incorporate certain top-tier exercises into fitness programming without any progressions or modifications of these particular movements. One of the most common mistakes fitness professionals make in exercise selection is that they try to fit their clients into a program with specific, must-do exercises. Instead, they should do exactly the opposite and fit exercises to their clients. When working with individuals who have excess weight, exercise professionals should know how to address the following three scenarios concerning proper, pain-free exercise selection.

Scenario 1

- *Observation:* An exercise increases pain and movement limitations.
- *Action:* Avoid, or apply a modification (regression) to, the prescribed exercise.

Scenario 2

- *Observation:* The client feels safe, but the execution of the exercise needs some improvement.
- *Action:* Focus on the quality of the movement without adding resistance.

Scenario 3

- *Observation:* The client feels good, and the execution is acceptable.
- *Action:* Train the movement pattern with progressive overload.

Flexibility and Mobility

Flexibility and mobility exercises should be included in both the warm-up and cool-down phases of a workout (see chapters 7 and 11). These exercises are critically important for sedentary clients with excess weight, who may have a limited range of motion in most or all joints as well as musculoskeletal health disorders (Sabharwal and Root 2012; Wearing et al. 2006). In general, flexibility or mobility exercises should be performed at least two to three days a week. For sedentary adults and older adults with overweight or obesity, these exercises can be performed daily to enhance critical aspects of musculoskeletal fitness, commonly defined as one of the weak links in the fitness profile of clients with overweight or obesity (Pataky et al. 2014; Sabharwal and Root 2012).

In particular, static, dynamic, or proprioceptive neuromuscular facilitation (PNF) stretches are recommended, targeting all major muscle–tendon groups. For static stretches, the volume should be 1 or 2 sets (15-60 s per stretch) for each muscle group, while PNF stretches should use a 6-second isometric contraction, followed by a 10- to 30-second passive stretch.

Partner-assisted or self-myofascial release also can be applied, although with caution, given that clients with overweight or obesity may find this technique somewhat painful and uncomfortable. Exercise professionals should consider the positive and negative points in each client's case and act accordingly, since foam rolling is a proven method for promoting mobility and recovery in various populations (Wiewelhove et al. 2019). Specifically, foam rolling increases blood flow, which is a positive technique to massage tight, overactive, stiff, and sore muscles either during the warm-up (for greater mobility and neuromuscular performance) or the cool-down (for greater flexibility and recovery). Typically, 1 or 2 sets of foam rolling (20-30 s per set) should be used on a particular muscle group to be a feasible and tolerant stimulus for individuals with excess weight.

Neuromotor Fitness

Neuromotor exercise is an important component of a workout tailored for clients with excess weight, because this population is likely to have poor functional capacity (Pataky et al. 2014), which adversely affects activities of daily living and health-related quality of life (Sabharwal and Root 2012; Warburton et al. 2001). Neuromotor exercises should take place for 5 to 10 minutes at the beginning of the conditioning phase of a workout in order to ensure a fresh central nervous system before undertaking demanding tasks related to resistance training. Neuromotor exercises for people with overweight or obesity of all ages and fitness levels do not have to be technically and physically demanding. Instead, low-intensity, low-skill drills are suggested for enhancing agility, balance, coordination, gait, and proprioception among people with impaired motor skills and common physical limitations. Such an exercise approach teaches important technical basics that every physically inactive client with excess weight should know, aiming to achieve better functionality, physical independence, and injury prevention (Donnelly et al. 2009; Piercy et al. 2018; Warburton et al. 2001; Wearing et al. 2006).

How and When to Use Neuromotor Fitness Modalities

Exercises for improving neuromotor fitness should be performed two to three days a week. Postmenopausal women and older adults with excess weight should particularly emphasize functional fitness training since these populations are at higher risk of falls and of fall-related fractures due to their higher chance of developing osteopenia and osteoporosis. Neuromotor and functional exercises are crucial for independence and longevity, and therefore, these exercises should be a foundational piece of the exercise programming puzzle for older adults with overweight or obesity. Examples of locomotor movements aiming to enhance motor skills include foot and ankle work, high and low knees, zigzags, skipping in various directions, and using a speed ladder (see chapter 9). By practicing these movements, clients with excess weight will improve motor control, resulting in reduced risk of injury, while enhancing their motor efficacy in daily tasks. This short workout phase may act as an extension of the dynamic warm-up phase, promoting greater neuromuscular activation and greater exercise engagement in clients with overweight or obesity who have no training experience and impaired musculoskeletal fitness (Donnelly et al. 2009). In addition, specific tasks simulating activities of daily living, such as bending and lifting, getting up from the floor, carrying heavy things, loading and unloading the car, and torso rotation, should be regularly trained, aiming to induce improvements in functional abilities among individuals with excess weight (Pataky et al. 2014).

Mind–Body Fitness Modalities

Adapted mind–body fitness activities, such as Pilates, yoga, and tai chi, may be used as an adjunct exercise tool for promoting functional benefits among people with impaired functional capacity (Batrakoulis 2022c). Yoga, tai chi, and qi gong are mind–body practices combining physical movement with proper breathing patterns and mental awareness. Such meditative, movement-based activities have been reported as effective exercise solutions for people with overweight or obesity (Batrakoulis 2022a, 2022b). However, exercise professionals seeking to incorporate these mind–body fitness modalities, or components of them, into a client-centered exercise program must be qualified and learn how to tailor these alternative modalities for individuals with excess weight to avoid any inconvenience, discomfort, or injury (Batrakoulis 2022c).

Muscular Fitness

The influence of resistance training on metabolic health has been widely reported, underlining the importance of including muscle-strengthening activities in every weight management program (American College of Sports Medicine et al. 2021). Interestingly, even low- to moderate-intensity resistance exercise (50%-75% of the 1-RM) induces beneficial changes in muscle protein remodeling and mitochondrial oxidative capacity (Lopez et al. 2022) while lowering the risk of mortality (Shailendra et al. 2022). However, resistance training alone seems to be less effective than combined training, moderate-intensity continuous training (MICT), and high-intensity interval training (HIIT) for reducing visceral adipose tissue (Chen et al. 2024), although it appears superior to MICT for improving glycolipid metabolism in individuals with overweight or obesity (Strasser and Schobersberger 2011). Collectively, muscular fitness activities should be a critical piece of the exercise programming puzzle, playing an adjunct role in obesity treatment (Paluch et al. 2024).

From a program design standpoint, although the interference effect (i.e., a decrease in overall training effectiveness when endurance and strength training exercises are combined in a single workout) is not common in people working out with low to moderate volume and intensity, completing muscle-strengthening activities before cardiorespiratory ones not only avoids any significant interference but also ensures that less demanding tasks for the central nervous system are performed at the end of an exercise session. Thus, to optimize neuromuscular adaptations, resistance training should be performed at the beginning of a workout, because performing aerobic exercise first may compromise the quality and safety of subsequent resistance training (Fyfe et al. 2014).

To optimize muscular fitness, functional performance, and injury prevention, it is important to focus on mastering the following foundational movement patterns:

- Squat (bilateral and unilateral)
- Hinge (bilateral and unilateral)

- Lunge (static and dynamic)
- Push (horizontal, vertical, and diagonal)
- Pull (horizontal, vertical, and diagonal)
- Carry (three types of lever)
- Rotation (horizontal and diagonal)

Implementing Manual Resistance Training

Exercise professionals should carefully consider the following special instructions when designing personalized manual resistance training workouts for clients with excess weight (Baffour-Awuah, Pearson, Dieberg, and Smart 2023; Baffour-Awuah, Pearson, Dieberg, Wiles, et al. 2023; Lum and Barbosa 2019):

- Normal breathing patterns should be used while performing isometric holds to avoid a significant elevation in blood pressure. The Valsalva maneuver should be avoided.
- To ensure normal blood pressure levels and proper joint stability throughout the isometric holds, intensity should not exceed 70% of the maximum voluntary isometric contraction.
- The recommended duration to maintain isometric tension for a strengthening effect should range from 3 to 10 seconds per repetition.
- One exercise is recommended per major muscle group (i.e., chest, back, shoulders, triceps, biceps, quadriceps, hamstrings, and core).
- A total contraction time of 15 to 30 seconds per major muscle group is recommended to induce muscular adaptations.
- The total contraction time should be achieved by a given number of repetitions with a selected hold duration per repetition.
- The work-to-rest ratio should be gradually progressed from 1:2 to 1:1.
- Manual resistance should be used in combination with dynamic (also known as isotonic) exercises using concentric and eccentric contractions, aiming to provide optimal muscular fitness improvements.

The Holistic Core-Training Concept

Trunk flexion, lateral flexion, and extension should be avoided among individuals with excess weight, with regard to the poor functional capacity, physical limitations, and reduced mobility commonly observed in this population. Clients with overweight or obesity may feel embarrassed and uncomfortable while performing these particular movement patterns, and exercise professionals should pay attention to safety and training considerations when designing personalized core-training routines for these individuals. Muscle-strengthening core exercises should acknowledge the client's biomechanics and functionality and aim to provide pain-free, effective, and engaging fitness experiences in various supervised or unsupervised exercise settings.

Taking this into account, exercise professionals should not prescribe dynamic spinal flexion and extension exercises to clients with overweight or obesity, given that this population is likely to have common musculoskeletal disorders and postural instability (Pataky et al. 2014; Warburton et al. 2001; Wearing et al. 2006). Integrated core exercises promote greater muscle activation than isolation exercises while eliciting a complete core-training stimulus (Gottschall et al. 2013; Lee and McGill 2015). The resulting lumbar spine stability is associated with a lower risk of developing chronic back pain (Calatayud et al. 2019). However, a holistic core-training concept appears to be a suitable and effective strategy for inducing favorable changes in lumbar spine stability among individuals with excess weight. This training concept should incorporate the following movements into a multicomponent workout (see a sample workout in chapter 13):

- Antiflexion
- Antiextension
- Anti–lateral flexion
- Antirotation
- Rotation

In summary, a holistic core-training workout encompasses various antimotion static and dynamic core exercises performed in all planes of motion. This is important because multiplanar movements support a client's functionality in activities of daily living, resulting in improved health-related quality of life, injury prevention, and physical performance (Calatayud et al. 2019; Gottschall et al. 2013; Lee and McGill 2015).

Core-Training Mistakes

Exercise professionals should avoid the five most common mistakes in designing core-training programs for people with overweight or obesity:

1. Emphasizing only one pattern, movement, or position while underestimating others
2. Not emphasizing movement quality, safety, and functional performance
3. Overestimating the exercise intensity (loads are too heavy) and volume (there are too many sets and repetitions)
4. Underestimating the involvement of the core in other resistance training exercises
5. Implementing an extremely high volume of spot-reduction exercises to target fat loss in the abdominal region

Progressions and Modifications
of Fundamental Movement Patterns

The program design strategies presented in this part of the chapter with regard to progressions and modifications of fundamental movement patterns in resistance training combine the professional experience of this book's editor with established exercise prescription guidelines for individuals with overweight or obesity (American College of Sports Medicine 2009; American College of Sports Medicine et al. 2021; Donnelly et al. 2009). Particularly, once the client's performance fully meets four specific criteria, the exercise professional should consider implementing a progression without changing the prescribed movement pattern. Such a strategy helps clients with excess weight to gradually progress in more advanced muscle-strengthening exercises and obtain physiological and functional benefits through pain-free resistance training sessions. The four key criteria are as follows:

1. Acceptable form, ensuring safety and effectiveness
2. No pain throughout the movement, ensuring an injury-free experience and exercise engagement
3. Completion of at least 12 to 15 repetitions, ensuring muscular endurance adaptations
4. No muscle failure, ensuring low increases in acute inflammation markers and faster recovery

Considering the exercise recommendations presented in this chapter, linear and nonlinear (undulating) periodized resistance training appear to be effective program design approaches for improving muscular fitness in adults with overweight or obesity (Donnelly et al. 2009). These strategies are characterized by progressive overload and aim to provide a beneficial muscle-strengthening experience in a gym setting, acknowledging the health and fitness status of individuals with metabolic health impairments and respecting any potential physical limitations in this population (Batrakoulis, Jamurtas, and Fatouros 2022). Linear periodization can be used with clients of all fitness and training experience levels because it gradually increases the intensity and decreases the volume of a training program over a long period of time. On the other hand, undulating periodization may be more suitable for advanced clients because it involves frequent changes in training intensity and volume (American College of Sports Medicine 2009). From a workout-schedule perspective, two to three whole-body routines are preferred on a weekly basis; however, routines split between upper- and lower-body exercises can also be used, especially for intermediate and advanced clients able to engage in four sessions per week. Six-month linear and undulating (nonlinear) periodized resistance training plans tailored for people with overweight or obesity are provided in tables 12.3 and 12.4.

Table 12.3   Linear Periodized Resistance Training Plan

Period	Frequency, d/wk	Intensity, % 1-RM	Volume and rest time	Muscle groups used in fundamental movement patterns*	Equipment
Weeks 1-6	2-3	40-59	1-2 sets of 12-15 reps (6 exercises); 60 s of rest per set	Quadriceps, hamstrings, back, chest, shoulders, core	Weight machines, free weights, resistance bands, and body weight
Weeks 7-12	2-3	60-69	1-2 sets of 10-12 reps (8 exercises); 75 s of rest per set	Quadriceps, hamstrings, back, chest, shoulders, triceps, biceps, core	
Weeks 13-18	2-3	70-74	2-3 sets of 8-10 reps (8 exercises); 90 s of rest per set	Quadriceps, hamstrings, back, chest, shoulders, triceps, biceps, core	
Weeks 19-24	2-3	75-85	2-3 sets of 6-8 reps (10 exercises); 120 s of rest per set	Quadriceps, hamstrings, glutes, calves, back, chest, shoulders, triceps, biceps, core	

Note: 1-RM = 1-repetition maximum.
*Fundamental movement patterns include squats, hinges, lunges, pushes, pulls, carries, and rotations.

Table 12.4   Undulating (Nonlinear) Periodized Resistance Training Plan

Period	Frequency, d/wk	Intensity, % 1-RM	Volume and rest time	Muscle groups used in fundamental movement patterns*	Equipment
Weeks 1-6	Day 1 (Monday)	40-59	1-2 sets of 12-15 reps (6 exercises); 60 s of rest per set	Quadriceps, hamstrings, back, chest, shoulders, core	Weight machines, free weights, resistance bands, and body weight
Weeks 1-6	Day 2 (Wednesday)	60-69	1-2 sets of 10-12 reps (8 exercises); 75 s of rest per set	Quadriceps, hamstrings, back, chest, shoulders, triceps, biceps, core	
Weeks 1-6	Day 3 (Friday)	70-74	2-3 sets of 8-10 reps (8 exercises); 90 s of rest per set	Quadriceps, hamstrings, back, chest, shoulders, triceps, biceps, core	
Weeks 1-6	Day 4 (Monday)	75-85	2-3 sets of 6-8 reps (10 exercises); 120 s of rest per set	Quadriceps, hamstrings, glutes, calves, back, chest, shoulders, triceps, biceps, core	

Note: 1-RM = 1-repetition maximum.
*Fundamental movement patterns include squats, hinges, lunges, pushes, pulls, carries, and rotations.

The Circuit Training Concept

Circuit weight training may promote positive changes in cardiorespiratory fitness, even without adding aerobic-based stations (Gotshalk et al. 2004). Such a training program encompasses a group of resistance training exercises that are performed consecutively and target all major muscle groups. In circuit weight training, the exercise at each station is performed for either a specified number of repetitions or a set time before a short recovery interval; then the client moves on to the next exercise station. The round can be repeated multiple times (typically two to five), depending on the client's tolerance. Suggestions for designing a circuit training program for clients with overweight or obesity of any fitness level are shown in tables 12.5 through 12.7.

Table 12.5 Beginner Circuit Training Program

Structure	Frequency	Intensity	Volume and time	Exercise type	Rest
Lower body: compound • Squat • Hinge	2 weekly sessions on nonconsecutive days	40%-60% of 1-RM (RPE of 11-13: fairly light to somewhat hard)	8-12 reps (30-40 s) per exercise	4-5 compound (foundational lifts) and 2-3 isolation (for small muscle groups); 6-8 total	20-30 s per exercise for 2 rounds
Upper body: compound • Push • Pull Upper body: isolation • Triceps • Biceps					
Core • Anti–lateral flexion • Antiflexion or extension					

Note: 1-RM = one-repetition maximum; RPE = rating of perceived exertion.

Table 12.6 Intermediate Circuit Training Program

Structure	Frequency	Intensity	Volume and time	Exercise type	Rest
Lower body: compound • Squat • Hinge • Lunge	2-3 weekly sessions on nonconsecutive days	40%-60% of 1-RM (RPE of 13-15: somewhat hard to hard)	12-15 reps (40-50 s) per exercise	8-10 compound (foundational lifts)	10-20 s per exercise for 2-3 rounds
Upper body: compound, horizontal • Push • Pull Upper body: compound, vertical • Push • Pull					
Core • Antiflexion or extension • Anti–lateral flexion or antirotation • Rotation					

Note: 1-RM = one-repetition maximum; RPE = rating of perceived exertion.

Table 12.7   Advanced Circuit Training Program

Structure	Frequency	Intensity	Volume and time	Exercise type	Rest
Lower body: compound • Squat • Hinge • Lunge	3 weekly sessions on nonconsecutive days	40%-60% of 1-RM (RPE of 15-17: hard)	15-20 reps (50-60 s) per exercise	10-12 compound (foundational lifts)	0-10 s per exercise for 3 rounds
Upper body: compound, horizontal • Push • Pull Upper body: compound, vertical • Push • Pull Upper body: compound, vertical or horizontal • Push • Pull					
Core • Antiflexion or extension • Anti–lateral flexion or antirotation • Rotation					

Note: 1-RM = one-repetition maximum; RPE = rating of perceived exertion.

Cardiorespiratory Fitness

As part of a basic, multicomponent workout structure, aerobic training should be performed at the end of the conditioning phase. This program design strategy is supported by research findings indicating interference between concurrent resistance and endurance exercise, because these two types of training create competing influences at the molecular level (Fyfe et al. 2014). However, this phenomenon occurs most often in well-trained athletes undertaking high volumes of both training modalities rather than in general and clinical populations.

That said, the order of exercise types can be chosen based on a client's personal preferences and what keeps them engaged in structured, gym-based exercise because both training modalities are highly recommended for populations with excess weight (Donnelly et al. 2009). In a cardioresistance training program, however, this general guideline cannot be fully met. Therefore, the exercise intensity used in such nontraditional workouts is not ranged at high levels, because the exercise approach does not target optimum cardiovascular adaptations or neuromuscular adaptations alone through single-component (aerobic or resistance) or combined (aerobic and resistance) exercise sessions (American College of Sports Medicine 2009).

Continuous Training

People with overweight or obesity are likely to have an insufficient physical activity level and poor functionality capacity and may also have cardiometabolic complications. Therefore, a progressive, continuous aerobic training plan is highly recommended, providing these clients with an applicable and effective cardiorespiratory fitness solution. MICT has been widely reported as a feasible and safe exercise programming option for individuals with impaired metabolic health (Batrakoulis, Jamurtas, and Fatouros 2022). A 6-month, progressive aerobic training plan is provided in table 12.8.

Table 12.8 Progressive Aerobic Training Plan

Phase	Period	Frequency, d/wk	Intensity, %HRmax / RPE	Time, min/ session*	Type (nonimpact or low-impact)
1	Weeks 1-6	2-3	55-60 / 9-10	15-20	Treadmill walking
					Stationary cycling
2	Weeks 7-12	3-4	60-65 / 11-12	20-30	Stair climbing
					Elliptical training
					Stationary rowing
3	Weeks 13-18	4-5	65-70 / 12-13	30-45	Swimming
					Water-based exercise
4	Weeks 19-24	5-6	70-75 / 13-14	45-60	

Note: 1-RM = one-repetition maximum; HRmax = maximum heart rate; RPE = rating of perceived exertion.
*Gradually increase by 10% to 20% per week.

Interval Training

Once clients with excess weight have established a sufficient aerobic base after implementing a progressive aerobic plan, they can combine MICT and moderate-intensity interval training (MIIT) as well as HIIT. Such an approach helps clients gradually incorporate some vigorous-intensity work into a weekly routine (Batrakoulis et al. 2021). Various nonimpact or low-impact cardiorespiratory fitness activities are preferred, such as treadmill walking, stationary cycling, stair climbing, elliptical training, stationary rowing, swimming, or water-based exercise. Importantly, interval training does not have to be all-out to evoke significant improvements in body composition, physical fitness, and glucose control in adults with impaired metabolic health (Karstoft et al. 2013). Also, both HIIT and MICT significantly enhance maximum fat oxidation in adults with overweight or obesity (Yin et al. 2023), highlighting that there is no magic bullet in aerobic exercise with respect to substantial body-composition improvements. Interestingly, HIIT-type protocols are applicable for adults with insufficient physical activity and generally show lower attrition rates than are commonly reported for MICT programs (Reljic et al. 2019). These observations are important for exercise professionals working with beginners and previously inactive individuals with excess weight, because a proper program design strategy may provide these clients with the possibility of engaging in interval training smoothly and safely. Taking this into account, exercise professionals should pay more attention to MIIT, aiming to promote feasible, interval-type exercise experiences among clients with excess weight. A 6-month, progressive plan combining MICT, MIIT, and HIIT is shown in table 12.9.

Table 12.9 Progressive Combined Continuous and Interval Training Plan

Phase	Period	Mode	Frequency, d/wk	Intensity, %HRmax / RPE	Time*	
1	Weeks 1-6	MICT	3-5	55-69 / 11-13	20-60 min/session	150-300 min/wk
2	Weeks 7-12	MIIT	2-3	70-84 / 13-15	30-40 min/session	75-150 min/wk
3	Weeks 13-18	HIIT	1-2	≥85 / 15-16	15-25 min/session	15-50 min/wk
4	Weeks 19-24	HIIT	1-2	≥90 / 16-17	10-20 min/session	10-40 min/wk

Note: HIIT, high-intensity interval training; HRmax = maximum heart rate; MICT, moderate-intensity continuous training; MIIT, moderate-intensity interval training; RPE = rating of perceived exertion.
*Gradually increase by 10% to 20% per week.

Traditional and Hybrid Interval Training

In general, protocols based on intermittent exercise appear to have an effect on various cardiometabolic health-related indicators, including maximal aerobic capacity among populations with metabolic dysregulation (Cassidy et al. 2017; Sabag et al. 2022). Importantly, HIIT induces a similar or even greater increase in cardiorespiratory fitness compared with MICT while provoking favorable alterations in several cardiovascular disease risk factors commonly observed among physically inactive people with overweight or obesity (Batacan et al. 2017). Such positive adaptations occur more efficiently compared to MICT because HIIT requires 40% less of a weekly time commitment (Wewege et al. 2017). Thus, HIIT seems to be an attractive exercise solution in the health and fitness industry (Newsome et al. 2024).

As described in detail in chapter 10, intermittent-based workout routines, both traditional and hybrid-type, can be applied for improving cardiorespiratory fitness in individuals with overweight or obesity. Generally, HIIT-type protocols have been documented as a practicable, injury-free, effective, and pleasant exercise mode for populations with metabolic dysregulation, including for individuals with excess weight (Batrakoulis et al. 2021). Exercise professionals should consider implementing either traditional, single-component or hybrid-type, multicomponent interval training programs for clients with overweight or obesity in a gym setting, using the program design recommendations in tables 12.10 and 12.11.

Table 12.10 Traditional, Single-Component Interval Training Program

Phase	Training parameters	Modality
Warm-up	3 min at 55%-70% of HRmax (RPE of 9-11) plus dynamic stretching	Walking Running Stair climbing Elliptical Rowing Swimming
Conditioning	4-5 work intervals of 3-4 min at 85%-95% of HRmax (RPE of 15-16) 3-4 recovery intervals of 2-3 min at 60%-70% of HRmax (RPE of 11-13) Progression of work-to-rest ratios: • 0.75:1 (weeks 1-6) • 1:1 (weeks 7-12) • 1:0.75 (weeks 13-16)	
Cool-down	2 min at 50%-60% of HRmax, plus static stretching and foam rolling	

Note: HRmax = maximum heart rate; RPE = rating of perceived exertion.

Table 12.11   Hybrid-Type, Multicomponent Interval Training Program

Phase	Training parameters	Modality
Warm-up	5 min at 55%-70% of HRmax (RPE of 9-11) Movement preparation and dynamic stretching	Brisk walking
Conditioning	6-12 work intervals of 30-60 s (≥85% HRmax; RPE of 15-17) 5-11 recovery intervals of 30-60 s (passive) Volume: 2-3 rounds (2-3 min rest per round) Progression of work-to-rest ratios: • 1:3 (weeks 1-6) • 1:2 (weeks 7-12) • 1:1 (weeks 13-16)	Integrated neuromuscular exercises and locomotor movements*
Cool-down	2 min at 50%-60% HRmax, plus static stretching and foam rolling	Easy walking

Note: HRmax = maximum heart rate; RPE = rating of perceived exertion.

*Combined resistance-based exercises (e.g., bending, lifting, pushing, pulling, carrying, single-leg, and twist) and locomotor movements (e.g., low-knee skips, hops in place, jogging in place, jumping jacks, split jacks, ice skaters, mountain climbers, and burpees). Two exercises can also be combined into a single exercise (i.e., squat to overhead press or sumo deadlift high pull).

CHAPTER SUMMARY

This chapter touched on basic training principles—namely overload, specificity, and reversibility. It also discussed exercise prescription principles (frequency, intensity, time, and type) along with progression. In addition, components of a tailored workout and exercise engagement strategies were analyzed. Exercise recommendations, special considerations, and precautions for patients following bariatric surgery were presented. Feasible, effective, and safe multicomponent exercise programming solutions for clients with excess weight were also provided, including plans for muscular, neuromotor, and cardiorespiratory fitness activities.

KEY POINTS

- There are six key principles of exercise training—overload, reversibility, progression, individualization, periodization, and specificity.
- The FITT (frequency, intensity, time, and type) principles are fundamental components of exercise prescription and are used to design and modify exercise programs.
- A multicomponent exercise program is suggested for people with overweight or obesity to target various health and fitness aspects through pain-free, pleasant, and tailored exercise.
- Periodized resistance training plans should be applied, aiming to gradually manage long-term training parameters and achieve muscular fitness goals.
- Progressive MICT, MIIT, and HIIT should be adapted to the physiological and psychological profile of a client with excess weight, aiming to obtain cardiorespiratory fitness improvements.

CHAPTER QUIZ

Quiz answers can be found in the appendix.

1. Is medical clearance mandatory for inactive individuals with obesity and type 2 diabetes but without signs or symptoms of additional cardiovascular, pulmonary, or renal disease before participating in light- to moderate-intensity exercise programs?

   a. yes

   b. no

   c. it depends on the obesity-related comorbidities

   d. it depends on the client's age

2. Which of the following aerobic training options is the most appropriate for previously inactive clients with obesity during the first month?

   a. moderate-intensity continuous training 3 to 4 times per week at 70% to 85% of the HRmax

   b. high-intensity interval training 1 to 2 times per week

   c. moderate-intensity interval training 2 to 3 times per week

   d. moderate-intensity continuous training 3 to 4 times per week at 55% to 70% of the HRmax

3. Which of the following resistance training options is the most appropriate for previously inactive clients with obesity during the first month?

   a. compound lifts at 75% to 85% of the 1-RM

   b. bodyweight and dumbbell exercises, but not to muscle failure

   c. machine-based exercises: 3 sets of 8 repetitions to muscle failure

   d. isolation exercises at 40% to 50% of the 1-RM

4. Which of the following exercises may NOT be the most appropriate for clients with overweight or obesity due to their large body size?

   a. standing cable row

   b. diagonal leg press machine

   c. stepping up and down

   d. chair squat

5. Based on the physical limitations of a client with overweight or obesity, which of the following machine-based, muscle-strengthening exercises is the most appropriate?

   a. pec deck machine

   b. lying leg-curl or knee-curl machine

   c. seated abdominal machine

   d. standing high pulley cable row

6. Which of the following aerobic training modalities is the most feasible for clients with overweight or obesity?

   a. high-knee skipping

   b. treadmill walking

   c. stationary rowing

   d. treadmill running

7. Which of the following exercise engagement strategies is the most appropriate for inactive adults with overweight or obesity?

   a. Apply a gradual process and keep the workouts simple and fun.

   b. Gradually modify the fitness program and focus only on aerobic training.

   c. Gradually modify the fitness program and use only machine-based exercises.

   d. Apply a gradual process and focus only on resistance training.

8. For a client who has undergone bariatric surgery, what should the exercise volume and intensity be in a workout routine during the first 6 months after the operation?

   a. high volume and high intensity

   b. low volume and low intensity

   c. high volume and low intensity

   d. low volume and high intensity

9. Which of the following assessment methods for aerobic exercise intensity is NOT applicable when supervising a client with overweight or obesity who does not have obesity-related health conditions?

   a. heart rate monitoring
   b. rating of perceived exertion
   c. blood pressure monitoring
   d. talk test

10. Which of the following exercise training strategies may induce the most comprehensive health and fitness benefits in beginner clients with overweight or obesity?

    a. exercise (movement) snacks and HIIT
    b. resistance training and HIIT
    c. cardioresistance and flexibility or mobility training
    d. concurrent aerobic and resistance training

CASE STUDY

Case study answers can be found in the appendix.

Mary, a motivated, 60-year-old postmenopausal woman with a height of 5 ft 2 in. (158 cm), has obesity and physical limitations (osteoarthritis in the hip) that make exercise challenging. Over the past 7 years, she has gained 44 lb (20 kg) and is now the heaviest she has ever been in her life at 198 lb (90 kg). She is retired and has insufficient physical activity levels (<5,000 steps/d) on a regular basis. Before menopause and osteoarthritis, she was physically active, doing daily walks with friends, taking the stairs, and riding her bicycle several times per week. Currently, she misses her former health, fitness, physical independence, and functionality. Mary wants to control her weight, but more importantly, she seeks to return to her previously active lifestyle. She has been medically cleared and encouraged to participate in supervised exercise by her physician, with adjustments and caution regarding the pain linked to the hip osteoarthritis, which should be considered, but not feared, concerning activities of daily living and structured exercise. Mary has no other obesity-related complications; however, she demonstrates poor functional capacity and mobility in the lower extremities. She is interested in working with an exercise professional two to three times per week in a commercial gym setting while engaging in outdoor physical activity on the other days of the week.

1. What mode of training should Mary perform to meet her cardiorespiratory, muscular, and neuromotor and functional needs, priorities, and goals, from both a physiological and psychological perspective?

2. How would you design her aerobic and muscle-strengthening routine in terms of the number of exercises, volume, intensity, rest intervals, and type of equipment?

3. What type of physiological responses might Mary expect when performing a comprehensive exercise routine?

4. What should be a priority for Mary with respect to her health and fitness profile, especially regarding her behavior outside the gym? Suggest client-centered program design strategies.

5. Besides biological benefits, what psychological and mental benefits might Mary experience from a personalized exercise routine?

CHAPTER 13

Sample Workouts

After completing this chapter, you will be able to

- access progressive workout templates for various training goals, settings, and exercise modes;
- use each of the 21 workouts to help clients meet individual goals; and
- design diverse workouts in personal training, small group training, and group fitness formats.

The prevalence of obesity in the Western world is a significant public health concern, affecting a large proportion of the adult population. The provision of exercise training for individuals with obesity is a complex undertaking, requiring not only the expertise of fitness professionals but also a comprehensive understanding of the challenges associated with combating the twin epidemics of inactivity and obesity. This chapter provides 21 sample workouts to serve as a valuable resource for exercise professionals seeking to develop tailored training regimens for individuals with excess body weight or adiposity. The sample workouts encompass diverse training objectives, settings, and modalities and are accompanied by detailed insights into their implementation. Additionally, the chapter presents practical solutions for exercise professionals striving to create safe, feasible, effective, and enjoyable exercise experiences. An understanding of the sample workouts included in this chapter, together with an exploration of the numerous training concepts for clients with overweight or obesity, can assist exercise professionals in adopting proven practical examples of evidence-based training programs for their clients with excess weight. In particular, the following sample workouts are included:

Specific Populations

1. Training Clients With Obesity and Arthritis
2. Training Clients With Obesity and Lower-Extremity Joint Pain
3. Training Clients With Obesity and Chronic Low-Back Pain
4. Training Clients With Obesity and Osteoporosis
5. Training Clients With Obesity, Frailty, and Sarcopenia
6. Training Clients With Obesity and Postural Instability
7. Training Preadolescents With Obesity

Specific Training Modalities

1. Circuit Bodyweight Training
2. Dance Fitness
3. Progressive High-Intensity Functional Training for Experienced Clients
4. Hybrid-Type, Multicomponent Interval Training
5. Clinical High-Intensity Interval Training
6. Conventional High-Intensity Interval Training
7. Holistic Core Training
8. Progressive Resistance Training for Inexperienced Clients
9. Seated Core Foundation
10. Step Aerobics
11. Yoga

Specific Exercise Settings

1. Gym or Studio Full-Body Workout 1
2. Gym or Studio Full-Body Workout 2
3. At-Home Full-Body Workout

Training Clients With Obesity and Arthritis

Christine M. Conti, MEd

When working with a client who has overweight or obesity and one or more forms of arthritis, it is important to understand that arthritis is a condition that cannot be healed through exercise but can be managed through a safe and effective exercise program (Barrow et al. 2019). Fitness professionals who work with this demographic need to have a basic understanding of the various forms, causes, and symptoms of arthritis that affect the human body. Also, the strong link between hip or knee osteoarthritis and obesity should be carefully considered. Fortunately, regular, combined aerobic and strength training seems to be a protective strategy against osteoarthritis, resulting in positive changes in musculoskeletal and cardiorespiratory fitness as well as in body composition and metabolic health among people with obesity and osteoarthritis (Kraus et al. 2019).

Once the fitness professional understands the basic types and symptoms of arthritis, it is time to provide the client with a comprehensive client intake form. For example, very specific questions need to be addressed, such as the following:

1. Are you experiencing any stiffness, swelling, or pain in any joints?
2. Where is the exact location of your discomfort?
3. When do you feel most stiff? In the morning? After sitting? After exercise?
4. Are you currently taking any medications? Are you experiencing any side effects?

These answers will provide the foundation for creating a safe, effective, and progressive exercise program to best suit the needs of the client. Afterward, the fitness professional should conduct a full-body assessment to examine joint mobility and range of motion (ROM) before beginning any exercise regimen. The client should be led through the following movements as the trainer observes all major joints in the body and gains feedback regarding any pain, stiffness, or swelling. This initial assessment will provide a baseline for tracking any future improvements in joint mobility and motion.

Standing Full-Body Joint Assessment

1. Head and neck rolls
2. Shoulder rolls and shrugs
3. Hands to shoulders to overhead reach
4. Bear hug to open arms: spinal flexion to extension
5. Hip rotations and circles
6. Shallow squats
7. Alternating knee lifts
8. Single-leg standing alternating ankle rotations
9. Spreading fingers wide to making a fist and spreading toes wide to squeezing together
10. Wrist circles

This assessment also serves as the daily warm-up and cool-down for clients with obesity and arthritis. Because arthritis symptoms change daily, it is important to conduct a full-body assessment both before and after each exercise session. Ultimately, the goal is for clients to better understand and self-assess their bodies when they are not with the trainer.

Special Exercise Considerations

When working with clients with one or more forms of arthritis, it is important to understand that your prior knowledge of program design may not be safe for this demographic. For example, a client with arthritis should never have an arm day or a leg day that consists of using weights or movements targeting back-to-back opposing muscle groups. If the client has arthritis in their elbow, a biceps curl immediately followed by triceps kickback will overload the elbow joint. In addition, leg extensions followed by hamstring curls will put excess stress on an arthritic knee. The rule of thumb when designing an exercise program for clients with overweight or obesity and arthritis is the same for all clients with arthritis. If one exercise uses joints in the upper body, then the next exercise should target joints in the lower body. Imagine the body as having a top half and a lower half to create the most safe and effective programs for this demographic. Collectively, fitness professionals serving individuals who have both excess weight and arthritis should design a tailored, supervised, progressive, and pain-free training plan for these clients (Barrow et al. 2019; Kraus et al. 2019). See table 13.1 for a sample exercise program for joint care and table 13.2 for suggested mobility and muscle-strengthening exercises.

Table 13.1   Sample Exercise Programming for Joint Care

Training parameter	Cardiorespiratory fitness	Muscle strengthening	Flexibility
Frequency	3-5 d/wk	2-3 d/wk	3-5 d/wk
Intensity	50%-60% of HRmax RPE of 5-6 out of 10	RPE of 5-6 out of 10	Stretch without pain
Time	15-30 min/d (progressively increase to 150 min/wk through multiple shorter [10-15 min] daily bouts)	10-20 min/d	Dynamic stretching (warm-up): 5-10 reps per movement Static stretching (cool-down): 2-4 sets of 15-30 s per muscle group
Type	Full or partial weight-bearing exercise, including walking, aquatic activities, and biking	Multijoint exercises using bands, machines, or free weights for the upper body, lower body, and trunk	Combined dynamic and static stretching with a focus on muscles crossing affected joints

Note: HRmax = maximum heart rate; RPE = rating of perceived exertion scale (1-10).

Table 13.2   Suggested Mobility and Muscle-Strengthening Exercises

Movement pattern	Purpose	Sets/reps	Intermediate level	Advanced level
Ear-to-ear neck roll	Cervical spine mobility	1 set of 4-8 reps	—	—
Shoulder shrug	Shoulder and neck mobility	4-8 sets of 10 reps	Hold light hand weights	Use heavier weights and hold at the highest point for 3 s
Shoulder roll	Shoulder and neck mobility	1 set of 4-8 reps	Hold light hand weights or water bottles	Hold 10-20 lb (5-10 kg) hand weights
Front arm raise, lateral arm raise	Shoulder strength, mobility	2-3 sets of 8 reps	Hold light hand weights or water bottles	4-count raise and 4-count lower (hold light to medium weights)
Ball squeeze (tennis ball or small rubber ball)	Grip strength, forearm strength	3 sets of 30 s with each hand	Squeeze the ball for 3-4 breaths each rep	Squeeze the ball for 4 breaths while rotating wrists (palms up, then down)
Triceps kickback	Arm strength, stabilization of shoulder and elbow joints	3 sets of 8-10 reps or until form is compromised due to fatigue	Slow the movement backward and forward to 4 counts each	1. Increase weight and slow movement to 4 counts forward and back 2. Combine triceps kickback with a biceps curl

(continued)

Table 13.2 Suggested Mobility and Muscle-Strengthening Exercises *(continued)*

Movement pattern	Purpose	Sets/reps	Intermediate level	Advanced level
Supported body-weight squat or chair squat	Leg and hip strength, fall-risk reduction, functionality	3 sets of 8-10 reps (if the form becomes compromised, reduce reps)	Slow squat (3 counts down and up), body-weight only without an assist	Hold hand weights or a weighted bar for additional resistance and perform until reps are completed or form becomes compromised
Biceps curl	Arm strength, shoulder and elbow stabilization	3 sets of 8-10 reps or until form becomes compromised	Slow the movement up and down to 4 counts each	1. Increase weight and slow movement to 4 counts up and down 2. Advanced II: combine triceps kickback with a biceps curl*
Bodyweight forward lunge	Leg and hip strength, flexibility, mobility, functionality, fall-risk reduction	3 sets of 8 reps or until form becomes compromised	Add 1-2 pulses in each lunge position without any assistance	Hold hand weights or a bar for more resistance
Standing knee	Core strength	3 sets of 8-10 reps	Place hands behind the head to add an element of balance	Slow the movements to add longer muscle contraction and balance
Alternating bodyweight lateral lunges	Hip mobility, flexibility, and mobilization and stabilization of the lower body	3 sets of 10 reps	Add a pulse or slow the movement for longer muscle contractions	Use hand weights or a weighted bar for added resistance
Flex to extend and heel-to-toe raise	Foot and ankle mobility and stability	3 sets of 10 reps	Stand up and complete this exercise	Stand on a step with the heels hanging off the step; lower heels below the step

*Proceed with caution when training clients with elbow arthritis.

Circuit Bodyweight Training Workout for Clients With Overweight or Obesity

Alexios Batrakoulis, PhD

This section describes a circuit bodyweight training program designed to provide a progressive exercise approach for previously inactive clients with overweight or obesity in various settings (tables 13.3-13.5). This workout aims to increase cardiorespiratory and muscular fitness through a time-efficient routine incorporating only bodyweight exercises into a circuit-based session. Alternatively, the circuit training workout program may be performed with stationary weight machines, free weights, elastic resistance, calisthenics, or any combination of these. Circuit resistance training may induce favorable alterations in cardiovascular endurance, even without adding aerobic-based stations (Gotshalk et al. 2004). Specifically, this exercise approach includes muscle-strengthening exercises of all the major muscle groups, which are completed consecutively.

In this workout, each exercise is performed for a specified number of repetitions or for a set time, in seconds, before a brief rest. The client then moves on to the next exercise. The circuit can be repeated two to five times, depending on the client's physical fitness level (Klika and Jordan 2013).

Training Considerations

- Medical clearance to participate in vigorous-intensity circuit training is highly recommended for all clients with excess weight, regardless of their physical fitness level.

- All training parameters should be gradually progressed, with consideration of the client's physical fitness and overall health status.

Table 13.3   Beginner Circuit Bodyweight Training Workout

EXERCISES	
Body area	**Movement**
Lower body	Assisted squat
Upper body (push)	Incline push-up
Upper body (pull)	Close-grip inverted row
Core	Incline plank
TRAINING PARAMETERS	
Frequency	2 sessions per week on nonconsecutive days
Intensity	40%-60% of 1-RM; OMNI-RES of 3-4 out of 10
Time	8-12 reps (30-40 s) per exercise; rest of 20-30 s per exercise 2 rounds (3 min rest per round)
Type	4 bodyweight exercises

Note: 1-RM = 1-repetition maximum; OMNI-RES = OMNI resistance exercise scale of perceived exertion.

Table 13.4   Intermediate Circuit Bodyweight Training Workout

EXERCISES	
Body part	**Movement**
Lower body	Chair squat
Upper body (push)	Incline push-up
Upper body (pull)	Close-grip inverted row
Core	Incline plank
Lower body	Static lunge
Upper body (push)	Kneeling push-up
Upper body (pull)	Quadruped arm raise
Core	Modified side plank
TRAINING PARAMETERS	
Frequency	2-3 sessions per week on nonconsecutive days
Intensity	40%-60% of 1-RM; OMNI-RES of 5-6 out of 10
Time	12-15 reps (40-50 s) per exercise; rest of 10-20 s per exercise 2-3 rounds (2.5 min rest per round)
Type	8 bodyweight exercises

Note: 1-RM = 1-repetition maximum; OMNI-RES = OMNI resistance exercise scale of perceived exertion.

Table 13.5   Advanced Circuit Bodyweight Training Workout

EXERCISES	
Body part	**Movement**
Lower body	Bodyweight squat
Upper body (push)	Incline push-up
Upper body (pull)	Inverted row
Core	Incline plank
Lower body	Dynamic reverse lunge
Upper body (push)	Kneeling push-up
Upper body (pull)	Quadruped arm raise
Core	Modified side plank
Lower body	Bodyweight hip thrust
Upper body (push)	Incline close-grip push-up
Upper body (pull)	Wide-grip inverted row
Core	Bodyweight wood chop
TRAINING PARAMETERS	
Frequency	3 sessions per week on nonconsecutive days
Intensity	40%-60% of 1-RM; OMNI-RES of 7-8 out of 10
Time	15-20 reps (50-60 s) per exercise; rest of 0-10 s per exercise 3 rounds (2 min rest per round)
Type	12 bodyweight exercises

Note: 1-RM = 1-repetition maximum; OMNI-RES = OMNI resistance exercise scale of perceived exertion.

Dance Fitness Workout for Clients With Overweight or Obesity

Summer Sides

Designing a dance fitness workout tailored for individuals managing obesity requires a thoughtful approach that prioritizes safety, inclusivity, and enjoyment. By understanding the unique needs of this demographic, instructors can create a purposeful dance fitness class. The suggested sample workout (table 13.6) considers the following principles to craft a fun, inclusive, and well-rounded dance fitness class:

- *Joint-friendly movements:* Focus on low-impact maneuvers that place little stress on joints.
- *Simplicity and accessibility:* Make movements easy to follow so participants can enjoy the workout rather than struggle with intricate choreography.
- *Simplicity with dance flair:* Add arm, head, or hip movements without increasing complexity to maintain simplicity while increasing the intensity and fun.
- *Smooth transitions:* Design movement sequences that flow effortlessly from one to the next, reducing the risk of injury and confusion for participants.

Table 13.6   Sample Dance Workout: Balance Blast

Time	45-60 min 1. Warm-up: 10 min 2. Conditioning: 30-40 min 3. Cool-down: 5-10 min
Music tempo	120 bpm 32-count continuous play
Equipment	None
Purpose	Create a simple, inclusive, and well-rounded dance fitness class that emphasizes balance and posture while using traditional 32-count music to build 3 combinations that come together in a final routine

Warm-Up: 10 Minutes

Tables 13.7 to 13.9 provide different combinations of warm-up exercises that focus on the movements featured in the workouts that follow.

Table 13.7   Dance Warm-Up Combo A: Mobilization (64 Counts)

Base movement	Add dance flair	Reps	Counts
Inhale, arms up; exhale, arms down	Flex knees	2	16
Look up, down, right, left	—	2	16
Shoulder roll (right, left)	Look over shoulder	2	8
Double shoulder roll	—	2	8
Hip circle (right) with ankle circle	—	4	8
Hip circle (left) with ankle circle	—	4	8
Heel lift (right, left)	Toe stretch	4	16

When transitioning from warm-up combo A to B, do the mobilization flow as many times as feels good. The first time could be with the music at half count, and then speed it up a bit. This is meant to prepare the body for the workout ahead.

Table 13.8 Dance Warm-Up Combo B: Rehearsal Movements (64 Counts)

Base movement	Reps	Counts
March (right, left)	4	16
Walk forward and backward	2	16
Single side-step (right, left)	4	16
Double side-step (right, left)	2	16

When transitioning from warm-up combo B to C, the sequence can be repeated four or five times if the fitness professional wants to cut down on the number of repetitions as participants get more comfortable. This is a way to start building the intensity (both physically and mentally).

Table 13.9 Dance Warm-Up Combo C: Dynamic Stretches (32 Counts)

Base movement	Cues	Reps	Counts
Lunge lateral side shift (right, left)	—	4	16
Torso twist (right, left)	Hips and feet stay in place	2	16
Single-leg hip circle (right, left)	Like you're stepping over a fence	4	16
Torso twist with foot rotation (right, left)	Turn your entire body to the side	2	16

As an optional warm-up transition, if the fitness professional wants to kick class off with participants seeing how combinations will be built, then once the done warm-up combos have been done individually, they can be put together for one full combination that moves from A to B to C with flow.

Conditioning: 30 to 40 Minutes

Tables 13.10 to 13.12 provide different combinations of conditioning exercises intended to strengthen the muscles while improving cardiovascular fitness and balance coordination.

Table 13.10 Dance Conditioning Combo A (64 Counts)

Base movement	Add dance flair	Reps	Counts
March (right, left)	—	4	8
Single side-step (right, left)	Rib cage movement	2	8
Double side-step (right, left)	Rib cage movement	2	16

Base movement	Add dance flair	Reps	Counts
Heel dig, front (right, left)	Low V arms and snaps	2	8
Toe tap, side (right, left)	Low V arms and snaps	2	8
Heel dig, front (right, left)	Low V arms and snaps	2	8
Calf raise	Low arm press-back scapula retractions	2	8

When transitioning from conditioning combo A to B, after completing calf raises in combo A, perform 32 to 64 counts of hip sways with torso movement while slowly bringing the arms up in a dramatic arc to set the mood for combo B.

Table 13.11 Dance Conditioning Combo B (64 Counts)

Base movement	Add dance flair	Reps	Counts
Grapevine (right) with hip roll	The hip roll is the flair	1	8
Slow V-step (right)	Pump arms overhead	1	8
Repeat grapevine with slow V-step	—	1	16
Grapevine (right, left)	Rib cage movement	2	16
Wide-leg march	Hip sways	1	8
Standing still—look up, down, right, left	—	1	8

When transitioning from conditioning combo B to C, after completing the wide-leg march in combo B, give participants 32 counts of free movement to help them have fun and get ready for combo C.

Table 13.12 Dance Conditioning Combo C (64 Counts)

Base movement	Add dance flair	Reps	Counts
Kick-ball-change (right)	Freestyle movements with arms	2	6
Step out (right)	Balance hold	1	2
Kick-ball-change (left)	Arms	2	6
Step out (left)	Balance hold	1	2
Repeat kick-ball-change with step out (right, left)	—	—	16
Scoop front	Shoulders	4	8
Scoop back	Shoulders	4	8
Wide-leg double stomp (right, left)	Fist pumps, high and low	2	16

The wide-leg double stomp in conditioning combo C transitions easily back to the march in conditioning combo A. However, it can also be great to give participants a water break before coaching combo A, B, and C back-to-back.

Cool-Down: 5 to 10 Minutes

Tables 13.13 to 13.15 provide different combinations of cool-down exercises that bring the heart rate down and prevent muscle cramping and soreness.

Table 13.13   Dance Cool-Down Combo A: Lower Heart Rate

Base movement	Reps	Counts
Slow march (right, left)	4	16
Slow single side-step	2	16
Slow heel dig, front (right, left)	2	8
Calf raise	2	8

Repeat the transition from cool-down combo A to B as many times as appropriate to lower participants' heart rate. Spend longer than the designated counts for each movement, as necessary.

Table 13.14   Dance Cool-Down Combo B: Standing Core

Base movement	Notes	Reps	Counts
Wide-leg standing oblique crunch (right)	Reach the arm toward the knee	8	32
Standing high-pull scapula retraction	Reach and pull	8	32
Inhale, arms up; exhale, arms down	Make the breaths slow and deep	4	32
Repeat on left	—	—	64

Table 13.15   Dance Cool-Down Combo C: Standing Stretches

Base movement	Counts
Wide-leg lateral lunge with hold (right, left)	30 s/side
Fingertips behind ears, elbows wide, chest open	30 s
Lateral side-body stretch	30 s/side
Final inhale and exhale to finish class	30 s

Gym or Studio Full-Body Workout for Clients With Overweight or Obesity (Program 1)

Jonathan Mike, PhD

The proposed full-body exercise program (table 13.16) is designed to cater to all fitness levels—beginner, intermediate, and advanced—in a commercial gym or studio setting. This workout aims to engage all major muscle groups, improve cardiovascular health, enhance flexibility, and support overall weight management through a balanced mix of aerobic, resistance, and flexibility training. The training plan follows a weekly frequency of 2 days, with each session lasting approximately 60 minutes. This duration includes time for warm-up and cool-down phases. The intensity of the workouts is progressive, ensuring that individuals can advance through different training levels as their fitness improves.

Table 13.16   Gym or Studio Full-Body Workout 1 Sample Program

Warm-up (10-15 min)	Goal: Increase heart rate, warm up muscles, and prevent injury Activities: Light aerobic exercises (e.g., walking, cycling, or dynamic stretching)
Conditioning (35-40 min)	The core of the workout involves aerobic and resistance training; the progressive overload principle is applied to enhance intensity over time • Aerobic exercises (e.g., brisk walking, jogging, or cycling) • Resistance training involving bodyweight exercises, free weights, or machines
Cool-down (5-10 min)	Goal: Bring the body back to a resting state Activities: Low-intensity exercises (e.g., walking, static stretching) to improve flexibility
Frequency	2 d/wk

Progressive Training Plan

- *Beginner level:* Focus on low-intensity aerobic activities and basic resistance exercises with light weights or body weight (table 13.17).
- *Intermediate level:* Increase aerobic intensity (e.g., faster walking, light jogging) and resistance training with moderate weights (table 13.18).
- *Advanced level:* High-intensity aerobic exercises (e.g., running, high-intensity interval training [HIIT]) and advanced resistance training with heavier weights (table 13.19).

Table 13.17   Beginner Gym or Studio Full-Body Workout 1

Phase	Activity	Duration	Intensity
Warm-up	Treadmill walking	10 min	Low
Conditioning	Machine weights, bodyweight workout (leg press, chest press, lat pull-down) 2-3 sets of 12-15 reps; 1-2 min rest per set	20 min	Low
	Stationary bike	15 min	Low
Cool-down	Static stretching	5 min	Low

Table 13.18   Intermediate Gym or Studio Full-Body Workout 1

Phase	Activity	Duration	Intensity
Warm-up	Brisk walking	10 min	Moderate
Conditioning	Free-weight exercises (kettlebell goblet squat, kettlebell sumo deadlift, bench press, one-arm dumbbell row) 2-3 sets of 10-12 reps, 1-2 min rest per set	20 min	Moderate
	Light cardiovascular session (elliptical)	15 min	Moderate
Cool-down	Yoga or Pilates	10 min	Low

Table 13.19   Advanced Gym or Studio Full-Body Workout 1

Phase	Activity	Duration	Intensity
Warm-up	Dynamic movement preparation	15 min	High
Conditioning	Resistance training (squat, lunge, lat pull-down, cable row, chest press, and fly machine) 2 sets of 8-10 reps; 1-2 min rest per set	20 min	High
	High-intensity interval training (battle ropes, sled work, metabolic resistance training) 8 sets of 60 s; 60 s passive recovery per set	15 min	High
Cool-down	Comprehensive stretching	10 min	Low

Gym or Studio Full-Body Workout for Clients With Overweight or Obesity (Program 2)

Melody Schoenfeld, MS

This is a 12-week, full-body exercise program designed for use in a commercial gym or studio setting (tables 13.20-13.31). It is intended to cater to all fitness levels, from beginner to advanced, and is suitable for use in a gym or studio environment. The objective of this exercise program is to activate all major muscle groups, elevate cardiorespiratory fitness, improve mobility and flexibility, and enhance weight loss through a comprehensive exercise plan, including aerobic, resistance, and mobility or flexibility training. The training plan comprises 3 days of exercise per week, with each session lasting no more than 1 hour, including the warm-up and cool-down phases. The intensity of the training program is designed to increase progressively every 4 weeks, thereby enabling clients to advance through different training levels in accordance with their improvement in fitness.

Beginner Level (Weeks 1-4)

Table 13.20   Beginner Gym or Studio Full-Body Workout 2: Warm-Up

TRAINING PARAMETERS	
Frequency	3 d/wk (same routine for each workout)
Intensity	• Aerobic activity: 50%-60% of HRmax; RPE of 2-3 out of 10 • Dynamic stretching: Reach the joints' full ROM in a controlled way • Movement preparation: Perform basic movement patterns in a controlled way
Time	• Aerobic activity: 5 min • Dynamic stretching: 5 min (1 set of 8-12 reps per movement) • Movement preparation: 5 min (1 set of 8-12 reps per movement)
Type	• Low-impact aerobic activity: Treadmill walking or stationary cycling • Foam rolling: Focus on stiff, overactive, or sore muscles • Movement preparation: Mimic the movement patterns of the muscle-strengthening activities

Note: HRmax = maximum heart rate; ROM = range of motion; RPE = rating of perceived exertion scale (1-10).

Table 13.21   Beginner Gym or Studio Full-Body Workout 2: Conditioning

TRAINING PARAMETERS	
Frequency	3 d/wk
Intensity	60%-70% of maximal effort; OMNI-RES of 3-5 out of 10
Time	2-3 sets × 12-15 reps per exercise; 60 s rest per set
Type	Bodyweight exercises
Exercises (days 1-3)	• Incline push-up (using a bench or suspension strap) • Suspended row • Feet-elevated hip raise • Bodyweight squat • Alternating backward lunge

Note: OMNI-RES = OMNI resistance exercise scale of perceived exertion.

Table 13.22   Beginner Gym or Studio Full-Body Workout 2: Cardiorespiratory Fitness

TRAINING PARAMETERS	
Frequency	3 d/wk (same routine for each workout)
Intensity	60%-70% of HRmax; RPE of 3-5 out of 10
Time	20-30 min
Type	Continuous endurance training (brisk treadmill walking or stationary cycling)

Note: HRmax = maximum heart rate; RPE = rating of perceived exertion scale (1-10).

Table 13.23   Beginner Gym or Studio Full-Body Workout 2: Cool-Down

TRAINING PARAMETERS	
Frequency	3 days per week (same routine for each workout)
Intensity	Stretching: Stretch to the point of feeling tightness or slight discomfort Self-myofascial release: Foam roll to a comfortable level of discomfort (moderate pressure)
Time	Static stretching (2-3 min): 1 set of 15-30 s per muscle group Foam rolling (2-3 min): 1 set of 15-30 s per side or position
Type	Static stretching: Focus on stiff, overactive, or sore muscles Foam rolling: Focus on stiff, overactive, or sore muscles

Intermediate Level (Weeks 5-8)

Table 13.24   Intermediate Gym or Studio Full-Body Workout 2: Warm-Up

TRAINING PARAMETERS	
Frequency	3 d/wk (same routine for each workout)
Intensity	• Aerobic activity: 50%-60 % of HRmax; RPE of 2-3 out of 10 • Dynamic stretching: Reach the joints' full ROM in a controlled way • Movement preparation: Perform basic movement patterns in a controlled way
Time	• Aerobic activity: 5 min • Dynamic stretching: 5 min (1 set of 8-12 reps per movement) • Movement preparation: 5 min (1 set of 8-12 reps per movement)
Type	• Low-impact aerobic activity: Treadmill walking or stationary cycling • Foam rolling: Focus on stiff, overactive, or sore muscles • Movement preparation: Mimic the movement patterns of the muscle-strengthening activities

Note: HRmax = maximum heart rate; ROM = range of motion; RPE = rating of perceived exertion scale (1-10).

Table 13.25   Intermediate Gym or Studio Full-Body Workout 2: Conditioning

TRAINING PARAMETERS	
Frequency	3 d/wk
Intensity	70%-80% of maximal effort (OMNI-RES of 5-6 out of 10)
Time	3-4 sets × 8-12 reps per exercise; 90 s rest per set
Type	Compound exercises
Exercises (days 1-3)	• Kettlebell suitcase deadlift • Supported bent-over row • Dumbbell bench press • Box squat (back squat or front squat) • One-arm overhead press (kettlebell or dumbbell) • Front plank (15-60 s) or modified side plank (15-60 s) • Cable wood chop (10 reps per side) or Pallof press (10 reps per side)

Note: OMNI-RES = OMNI resistance exercise scale of perceived exertion.

Table 13.26   Intermediate Gym or Studio Full-Body Workout 2: Cardiorespiratory Fitness

TRAINING PARAMETERS	
Frequency	3 d/wk (same routine for each workout)
Intensity	3-5 work intervals (3-5 min at 70%-80% of HRmax; RPE of 5-7 out of 10); 3-5 active recovery intervals (3-5 min at 50%-60% of HRmax; RPE of 1-2 out of 10)
Time	20-30 min
Type	Moderate-intensity interval training (brisk treadmill walking, stationary cycling, or elliptical training)

Note: HRmax = maximum heart rate; RPE = rating of perceived exertion scale (1-10).

Table 13.27 Intermediate Gym or Studio Full-Body Workout 2: Cool-Down

TRAINING PARAMETERS	
Frequency	3 d/wk (same routine for each workout)
Intensity	• Stretching: Stretch to the point of feeling tightness or slight discomfort • Self-myofascial release: Foam roll to a comfortable level of discomfort (moderate pressure)
Time	• Static stretching (2-3 min): 1 set of 15-30 s per muscle group • Foam rolling (2-3 min): 1 set of 15-30 s per side or position
Type	• Static stretching: Focus on stiff, overactive, or sore muscles • Foam rolling: Focus on stiff, overactive, or sore muscles

Advanced Level (Weeks 9-12)

Table 13.28 Advanced Gym or Studio Full-Body Workout 2: Warm-Up

TRAINING PARAMETERS	
Frequency	3 d/wk (same routine for each workout)
Intensity	• Aerobic activity: 50%-60% of HRmax; RPE of 2-3 out of 10 • Dynamic stretching: Reach the joints' full ROM in a controlled way • Movement preparation: Perform basic movement patterns in a controlled way
Time	• Aerobic activity: 5 min • Dynamic stretching: 5 min (1 set of 8-12 reps per movement) • Movement preparation: 5 min (1 set of 8-12 reps per movement)
Type	• Low-impact aerobic activity: Treadmill walking or stationary cycling • Foam rolling: Focus on stiff, overactive, or sore muscles • Movement preparation: Mimic the movement patterns of the muscle-strengthening activities

Note: HRmax = maximum heart rate; ROM = range of motion; RPE = rating of perceived exertion scale (1-10).

Table 13.29 Advanced Gym or Studio Full-Body Workout 2: Conditioning

TRAINING PARAMETERS		
Frequency	3 d/wk	
Intensity	75%-85% of maximal effort (OMNI-RES of 7-8 out of 10)	
Time	3-4 sets × 6-10 reps per exercise; 120 s rest per set	
Type	Compound exercises	
EXERCISES		
Day 1	Day 2	Day 3
Barbell or hex barbell deadlift	Single-leg dumbbell deadlift	Barbell or hex barbell deadlift
Pendlay row	Chest-supported dumbbell row	Bent-over reverse-grip row
Barbell bench press	Cable chest flies	Dumbbell bench press
Barbell squat (back squat or front squat)	Leg (knee) curl	Dumbbell alternating forward lunge
Two-arm overhead press (dumbbell or kettlebell)	Leg (knee) extension	Incline bench press

(continued)

Table 13.29   Advanced Gym or Studio Full-Body Workout 2: Conditioning *(continued)*

TRAINING PARAMETERS		
Stability ball roll-outs (10-12 reps)	Calf raise off platform	Cable wood chop (15 reps per side)
—	Biceps curl (barbell or dumbbell)	—
—	Triceps cable push-down	—
—	Modified side plank (30-60 s per side)	—

Note: OMNI-RES = OMNI resistance exercise scale of perceived exertion.

Table 13.30   Advanced Gym or Studio Full-Body Workout 2: Cardiorespiratory Fitness

TRAINING PARAMETERS	
Frequency	3 d/wk (same routine for each workout)
Intensity	3-5 work intervals (60-90 s at 80%-90% of HRmax; RPE of 6-8 out of 10) and 3-5 active recovery intervals (3-5 min at 60%-70% of HRmax; RPE of 3-4 out of 10)
Time	15-20 min
Type	High-intensity interval training (brisk treadmill walking, stationary cycling, or elliptical training)

Note: HRmax = maximum heart rate; RPE = rating of perceived exertion.

Table 13.31   Advanced Gym or Studio Full-Body Workout 2: Cool-Down

TRAINING PARAMETERS	
Frequency	3 d/wk (same routine for each workout)
Intensity	• Stretching: Stretch to the point of feeling tightness or slight discomfort • Self-myofascial release: Foam roll to a comfortable level of discomfort (moderate pressure)
Time	• Static stretching (2-3 min): 1 set of 15-30 s per muscle group • Foam rolling (2-3 min): 1 set of 15-30 s per side or position
Type	• Static stretching: Focus on stiff, overactive, or sore muscles • Foam rolling: Focus on stiff, overactive, or sore muscles

Progressive High-Intensity Functional Training for Experienced Clients With Overweight or Obesity

Michael Piercy, MS

The following circuit-based, high-intensity functional training (HIFT) workouts are suggested for clients with overweight or obesity who are physically active and have gym experience, particularly in functional or neuromotor fitness activities, and who do not have musculoskeletal or cardiometabolic health issues (tables 13.32-13.36).

Table 13.32   1-Week Progressive HIFT Programming

Level	Weeks	Rounds	Work	Rest	Rest per round
1	1-4	3	15-20 s	30-40 s	180 s
2	5-8	3	20-25 s	30-35 s	180 s
3	9-12	3	25-30 s	25-30 s	150 s
4	13-16	3	30-35 s	30-35 s	150 s
5	17-20	3	35-40 s	25-30 s	120 s
6	21-24	3	40-45 s	20-25 s	120 s

Table 13.33   Progressive HIFT Circuit A

Warm-up	Reverse lunge with twist
	Walking leg cradles
	Lying side raise
	Side-lying T-spine rotations
	Low side-to-side lunge
Conditioning	(1a) Quick feet
	(1b) Speed squat
	(2a) Traveling push-up
	(2b) Plank hollow hold
	(3a) High knees
	(3b) Alternating dumbbell single-leg RDL
	(3c) Bear crawl
	(3d) Plank rotation
	(4a) Shuffle cone touch
	(4b) Split squat
	(4c) Dumbbell chop
	(4d) Landmine antirotation
Cool-down	Static stretching and foam rolling (optional)

Note: RDL = Romanian deadlift.

Table 13.34   Progressive HIFT Circuit B

Warm-up	Rotational arm swing
	Split jack
	Wall slide
	Side-lying T-spine rotation
	Low side-to-side lunge

(continued)

Table 13.34 Progressive HIFT Circuit B *(continued)*

Conditioning	(1a) Alternating lateral squat
	(1b) Lunge curl press
	(1c) Straight-arm plank
	(1d) Suspended chest press
	(2a) Kneeling stability ball rollout
	(2b) Plank to hip raise
	(2c) Suspended Y-row
	(2d) Plank with rotation
Cool-down	Static stretching and foam rolling (optional)

Table 13.35 Progressive HIFT Circuit C

Warm-up	Rotational arm swing
	Split jack
	Wall slide
	Side-lying T-spine rotation
	Low side-to-side lunge
Conditioning	(1a) Scissor hop
	(1b) Stability ball push-up
	(2a) Speed squat
	(2b) Seal jack with cross
	(3a) Single-arm dumbbell row
	(3b) Medicine ball swing
	(3c) High-knee marching and back pedal
	(3d) Barbell hip thrust
	(3e) Reverse T-fly with band
Cool-down	Static stretching and foam rolling (optional)

Table 13.36 Progressive HIFT Circuit D

Warm-up	Knee hug
	Jumping jack
	High knees
	Side shuffle
	Gate swing

Conditioning	(1a) Squat thrust
	(1b) Stability ball push-up
	(1c) Stability ball rollout
	(1d) Squat with dumbbell press
	(2a) Rotational mountain climber
	(2b) Dumbbell renegade row to T-rotation
	(2c) TRX body saw
	(2d) Dumbbell farmer carry
	(3a) 180° jump squat
	(3b) Lunge matrix
	(3c) Stability ball Y-fly
	(3d) Plank with forward reach
Cool-down	Static stretching and foam rolling (optional)

Hybrid-Type, Multicomponent Interval Training Workout for Clients With Overweight or Obesity

Alexios Batrakoulis, PhD

This hybrid-type, multicomponent interval training program is designed to support previously inactive clients with overweight or obesity of all fitness levels (i.e., beginner, intermediate, and advanced) in a real-world fitness setting (tables 13.37-13.39). This nontraditional, high-intensity intermittent workout integrates foundational interval training principles and functional resistance accessory training into a single session. Such an exercise approach aims to provide both cardiorespiratory and musculoskeletal stimuli in a time-efficient fashion through a progressive, circuit-based exercise protocol tailored for clients with excess weight.

This workout is considered an attractive exercise mode among various populations, including those with overweight or obesity (Newsome et al. 2024). It is a multicomponent solution incorporating pleasant, injury-free, and effective aerobic and muscle-strengthening activities into a short workout. The training plan suggests a weekly frequency of three sessions, with a total time commitment of approximately 100 minutes per week. The intensity of the workouts is progressive, ensuring that previously inactive clients with excess weight can advance through different training levels as their physical fitness improves (Batrakoulis and Fatouros 2022; Batrakoulis, Jamurtas, et al. 2021; Batrakoulis et al. 2018; Batrakoulis 2022; Batrakoulis et al. 2023; Batrakoulis et al. 2020; Batrakoulis, Tsimeas, et al. 2021).

Safety and Training Considerations

- Medical clearance to participate in vigorous-intensity exercise is highly recommended for all clients with overweight or obesity, regardless of their physical fitness level.
- Clients with excess weight and impaired musculoskeletal health should avoid high-impact, aerobic-based activities.
- Medically cleared clients with overweight or obesity and complications should engage first in a familiarization training phase though supervised hybrid-type exercise protocols, using lower frequency, intensity, and time, as suggested previously.

Table 13.37 Beginner Hybrid-Type, Multicomponent Interval Training

EXERCISES	
1	Kettlebell goblet squat
2	Medicine ball overhead press
3	Suspended neutral-grip row
4	Kettlebell sumo deadlift
5	Front plank
6	Agility ladder low-knee skip
TRAINING PARAMETERS	
Frequency	3 sessions per week
Intensity	6 work bouts of 15-20 s at 75%-80% of HRmax and RPE of 4-5 out of 10; 5 passive recovery bouts of 45-60 s at 60%-70% of HRmax and RPE of 2-3 out of 10; work-to-rest ratio 1:3; rest interval per round: 3 min
Time	30 min per session, including the warm-up (3 min) and cool-down (2 min)
Type	Bodyweight exercises and loaded fundamental movement patterns

Note: HRmax = maximum heart rate; RPE = rating of perceived exertion.

Table 13.38 Intermediate Hybrid-Type, Multicomponent Interval Training

EXERCISES	
1	Medicine ball goblet squat to overhead press
2	Kettlebell swing
3	Diagonal medicine ball chest press
4	Suspended supinated-grip row
5	Front plank with alternating leg lift
6	Squat hops straddling an agility ladder
7	Medicine ball diagonal wood chop
8	Battle rope tsunami
TRAINING PARAMETERS	
Frequency	3 sessions per week
Intensity	8 work bouts of 20-30 s at 80%-85% of HRmax and RPE of 5-6 out of 10; 7 passive recovery bouts of 40-60 s at 60%-70% of HRmax and RPE of 2-3 out of 10; work-to-rest ratio 1:2; rest interval per round: 2.5 min
Time	35 min per session, including the warm-up (3 min) and cool-down (2 min)
Type	Bodyweight exercises and loaded fundamental movement patterns

Note: HRmax = maximum heart rate; RPE = rating of perceived exertion.

Table 13.39 Advanced Hybrid-Type, Multicomponent Interval Training

EXERCISES	
1	Medicine ball squat to diagonal press
2	Kettlebell snatch
3	Medicine ball hip thrust

4	Suspended T-, Y-, or I-row
5	Straight-arm plank shoulder taps
6	Agility ladder in-and-out steps
7	Standing medicine ball torso rotation
8	Alternating forward lunge with medicine ball chest press
9	Battle rope side-to-side wave
10	Agility ladder straddle jump
TRAINING PARAMETERS	
Frequency	3 sessions per week
Intensity	10 work bouts of 30-40 s at 85%-90% of HRmax and RPE of 6-7 out of 10; 9 passive recovery bouts of 30-40 s at 65%-75% of HRmax and RPE of 3-4 out of 10; work-to-rest ratio 1:1; rest interval per round: 2 min
Time	40 min per session, including the warm-up (3 min) and cool-down (2 min)
Type	Bodyweight exercises and loaded fundamental movement patterns

Note: HRmax = maximum heart rate; RPE = rating of perceived exertion.

Clinical High-Intensity Interval Training Workout for Clients With Overweight and Obesity

Alexios Batrakoulis, PhD

The proposed HIIT program is designed to serve clients with excess weight of all fitness levels (i.e., beginner, intermediate, and advanced) in a real-world fitness setting (table 13.40). This traditional HIIT workout aims to enhance cardiovascular endurance as a key component of the overall health and fitness status of people with excess weight. This workout is considered the most widely used HIIT-type protocol for clinical populations, including those with obesity (Taylor et al. 2019). Specifically, it is a single-component approach using feasible, pain-free, low-impact, aerobic-based activities for individuals with excess weight. The present training plan follows a weekly frequency of one (beginner), two (intermediate), or three (advanced) sessions, with each session lasting approximately 30 minutes, including the warm-up and cool-down time. The intensity of the workouts is progressive, ensuring that beginner clients can advance through different training levels as their cardiorespiratory fitness and functional capacity levels improve.

Training Considerations

- Medical clearance to participate in vigorous-intensity exercise is highly recommended for all clients with excess weight, regardless of their physical fitness level.
- All training parameters should be gradually progressed, considering the client's physical fitness and overall health status.
- Clients with excess weight who have musculoskeletal health disorders and physical limitations should avoid high-impact, aerobic-based activities.
- Medically cleared clients with overweight or obesity and comorbidities may engage in supervised traditional HIIT workouts using lower frequency, intensity, and time.

Table 13.40   Clinical HIIT Training Parameters

Frequency	1-3 sessions per week, depending on the client's fitness level
Intensity	3-4 work bouts of 4 min at 75%-95% of HRmax; RPE of 5-8 out of 10; 2-3 active recovery bouts of 3 min at 55%-70% of HRmax; RPE of 2-3 out of 10
Time	40 min per session, including the warm-up (3 min) and cool-down (2 min)
Type	Bodyweight exercises and loaded fundamental movement patterns

Note: HRmax = maximum heart rate; RPE = rating of perceived exertion.

Conventional High-Intensity Interval Training Workout for Clients With Overweight or Obesity

Alexios Batrakoulis, PhD

This HIIT program is designed to support clients with overweight or obesity of all fitness levels (i.e., beginner, intermediate, and advanced) in a gym environment (table 13.41). This traditional HIIT workout aims to increase cardiorespiratory fitness as a critical piece of the overall health and fitness status in adults with excess weight. This workout is considered one of the most popular HIIT-type protocols for general and special populations, including those with excess weight (Cress et al. 2015). Specifically, it is a single-component approach using feasible, pain-free, low-impact, aerobic-based activities for clients with overweight or obesity. The present training plan follows a weekly frequency of one (beginners), two (intermediate), or three (advanced) sessions, with each session lasting approximately 20 minutes, including the warm-up and cool-down time. The intensity of the workouts is progressive, ensuring that beginner clients can advance through different training levels as their cardiorespiratory fitness and functional capacity levels improve.

Training Considerations

- Medical clearance to participate in vigorous-intensity exercise is highly recommended for all clients with excess weight, regardless of their physical fitness level.
- All training parameters should be gradually progressed, considering the client's physical fitness and overall health status.
- Clients with excess weight who have musculoskeletal health disorders and physical limitations should avoid high-impact, aerobic-based activities.
- Medically cleared clients with overweight or obesity and comorbidities may engage in supervised traditional HIIT workouts using lower frequency, intensity, and time.

Table 13.41   Conventional HIIT Training Parameters

Frequency	1-3 sessions per week, depending on the client's fitness level
Intensity	8-10 work bouts of 60 s at 85%-95% of HRmax; RPE of 6-8 out of 10; 7-9 passive or active recovery bouts of 60 s at 60%-70% of HRmax; RPE of 2-3 out of 10
Time	20-25 min per session, including the warm-up (3 min) and cool-down (2 min)
Type	Aerobic-based activities (treadmill walking or jogging, stationary cycling, elliptical training, stair climbing, stationary rowing, and cross-country skiing)

Note: HRmax = maximum heart rate; RPE = rating of perceived exertion.

Holistic Core Training for Clients With Overweight or Obesity

Alexios Batrakoulis, PhD

This workout encompasses various antimotion static and dynamic core exercises, performed in all planes of motion (tables 13.42-13.44). The prescribed core exercises can be implemented either as straight sets with rest intervals per exercise (beginner level) or in a circuit fashion (intermediate to advanced level), focusing on the core stability and endurance enhancement among people with excess weight. This progressive core training plan can be an effective and feasible approach for clients with excess weight who have poor functional capacity, physical limitations, or common musculoskeletal health disorders (Contreras and Schoenfeld 2011). Practicing these techniques will support lumber spine stability while promoting functionality, coordination, and pain-free core exercise experiences (McGill 2001; Schoenfeld and Kolber 2016).

Safety and Training Considerations

- Medical clearance to participate in core training workouts is recommended for clients with excess weight who have spine conditions, regardless of their physical fitness level.

- All training parameters should be gradually progressed, considering the client's functional capacity and musculoskeletal health levels.

- Medically cleared clients with overweight or obesity and comorbidities may engage in supervised core training workouts using lower frequency, intensity, and time.

- Clients with excess weight who have musculoskeletal health disorders, physical limitations, or poor mobility should avoid dynamic spinal-flexion exercises.

- Clients with excess weight seeking postural correction and spine rehabilitation should focus on static core exercises enhancing stabilization rather than dynamic movements flexing the spine.

Table 13.42   Holistic Core Training Program: Beginner Level

EXERCISES	
Category	**Movement**
Antiflexion or antiextension	Kneeling plank
Anti–lateral flexion	Asymmetric loaded carry
Antirotation	Lateral-force resisting abdominal bracing
TRAINING PARAMETERS	
Frequency	2 times per week
Intensity	OMNI-RES of 3-4 out of 10
Time	2 sets of 8-10 reps (or 15-30 s); work-to-rest ratio of 1:2
Type	Antimotion exercises

Note: OMNI-RES = OMNI resistance exercise scale of perceived exertion.

Table 13.43 Holistic Core Training Program: Intermediate Level

EXERCISES	
Category	**Movement**
Antiflexion or antiextension	Incline plank
Anti–lateral flexion	Modified side plank
Antirotation	Banded half-kneeling Pallof press
Rotation	Landmine twist
TRAINING PARAMETERS	
Frequency	2-3 times per week
Intensity	OMNI-RES of 4-6 out of 10
Time	2-3 sets of 12-15 reps (or 30-45 s); work-to-rest ratio of 1:1
Type	Antimotion and spinal rotation exercises

Note: OMNI-RES = OMNI resistance exercise scale of perceived exertion.

Table 13.44 Holistic Core Training Program: Advanced Level

EXERCISES	
Category	**Movement**
Antiflexion or antiextension	Assisted plank or bear crawl isometric hold
Anti–lateral flexion	Asymmetric loaded carry (shoulder or overhead)
Antirotation	Landmine antirotation
Rotation	Rotational chop
Antiextension	Elevated glute bridge
TRAINING PARAMETERS	
Frequency	3 times per week
Intensity	OMNI-RES of 6-8 out of 10
Time	3 sets of 15-20 repetitions (or 45-60 s); work-to-rest ratio of 2:1
Type	Antimotion and spinal rotation exercises

Note: OMNI-RES = OMNI resistance exercise scale of perceived exertion.

At-Home Full-Body Workout for Clients With Overweight or Obesity

Lee Boyce

Training for the client with overweight or obesity requires a few specific considerations aside from the actual size and weight of the individual. It is important to select movement patterns that do not place unwanted stress on their cardiac system, blood pressure, or load-bearing joints (beyond what is intended). For that reason, this single workout is tailored to the client with overweight or obesity and is confined to only minimal equipment to be used to train at home. It is also possible to perform the current workout in a gym or studio setting, should there be a lack of access to stationary machines. The proposed full-body exercise program is designed to cater to all fitness levels—beginner, intermediate, and advanced—in a home setting (tables 13.45-13.47). This workout aims to engage all major muscle groups, improve cardiovascular health, enhance flexibility, and support overall weight management through a balanced mix of aerobic, resistance, and flexibility training. The plan follows a weekly frequency of two to three days, with each session lasting approximately 60 minutes, including the warm-up and cool-down phases. The intensity of the workouts is progressive, ensuring that individuals can advance through different training levels as their fitness improves.

Table 13.45   Beginner At-Home Full-Body Workout Plan

Warm-up	Arm circles—10 revolutions in each direction
	Hamstring sweeps—10 strides per leg
	Band pull-apart—15 reps
	Prone superman—12 reps
	Glute bridge—15 reps
Conditioning: 3 sets each, 60 s rest between supersets	(1a) Squat to box—15 reps
	(2a) Band-resisted lateral raise—15 reps
	(3a) March on the spot (active rest)—60 s
	(1b) Dumbbell RDL—12 reps
	(2b) Dumbbell incline bench press—12 reps
	(3b) Band-resisted biceps curl (active rest)—60 s
	(1c) Dumbbell overhead press—12 reps
	(2c) Medicine ball slam—12 reps
Cool-down	Treadmill incline walk—15 min at 70% HRmax Static stretching and foam rolling

Note: HRmax = maximum heart rate; RDL = Romanian deadlift.

Table 13.46 Intermediate At-Home Full-Body Workout Plan

Warm-up	Arm circles—10 revolutions in each direction
	Hamstring sweeps—10 strides per leg
	Band pull-apart—15 reps
	Prone superman—12 reps
	Glute bridge—15 reps
Conditioning: 3 sets each, 60 seconds rest between supersets	(1a) Assisted bench step-up—10 reps per leg
	(2a) Squat with front raise—12 reps
	(3a) March on the spot (active rest)—60 s
	(1b) Dumbbell hip thrust—12 reps
	(2b) Bench push-up—12 reps
	(3b) Band-resisted biceps curl (active rest)—60 s
	(1c) Dumbbell push-press—12 reps
	(2c) Medicine ball slam—12 reps
Cool-down	Treadmill incline walk—15 min at 70% HRmax Static stretching and foam rolling

Note: HRmax = maximum heart rate.

Table 13.47 Advanced At-Home Full-Body Workout Plan

Warm-up	Arm circles—10 revolutions in each direction
	Hamstring sweeps—10 strides per leg
	Band pull-apart—15 reps
	Prone superman—12 reps
	Glute bridge —15 reps
Conditioning: 3 sets each, 60 seconds rest between supersets	(1a) Bench step-up with slow eccentric—10 reps per leg
	(2a) Isometric wall sit with front raise—12 reps
	(3a) March on the spot (active rest)—60 s
	(1b) Dumbbell single-leg hip thrust—12 reps per leg
	(2b) Bench push-up—12 reps
	(3b) Band-resisted face pull (active rest)—60 s
	(1c) Single-arm dumbbell swing—8 reps
	(2c) Quadruped bird dog—12 reps
Cool-down	Treadmill incline walk—15 min at 70% HRmax Static stretching and foam rolling

Note: HRmax = maximum heart rate.

Training Clients With Obesity and Lower-Extremity Joint Pain

Lauren Shroyer, MS

Research evidence demonstrates the harmful effects of obesity on lower-extremity musculoskeletal disorders, increasing the risk of skeletal malalignments, joint stress, pain, and discomfort. Clients with excess body weight or adiposity commonly exhibit increased knee valgus in conjunction with an increased step width. The accompanying muscular dysfunctions impede their ability to compensate for these alterations, particularly in the frontal plane (Pataky et al. 2014). Obesity-related knee and hip pain is extremely common; individuals with a body mass index exceeding 36 kg/m² have been observed to exhibit a 14-fold increase in the prevalence of obesity-related knee and hip osteoarthritis (Jurado-Castro et al. 2022).

Obesity influences pain through several mechanisms, including mechanical loading, inflammation, and psychological status. The experience of pain in people with obesity is associated with a reduction in physical ability, adverse effects on health-related quality of life, and an increased risk of functional dependence. However, a mere 5% reduction in body weight can mitigate pain and enhance the safety of potential surgical procedures, such as joint replacement (Barrow et al. 2019). It seems that regular exercise, which combines cardiorespiratory and muscular fitness activities, represents an effective strategy for reducing lower-extremity joint pain (Zdziarski et al. 2015).

In programming workouts for the week, it is ideal to alternate cardiorespiratory and muscular fitness training days; a recovery day may be indicated. An example workout schedule is shown in table 13.48.

Table 13.48 Lower-Extremity Joint Workout Sample Program

Week 1	Week 2
Day 1: Cardiorespiratory fitness	Day 1: Cardiorespiratory fitness
Day 2: Muscular fitness	Day 2: Muscular fitness
Day 3: Recovery	Repeat sequence
Repeat sequence	—

Cardiorespiratory Fitness

When lower-extremity pain is present, aerobic exercise options for beginners should be non-weight-bearing (e.g., swimming, water-based activities, and seated bodyweight exercises, such as marches, in-and-out movements, and heel taps). As lower-extremity strength increases, adding low-impact weight-bearing exercise at a slow progression is favorable (e.g., biking, using a stationary bike or elliptical machine, walking, or low-impact dance).

Muscular Fitness

Programs for individuals with overweight or obesity who are struggling with lower-extremity joint pain should focus on strength building, with an effort to limit the number of repetitions that add stress to the painful joints. When engaging with an individual who is prone to pain or experiences increased pain during exercise, it is important to start with basic movements to better understand pain triggers, then progress the exercises as tolerated. Ask for feedback from the client when introducing a new exercise and throughout each set by using a pain scale.

In the workouts in tables 13.49 to 13.52, an alternate exercise is provided if the client reports a pain level of 5 or higher (on a scale of 10) during the recommended exercise. If the alternate option is also painful, discontinue the exercise and have the client do an additional set of the previous exercise or a stretch appropriate for that muscle group. In time, clients may advance to the exercises in the right-hand column. Nonetheless, it is crucial to consider specific injuries or conditions, because pain may persist and certain exercises may not be suitable. The choice of exercise should be guided by the individual's pain level.

Table 13.49 Static Stretching and Self-Myofascial Release

Goal	Improve passive ROM and achieve close to bilateral symmetry in ROM	
Volume	Foam rolling as tolerated, with a goal of 2 min per area; for plasticity change, hold stretches for 1-2 min	
Stretching or foam rolling	**Alternate option**	**Progression**
Foam roll: Quads and hip flexor	Self-massaging tool: Quads and hip flexor	N/A
Foam roll: IT band and tensor fascia latae	Self-massaging tool: IT band and tensor fascia latae	N/A
Foam roll: Piriformis and lower back	N/A	N/A
Standing quad stretch	Quad stretch with yoga strap while lying prone	Kneeling quad and hip flexor stretch
Figure-4 and piriformis stretches while lying supine	Standing pigeon pose with affected leg on massage table	Pigeon pose with yoga blanket under hip

Note: IT = iliotibial; N/A = not applicable; ROM = range of motion.

Table 13.50 Lower-Extremity Joint Care Warm-Up

Goal	Neuromuscular stimulation and multiplanar elasticity
Volume	The total time of each exercise should be 45-90 s; this can be broken up into multiple sets to accommodate individual needs

Exercise	Alternate option	Progression
High-knee walking (on floor)	High-knee marching in place with dowel for balance	High-knee walking (on floor) with heel raise
RDL, body weight only	Standing downward dog with hands on wall, Vinyasa style	Single-leg RDL
Wide-leg, stationary lateral lunge	Decrease ROM	Step to lateral lunge
Bodyweight half squat, holding suspension trainer straps or ballet bar for support	Bodyweight quarter squat, holding suspension trainer straps or ballet bar for support	Bodyweight squat
Standing rotation with medicine ball	Standing rotation without resistance	Rotation with medicine ball while lying supine
Smith bar push-up	Wall push-up	Bench push-up
Standing cable row	Seated cable row	Seated cable row with increased weight

Note: RDL = Romanian deadlift; ROM = range of motion.

Structuring the workout as a circuit allows for more rest time between sets taxing the same muscle group, which minimizes effects on painful areas.

Table 13.51   Lower-Extremity Joint Care Conditioning Circuit

Goal	Increased strength and stability	
Volume	1-5 circuits with 8-12 reps each set, as tolerated	
Exercise	**Alternate option**	**Progression**
RDL with dumbbells	RDL with body weight	RDL with barbell
Standing 1-arm cable press	Seated 2-arm machine chest press	Standing 1-arm cable press with rotation
Bodyweight squat, holding suspension trainer straps or ballet bar for support	Bodyweight chair sit-to-stand, holding suspension trainer straps or ballet bar for support	Squat with dumbbell or medicine ball
Standing 1-arm cable row	Seated 2-arm machine row	Standing 1-arm cable row with rotation
Agility ladder lateral walking in and out	Lateral marching	Agility ladder lateral walking in and out, increasing speed
Lat pull-down	Wide-grip cable lat pull-down	Lat pull-down with increased weight
Chest press with dumbbells	Seated 2-arm machine chest press	Chest press with dumbbells, increased weight
Lateral bodyweight lunge	Sumo squat	Lateral dumbbell lunge
Straight-arm lateral cable walks	Lateral cable torso rotation	Straight-arm lateral cable step and swing

Note: RDL = Romanian deadlift.

Table 13.52 Lower-Extremity Joint Care Cool-Down

Goal	Static stretching or self-myofascial release (foam rolling)	
Volume	For plasticity change, hold stretches for 1-3 min	
Exercise	**Alternate option**	**Progression**
Standing quad stretch	Quad stretch with yoga strap while lying supine	Kneeling quad and hip flexor stretch
Standing downward dog with hands on a wall	Single-leg seated hamstring stretch	Downward dog
Figure-4 and piriformis stretches while lying supine	Standing pigeon pose with affected leg on massage table	Pigeon pose with yoga blanket under hip
Foam roll, lying goalpost pectoral stretch	Standing doorway pectoral stretch	Foam roll, lying snow angels

Training Clients With Obesity and Chronic Low-Back Pain

Rodiel Kirby Baloy, DPT

Individuals with low-back pain demonstrate similar characteristics to those without this pathology when not experiencing serious back issues (American College of Sports Medicine 2021). An increase in body weight augments mechanical stress on the musculoskeletal structures of the back. To maintain equilibrium, the spine may undergo a compensatory tilt and uneven stress distribution (Frilander et al. 2015). Excessive abdominal adiposity can contribute to pelvic forward tilt, which increases lumbar lordosis and may exacerbate low-back discomfort. There is a correlation between obesity and an elevated risk of back pain. Furthermore, excess weight has been linked to herniated discs, osteoarthritis, and an extended recovery period following episodes of back pain (Walsh et al. 2018). Weight loss can reduce inflammation and decrease pressure on the spine, which may lead to a reduction in pain. Incorporating regular exercise into a weight loss plan may also result in stronger stomach and back muscles. This provides enhanced support for the spine and is beneficial for pain relief (Chen et al. 2022; Wasser et al. 2017). Table 13.53 outlines training parameters for individuals with chronic low-back pain.

Exercise Considerations and Suggestions for Warm-Ups

- Aerobic-type exercises are recommended and largely depend on positions or postures that may help relieve low-back symptoms.
- For individuals with low-back pain with an extension bias or extension relief, warm-ups such as treadmill walking or using an elliptical trainer may reduce the possibility of a back-pain flare during exercise.
- For individuals with low-back pain with a flexion bias or flexion relief, warm-ups such as using a stationary bike or stair climber may reduce the possibility of a back-pain flare during exercise.

Table 13.53   Training Parameters for Chronic Low-Back Pain

Fitness type	Frequency	Intensity	Time	Type
Cardiorespiratory	3-5 times per week	55%-70% of HRmax; RPE of 2-3 out of 10 (progressing to 70%-85% of HRmax; RPE of 4-5 out of 10)	15-30 min (progressing to 30-45 min) per session	Low-impact aerobic activities (e.g., treadmill walking, stationary cycling, elliptical training, stair climbing, swimming, aquatic exercise)
Muscular conditioning	2-3 times per week (on nonconsecutive days)	50%-60% of 1-RM; OMNI-RES of 5-6 out of 10 (progressing to 70%-80% of 1-RM; OMNI-RES of 7-8 out of 10)	1-2 sets of 12-15 reps per muscle group; 60 s rest between sets (progressing to 2-3 sets of 6-10 reps; 90 s rest between sets)	Multijoint exercises using stationary machines, free weights, elastic bands, or adjunct modalities (e.g., suspension straps, kettlebells, medicine balls) and bodyweight movements
Flexibility	2-3 times per week	Stretch to the point of feeling tightness or slight discomfort	1-2 reps with hold of 15-30 s (progressing to 30-60 s) per muscle group	Static stretching with an emphasis on hamstrings, glutes, hip flexors, and back extensors

Note: 1-RM = 1-repetition maximum; HRmax = maximum heart rate; OMNI-RES = OMNI resistance exercise scale of perceived exertion; RPE = rating of perceived exertion.

Adapted from Franz et al. (2017); Surkitt et al. (2012); and Yarznbowicz and Tao (2018).

Exercise Considerations and Suggestions for Muscular Conditioning

- Begin with bodyweight exercises for a duration of 20 to 30 minutes, targeting the larger muscle groups through whole-body sessions.
- At the outset of the exercise program, participants should engage in bodyweight exercises at a level that is both tolerable and comfortable and then progress as appropriate (table 13.54). The initial objective is to devise a schedule that can be practically maintained throughout the week.
- Some exercise-related soreness is expected but should resolve in 24 hours. Should a conditioning regimen cause prolonged soreness, changes must be made to allow for earlier resolution.
- A consistently performed regimen with minimal to no soreness will increase program protocol adhesion as well as consistency.
- It is inadvisable to prioritize dynamic spinal-flexion exercises, such as sit-ups, crunches, and reverse crunches, as a means of core activation.
- Static core exercises enhancing stabilization (e.g., planks, bridges, and bird dogs) seem to be superior to dynamic movements flexing the spine.

Exercise Considerations and Suggestions for Cool-Down

- Cool-downs partially inhibit depression of the immune system after strenuous exercise. They also help accelerate the recovery of the cardiopulmonary system after training.
- Active cool-downs are significantly more effective than passive activities.

Table 13.54   Muscular Conditioning Exercises for Chronic Low-Back Pain

Beginner	Intermediate	Advanced
Supported squat	Chair squat	Bodyweight squat
Supported lunge	Static bodyweight lunge	Dynamic bodyweight lunge
Inverted row	Suspended row	Single dumbbell row
Incline bench push-up	Floor push-up	Decline bench push-up
Elevated front plank	Straight-arm front plank	Front plank with feet elevated
Half-kneeling Pallof press	Kneeling Pallof press	Standing Pallof press
Floor glute bridge	Elevated glute bridge	Single-leg glute bridge

Adapted from Schoenfeld and Kolber (2016).

Low-back pain is divided into three categories:

1. Low-back pain with pathology such as cancer or fractures
2. Low-back pain with neurological signs
3. Nonspecific low-back pain

Nonspecific low-back pain accounts for most cases of low-back pain, with estimates between 85% and 95% (Balagué et al. 2012). Table 13.55 offers a few methods of aerobic activities for specific types of back pain.

Table 13.55   Recommended Modalities for Chronic Low-Back Pain

Back pain caused by extension	Back pain caused by flexion
Stationary bike	Treadmill (walking)
Stair climber	Elliptical trainer

Adapted from Van Hooren and Peake (2018).

Situation-Specific Suggestions
- Many cases of low-back pain respond well to early mobility and activity and will show quick improvement.
- Exercising in the individual's preferred direction or pattern of motion is a good way to initiate activity without the risk of a symptom flare-up.

Training Clients With Obesity and Osteoporosis

Ryan Carver, BS

Osteoporosis is a chronic musculoskeletal disease adversely affecting body functionality and quality of life while requiring pharmacological interventions associated with several adverse effects. The presence of obesity along with osteoporosis is a complicated situation that increases cardiometabolic and musculoskeletal health impairments. However, regular exercise seems to be a powerful, noninvasive, and nonpharmacological tool for managing both conditions by promoting bone and muscle anabolism while limiting the formation and expansion of fat mass (Liu et al. 2023; Pagnotti et al. 2019). Tables 13.56 to 13.61 outline suggestions for beginner, intermediate, and advanced programming for individuals with osteoporosis.

Beginner Program

Table 13.56   Beginner 7-Day Schedule for Osteoporosis Care

Day	Monday	Tuesday	Wednesday	Thursday	Friday	Saturday	Sunday
Exercise	Resistance training, flexibility and mobility, agility	Aerobic training (walking)	Aerobic training (biking or swimming)	Resistance training, flexibility and mobility, agility	Off	Aerobic training (walking)	Off
Time	60 min	20-30 min	20-30 min	60 min	—	20-30 min	—

Note: This schedule meets minimum recommendations for muscle-strengthening activities.

Table 13.57   Beginner Sample Program for Osteoporosis Care

Phase	Modality	Method and targeted areas	Sets × reps or time
Warm-up	Power nasal breathing	Breathe in through the nose for 3-4 s, then out through the nose for 6-8 s	1 × 4-5
Mobility	Stick rolling	Thighs, glutes, hamstrings, IT band, calves, anterior tibialis, adductors	1 × 20 s each
	Elevated controlled articular rotations	Ankle, hip, shoulder, scapula, wrist	1 × 4-5 in each direction
Movement preparation	Movement patterns	Squat, hip hinge, elevated push-up, TRX row	1 × 8-10
Core activation	Ball dead bug squeezes	—	2 × 10 breaths
Power, speed, agility, and quickness	Box taps	—	2 × 20 s
Conditioning	(1a) Box or bench squat	—	2 × 8-12
	(1b) Single-arm dumbbell bent-over row	—	2 × 8-12
	(2a) Dumbbell RDL	—	2 × 8-12
	(2b) Dumbbell bench press	—	2 × 8-12
	(3a) Elevated bird dog (10 s hold)	—	2 × 5-6
	(3b) In-place cognitive agility*	—	2 × 8-12
	(4) Overhead dumbbell press	—	1-2 × 10-12
Cool-down	Breathing	Recovery position	2-3 min

IT = iliotibial.

*Challenge and emphasize one of the four cognitive domains: memory, executive function, attention, or processing speed (i.e., the client spells out certain names, places, or things while executing stationary exercises).

Note: The warm-up, mobility, and movement preparation exercises are great for helping low-back pain (a common complaint with obesity and osteoporosis). The core activation, power, and conditioning exercises target all major muscle groups, and the core exercises are designed to help stabilize and mitigate back pain.

Intermediate Program

Table 13.58   Intermediate 7-Day Schedule for Osteoporosis Care

Day	Monday	Tuesday	Wednesday	Thursday	Friday	Saturday	Sunday
Exercise	Resistance training, agility, flexibility and mobility	Aerobic training (walking or hiking)	Resistance training, agility, flexibility and mobility	Sports (pickleball)	Resistance training, agility, flexibility and mobility	Aerobic training (swimming, biking, or rowing)	Physical activity (easy walk)
Time	60 min	30-45 min	60 min	45-60 min	60 min	30-60 min	30-45 min

Note: Meets recommendations for improving overall fitness, for frequency of muscle-strengthening activities, and for 150 min/wk of moderate-intensity aerobic activity.

Table 13.59   Intermediate Sample Program for Osteoporosis Care

Phase	Modality	Method and targeted areas	Sets × reps or time	Tempo
Warm-up	Power nasal breathing	Breathe in through the nose for 3-4 s, then out through nose for 6-8 s	1 × 4-5	—
Mobility	Foot release with a ball	Thighs, glutes, hamstrings, IT band, calves, anterior tibialis, adductors	1 × 45 s	—
	Foam rolling	Calves, hamstrings, IT band, quads, glutes, upper back, latissimus dorsi, chest	1 × 20 s each	2-3 s per 1 in. (3 cm) area
	Controlled articular rotation[a]	Ankle, hips, shoulder, scapula, wrist	1 × 4-5 each direction	6-10 s per revolution
Movement preparation	Movement pattern[b]	Squat, hip hinge, TRX row, elevated push-up	1 × 8-10	2-3 s/rep
Core activation	Supine single-leg brace	—	2 × 3-4	5-10 s/rep
Power, speed, agility, quickness	Ladder drill: Forward-forward, back-back	—	2 × 30 s	As fast as possible

Phase	Modality	Method and targeted areas	Sets × reps or time	Tempo
Conditioning	(1a) Low elevated push-up	—	2-3 × 8-10	—
	(1b) Split squat	—	2-3 × 8-10	—
	(1c) Falling start	—	2-3 × 4-5 / each leg	—
	(2a) Cable lat pull-down	—	2-3 × 10-12	—
	(2b) Side leg lift or side plank from knees	—	2-3 × 4-5	5-10 s/rep
	(2c) Staggered-stance hip bridge	—	2 × 30 s[c]	—
	(3a) Ball leg curl	—	2-3 × 10-12	—
	(3b) Bent-over T-rows	—	2-3 × 12-15	—
	(3c) Elevated plank	—	2-3 × 4-5[c]	—
Cool-down	Breathing	Recovery position	2-3 min	—

Note: IT = iliotibial.

[a]Hip and shoulder rotations should be done in a quadruped position, as tolerated by the knees.

[b]All movements should be done with the eyes closed.

[c]Each set is 30 s leading with the left leg, then 30 s leading with the left leg.

Advanced Program

Table 13.60 Advanced 7-Day Schedule for Osteoporosis Care

Day	Monday	Tuesday	Wednesday	Thursday	Friday	Saturday	Sunday
Exercise	Resistance training, agility, flexibility, mobility	Resistance training, agility, flexibility, mobility	Sports (e.g., pickleball) or other aerobic training	Resistance training, agility, flexibility, mobility	Resistance training, agility, flexibility, mobility	Aerobic training (swimming, biking, or rowing)	Physical activity (easy walk)
Time	60 min	60 min	45-60 min	60 min	60 min	30-60 min	30-45 min
Exercise	Easy walk	—	—	Hill walking	—	—	—
Time	20-45 min	—	—	15-20 min	—	—	—

Note: Meets recommendations for improving overall fitness, for frequency of muscle-strengthening activities, for 150 min/wk of moderate-intensity aerobic activity, and for 75 min/week of vigorous-intensity aerobic activity.

Table 13.61 Advanced Sample Program for Osteoporosis Care

Phase	Modality	Method and targeted areas	Sets × reps or time	Tempo
Warm-up	Power nasal breathing	Breathe in through the nose for 4-5 s, then out through the nose for 8-10 s	1 × 4-5	—
Mobility	Foot release with the ball	Thighs, glutes, hamstrings, IT band, calves, anterior tibialis, adductors	1 × 45 s	—
	Foam rolling	Calves, hamstrings, IT band, quads, glutes, upper back, latissimus dorsi, chest	1 × 20 s each	2-3 s per 1 in. (3 cm) area
	Controlled articular rotation	Ankle, hip, shoulder, scapula, wrist	1 × 4-5 in each direction	6-10 s per revolution
Movement preparation	Movement pattern	Split squat, staggered hip hinge, TRX row, low elevated push-up	1 × 9	• 3 super slow (10 s each) • 3 medium speed (3-5 s each) • 3 fast (as fast as possible)
Core activation	Bird dog hold	—	2 × 4-5	Hold each rep 10 s
Power, speed, agility, and quickness	Cognitive agility drills[a]: • Spelling ladder[b] • Counting catches • Colored cones	—	2 × 20-30 s	—
Conditioning: Days 1 and 3	(1a) Goblet squat	—	3 × 8-10	—
	(1b) Standing banded stallion	—	3 × 12-15	—
	(1c) Banded speed row	—	3 × 15-20 s	Fast in, slow out
	(1d) Single-arm medicine ball chest throw	—	3 × 6-8	Fast
	(2a) Power step-up	—	3 × 6-8	Fast
	(2b) 2:1 bodyweight hip thrust (both legs up for the concentric phase and one leg down for the eccentric phase)	—	3 × 6-8 each	3 s down
	(2c) Lat pull-down	—	3 × 10-12	3 s pause at bottom
	(2d) Incline dumbbell press	—	3 × 10-12	—

Phase	Modality	Method and tar-geted areas	Sets × reps or time	Tempo
Condition-ing: Days 2 and 4	(1a) Overhead medicine ball slam	—	3-4 × 30:30	—
	(1b) Medicine ball squat and throw	—	3-4 × 30:30	—
	(1c) Speed squat	—	3-4 × 30:30	—
	(1d) Dumbbell skier swing	—	3-4 × 30:30	20-45 min
	(2a) Seated hammy tan-trum	—	3-4 × 30:30	—
	(2b) Standing speed chest press with band	—	3-4 × 30:30	Fast out, controlled in
	(2c) In-place reverse lunge with knee drive (right leg)	—	3-4 × 30:30	—
	(2d) In-place reverse lunge with knee drive (left leg)	—	3-4 × 30:30	—
	(2e) Pallof pulse (right side)	—	3-4 × 30:30	—
	(2f) Pallof pulse (left side)	—	3-4 × 30:30	Rest 1-2 min between rounds
Cool-down	Breathing	Recovery position	2-3 min	—

Note: IT = iliotibial.

[a]Challenge and emphasize one of the four cognitive domains (memory, executive function, attention, or process-ing speed).

[b]The client spells out certain names, places, or things while moving through various ladder exercises.

Progressive Resistance Training for Inexperienced Clients With Overweight or Obesity

Michael Piercy, MS

There is robust evidence showing that resistance training is pivotal in managing obesity. In light of this, the most recent exercise-prescription guidelines for individuals with excess body weight and adiposity advise a minimum of two to three muscle-strengthen-ing sessions per week (American College of Sports Medicine 2021). It can be reasonably deduced that progressive resistance training represents a fundamental exercise strategy for inexperienced clients with overweight or obesity (tables 13.62-13.82). This training approach has been demonstrated to provide multiple psychophysiological benefits to clients with obesity. Hence, resistance training, as a fundamental component of every weight management program, promotes beneficial alterations in body composition, cardiometabolic health, physical function, and mental health (Lopez et al. 2022).

The Foundation (Weeks 1-4)

Foundation A

Table 13.62   Progressive Resistance Training Foundation A (Weeks 1-4): Warm-Up

No.	Exercises	Sets	Reps	Rest
1	Knee hugs	1	8-12	30 s
2	In-and-out steps	1	8-12	30 s
3	High knees	1	8-12	30 s
4	Side shuffle	1	8-12	30 s
5	Gate swings	1	8-12	60 s

Table 13.63   Progressive Resistance Training Foundation A (Weeks 1-4): Conditioning

No.	Exercises	Sets	Reps or time	Rest
1a	Bodyweight squat	2	10-12	60 s
1b	Full-tension plank	2	3-10 s	60 s
2a	Glute bridge	2	12-15	60 s
2b	Modified push-up	2	12-15	60 s
3a	Stability ball leg curl	2	12-15	60 s
3b	Dumbbell row	2	10-12	60 s
4a	Inverted row	2	8-10	60 s
4b	Banded Y-row	2	12-15	60 s

Table 13.64   Progressive Resistance Training Foundation A (Weeks 1-4): Cool-Down

No.	Exercises*	Sets	Time	Rest
1	Static stretching	1	15-30 s	—
2	Foam rolling (optional)	1	15-30 s	—

*Per body part.

Foundation B

Table 13.65   Progressive Resistance Training Foundation B (Weeks 1-4): Warm-Up

No.	Exercises	Sets	Reps	Rest
1	Step and reach	1	8-12	30 s
2	In-and-out step	1	8-12	30 s
3	Frankenstein walk	1	8-12	30 s
4	Butt kick	1	8-12	30 s
5	Carioca	1	8-12	60 s

Table 13.66   Progressive Resistance Training Foundation B (Weeks 1-4): Conditioning

No.	Exercises	Sets	Reps	Rest
1a	Split squat	2	10-12	60 s
1b	Plank with shoulder tap	2	10-12	60 s
2a	Glute bridge with march	2	12-15	60 s
2b	Band chest press	2	12-15	60 s
3a	Incline plank leg raises	2	12-15	60 s
3b	Two-arm band row	2	12-15	60 s
4a	Band rotation	2	10-12 per side	60 s
4b	Stability ball knee tuck	2	12-15	60 s

Table 13.67   Progressive Resistance Training Foundation B (Weeks 1-4): Cool-Down

No.	Exercises*	Sets	Time	Rest
1	Static stretching	1	15-30 s	—
2	Foam rolling (optional)	1	15-30 s	—

*Per body part.

Foundation C

Table 13.68   Progressive Resistance Training Foundation C (Weeks 1-4): Warm-Up

No.	Exercises	Sets	Reps	Rest
1	March in place	1	8-12	30 s
2	World's greatest stretch	1	8-12	30 s
3	Reverse lunge with overhead reach	1	8-12	30 s
4	Arm circles	1	8-12	30 s
5	Lateral lunge with arm reach	1	8-12	60 s

Table 13.69   Progressive Resistance Training Foundation C (Weeks 1-4): Conditioning

No.	Exercises	Sets	Reps or Time	Rest
1a	Bodyweight lunge	2	10-12	60 s
1b	Vertical chest press machine	2	10-12	60 s
2a	Lateral band walks	2	10-12	60 s
2b	Kettlebell sumo deadlift	2	10-12	60 s
3a	Stability ball kneeling roll-out	2	12-15	60 s
3b	Inverted row	2	8-10	60 s
4a	Modified side plank	2	3-10 s per side	60 s
4b	Kneeling dumbbell curl to press	2	10-12	60 s

Table 13.70   Progressive Resistance Training Foundation C (Weeks 1-4):
Cool-Down

No.	Exercises*	Sets	Time	Rest
1	Static stretching	1	15-30 s	—
2	Foam rolling (optional)	1	15-30 s	—

*Per body part

Intensity and Strength (Weeks 5-8)

Intensification A

Table 13.71   Progressive Resistance Training Intensification A (Weeks 5-8):
Warm-Up

No.	Exercises	Sets	Reps	Rest
1	Rotational arm swing	1	8-12	30 s
2	In-and-out step	1	8-12	30 s
3	Wall slide	1	8-12	30 s
4	Side-lying T-spine rotation	1	8-12	30 s
5	Low side-to-side lunge	1	8-12	60 s

Table 13.72   Progressive Resistance Training Intensification A (Weeks 5-8):
Conditioning

No.	Exercises	Sets	Reps or time	Rest
1a	Dumbbell goblet squat	3	10-12	60 s
1b	Suspended high row	3	12-15	60 s
1c	Kneeling plank on a foam roller	3	30 s	60 s
2a	Kettlebell swing	3	10-12	60 s
2b	Suspended chest press	3	12-15	60 s
2c	Side plank with reach through	3	10-12	60 s
3a	Medicine ball chop	3	10-12	60 s
3b	Lateral lunge curl press	3	10-12	60 s
3c	Suspended incline plank	3	30 s	60 s

Table 13.73 Progressive Resistance Training Intensification A (Weeks 5-8): Cool-Down

No.	Exercises*	Sets	Time	Rest
1	Static stretching	1	15-30 s	—
2	Foam rolling (optional)	1	15-30 s	—

*Per body part.

Intensification B

Table 13.74 Progressive Resistance Training Intensification B (Weeks 5-8): Warm-Up

No.	Exercises	Sets	Reps	Rest
1	Bent reach to sky	1	8-12	30 s
2	Lunge with side bend	1	8-12	30 s
3	Shoulder circles	1	8-12	30 s
4	Air hurdle	1	8-12	30 s
5	Sumo squat T-stand	1	8-12	60 s

Table 13.75 Progressive Resistance Training Intensification B (Weeks 5-8): Conditioning

No.	Exercises	Sets	Reps	Rest
1a	Bodyweight walking lunge	3	8-10	60 s
1b	Dumbbell row	3	10-12	60 s
1c	Stability ball circles	3	12-15	60 s
2a	Kettlebell deadlift	3	8-10	60 s
2b	High incline dumbbell bench press	3	8-10	60 s
2c	Suspended plank	3	12-15	60 s
3a	Band core rotation	3	10-12 per side	60 s
3b	Single-leg balance touchdown	3	8-10	60 s
3c	Modified side plank with band row	3	8-10 per side	60 s

Table 13.76   Progressive Resistance Training Intensification B (Weeks 5-8): Cool-Down

No.	Exercises*	Sets	Time	Rest
1	Static stretching	1	15-30 s	—
2	Foam rolling (optional)	1	15-30 s	—

*Per body part.

Intensification C

Table 13.77   Progressive Resistance Training Intensification C (Weeks 5-8): Warm-Up

No.	Exercises	Sets	Reps	Rest
1	Walking leg cradles	1	8-12	30 s
2	High-knee marching	1	8-12	30 s
3	Lateral step-over	1	8-12	30 s
4	Side-to-side leg swing	1	8-12	30 s
5	Forward leg swing	1	8-12	60 s

Table 13.78   Progressive Resistance Training Intensification C (Weeks 5-8): Conditioning

No.	Exercises	Sets	Reps or time	Rest
1a	Barbell back squat	3	8-10	60 s
1b	Incline chest press on a Smith machine	3	10-12	60 s
1c	Bear crawl isometric hold	3	3-10 s	60 s
2a	Ball slam	3	12-15	60 s
2b	Kettlebell sumo deadlift	3	10-12	60 s
2c	Band Y-flys	3	10-12	60 s
3a	Barbell front squat	3	8-10	60 s
3b	Backward lunge	3	10-12	60 s
3c	Bird dog	3	12-15	60 s

Table 13.79   Progressive Resistance Training Intensification C (Weeks 5-8): Cool-Down

No.	Exercises*	Sets	Time	Rest
1	Static stretching	1	15-30 s	—
2	Foam rolling (optional)	1	15-30 s	—

*Per body part.

Intensification D

Table 13.80 Progressive Resistance Training Intensification D (Weeks 5-8): Warm-Up

No.	Exercises	Sets	Reps	Rest
1	Groiner	1	8-12	30 s
2	Over-under gate	1	8-12	30 s
3	Hand crossover	1	8-12	30 s
4	Neck rotation	1	8-12	30 s
5	Over-under shoulder stretch	1	8-12	60 s

Table 13.81 Progressive Resistance Training Intensification D (Weeks 5-8): Conditioning

No.	Exercises	Sets	Reps	Rest
1a	Dumbbell ski swing	3	10-12	60 s
1b	Suspended row	3	10-12	60 s
1c	Band Pallof press	3	12-15 per side	60 s
2a	Skater	3	12-15	60 s
2b	Dumbbell reverse lunge curl press	3	10-12	60 s
2c	Push-up to renegade row	3	8-10	60 s
3a	Assisted pull-up	3	8-10	60 s
3b	Suspended standing plank	3	12-15	60 s
3c	Medicine ball rotational slam	3	10-12	60 s

Table 13.82 Progressive Resistance Training Intensification D (Weeks 5-8): Cool-Down

No.	Exercises*	Sets	Time	Rest
1	Static stretching	1	15-30 s	—
2	Foam rolling (optional)	1	15-30 s	—

*Per body part.

Training Older Clients With Obesity, Frailty, and Sarcopenia

Keli Roberts

Sarcopenic obesity (SO) may be defined as having both sarcopenia (age-related loss of muscle mass and either low muscular strength or low physical performance) and obesity. Individuals with SO are at greater risk for the development of frailty and disability (Bouchonville and Villareal 2013). The functional implications of obesity in older populations are significant, because it can exacerbate the age-related decline in physical functions and mobility. Functional capacity, particularly mobility, is diminished in older adults with overweight and obesity as compared to adults of normal weight (Stenholm et al. 2009). Thus, regular physical activity and exercise can play a vital role in managing and reversing SO and promoting major psychophysiological benefits among older adults with SO (Sorace et al. 2024). Table 13.83 offers a sample combined training program for individuals with frailty and sarcopenia.

Table 13.83 Combined Training Program for Frailty and Sarcopenia

Frequency	Initially: 2-3 d/wk	Progression: 3-4 d/wk	Workouts should be planned on nonconsecutive days
General warm-up Dynamic warm-up	50%-60% of HRmax Mobility exercises	5 min (RPE of 2-3 out of 10) 5 min	Cycling or walking Movement preparation
Resistance exercise 1	Initially: 50%-60% of 1-RM (OMNI-RES of 4-5 out of 10) Progression: 60%-70% of 1-RM (OMNI-RES of 5-6 out of 10)	1-2 sets × 12-15 reps (1-2 min rest/set) 3 sets × 8-12 reps (1-2 min rest/set)	Leg press Goblet squat
Resistance exercise 2	Initially: 50%-60% of 1-RM (OMNI-RES of 4-5 out of 10) Progression: 60%-70% of 1-RM (OMNI-RES of 5-6 out of 10)	1-2 sets × 12-15 reps (1-2 min rest/set) 3 sets × 8-12 reps (1-2 min rest/set)	Incline or seated chest press Standing cable chest press
Aerobic exercise	Initially: 50%-59% HRmax RPE of 3-4 out of 10 Progression: 60%-75% HRmax RPE of 5-6 out of 10	3 min (client can comfortably talk) 5 min (client cannot comfortably talk)	Stationary bike or treadmill walk Elliptical trainer or incline treadmill walk
Resistance exercise 3	Initially: 50%-60% of 1-RM (OMNI-RES of 4-5 out of 10) Progression: 60%-70% of 1-RM (OMNI-RES of 5-6 out of 10)	1-2 sets × 12-15 reps (1-2 min rest/set) 3 sets × 8-12 reps (1-2 min rest/set)	Step-up right and left or knee extension machine

Resistance exercise 4	Initially: 50%-60% of 1-RM (OMNI-RES of 4-5 out of 10) Progression: 60%-70% of 1-RM (OMNI-RES of 5-6 out of 10)	1-2 sets × 12-15 reps (1-2 min rest/set) 3 sets × 8-12 reps (1-2 min rest/set)	Standing shoulder press or seated machine shoulder press
Aerobic exercise	Initially: 50%-59% HRmax RPE of 3-4 out of 10 Progression: 60%-75% HRmax RPE of 5-6 out of 10	3 min (client can comfortably talk) 5 min (client cannot comfortably talk)	Stationary bike or treadmill walk Elliptical trainer or incline treadmill walk
Resistance exercise 5	Initially: 50%-60% of 1-RM (OMNI-RES of 4-5 out of 10) Progression: 60%-70% of 1-RM (OMNI-RES of 5-6 out of 10)	1-2 sets × 12-15 reps (1-2 min rest/set) 3 sets × 8-12 reps (1-2 min rest/set)	Hip hinge or deadlift with a kettlebell or dumbbells, or hamstring curl machine
Resistance exercise 6	Initially: 50%-60% of 1-RM (OMNI-RES of 4-5 out of 10) Progression: 60%-70% of 1-RM (OMNI-RES of 5-6 out of 10)	1-2 sets × 12-15 reps (1-2 min rest/set) 3 sets × 8-12 reps (1-2 min rest/set)	Seated row or standing bilateral cable row
Aerobic exercise	Initially: 50%-59% HRmax RPE of 3-4 out of 10 Progression: 60%-75% HRmax RPE of 5-6 out of 10	3 min (client can comfortably talk) 5 min (client cannot comfortably talk)	Stationary bike or treadmill walk Elliptical trainer or incline treadmill walk
Core training	Initially: 1-2 sets × 8-12 reps (20-30 s) Progression: 2-3 sets × 12-15 reps (30-60 s)	Work-to-rest ratio: 1:2 1:1	Kneeling plank, side plank, and Pallof press Plank, side plank, and standing Pallof press
Flexibility training	Static stretching (passive and active)	3-5 min (hold stretches for 15-30 s)	All major muscle groups and overactive areas
Cool-down	SMR and diaphragmatic breathing	3-5 min	Foam rolling on stiff and overactive muscles

Notes:
• Warm-up: Pain-free dynamic stretching exercises for stability and mobility should be used.
• Aerobic training: Start with non-weight-bearing movements, such as cycling, before progressing to walking. Swimming or water-based exercise also offers good non-weight-bearing options.
• Resistance training: Progress to free weights and cables in weight-bearing positions to emphasize balance, gait, and functional movements.
• Flexibility training: Stretch to the point of tightness or slight discomfort.
• Cool-down: Foam rolling may be avoided in case of extreme pain or low intolerance.

1-RM = 1-repetition maximum; OMNI-RES = OMNI resistance exercise scale of perceived exertion; RPE = rating of perceived exertion; SMR = self-myofascial release.

Seated Core Foundation for Clients With Overweight or Obesity

Grace DeSimone, BA

The exercises in this workout are influenced by Pilates and yoga and are designed to develop muscular endurance, flexibility, coordination, balance, improved posture, and body awareness with a special emphasis on the core. Learning these techniques will enhance the mind–body connection, increasing the participant's functionality and confidence. This workout can be done up to three times a week as tolerated.

Setup
Use a sturdy chair without arms that allows the hips and knees to flex at approximately a 90° angle. The client should let their body be their guide for comfort. Similar to adjusting a car seat to one's preferences, creating the best seating environment for exercise will lead to the best outcomes. Participants with longer limbs may want to use yoga blocks or books on the chair seat to adapt to comfortable hip and knee angles. Participants with shorter limbs may prefer to use yoga blocks or books on the floor to elevate their feet. Ideally, sitting with the feet hip-width apart is suggested, but participants may adjust to a wider stance for stability and comfort as needed.

Posture and Breath Work

Primary Muscles Worked
- Trunk
- Hip
- Leg stabilizers

Note that these postural muscles will always be working while performing the seated exercises described in this workout.

Instructions
1. Sit in the center of the seat with the feet firmly planted on the floor.
2. Lengthen the spine to sit tall. Aim for good posture by keeping the spine from touching the back of the chair.
3. Using a finger, gently press the chin back to avoid a forward neck posture.
4. Press the shoulder blades together to prevent rounding the upper back.
5. Avoid shrugging the shoulders.
6. Maintain a natural curve in the lower back. This is known as neutral spine and is unique to each individual. Avoid flattening or rounding the back.
7. Inhale for a count of five. While inhaling, feel the sides of the body expand.
8. Exhale for a count of five, and feel the sides of the body coming to a rest. Imagine the belly deflating like a balloon.
9. Repeat 3 to 5 rounds of breathing, maintaining postural awareness.

Variations

- A rolled towel can be placed against the small of the back to assist in maintaining a neutral spine.
- Participants may progress to standing with the knees slightly flexed.

Coaching Cues

- The participant should sit *on* the chair, not *in* the chair. Encourage them to sit upon the chair while imagining a string at the top of their head, lifting and lengthening their torso and spine.
- All exercises referenced in this workout begin in good posture, as described in steps 1 to 6.

Cat–Cow

Primary Muscles Worked

- Spinal flexors
- Extensors

Instructions

1. Place the hands on the thighs, inhale, and gently lean forward while casting the gaze up, allowing the spine to arch and lengthen.
2. Pause for a moment.
3. Exhale and round the back while casting the gaze down.
4. Repeat, lengthening (extending) the spine and rounding (flexing) the spine, four to five times or as comfort permits.

Variations

- To reduce the intensity, minimize the ROM.
- To increase the intensity, stand facing a chair, with the hands on the chair seat, the knees slightly flexed, and the spine in a neutral position.

Coaching Cues

- During the inhale, keep the tail and eyes up; during the exhale, keep the tail and eyes down.
- Feel the spine articulating one vertebra at a time without pain or discomfort. If discomfort occurs, accommodate the movement pattern and maintain a comfortable ROM.
- Avoid overstretching at each end point.

Spinal Twist

Primary Muscles Worked
- Spinal rotators

Instructions
1. Sit sideways at the edge of a chair, with the left side close to the chair's back.
2. Turn to the left and bring the left hand to the back of the chair, allowing the spine to twist.
3. If preferred, keep the right hand on the right thigh for leverage or bring the right hand to the back of the chair as well. This will be a personal choice, based on comfort and flexibility.
4. When a comfortable end point on the twist has been reached, look over the left shoulder and inhale, feeling the sides of the body expand. Then exhale, relaxing the ribs.
5. Unwind and return to the start position.
6. Complete 5 repetitions, then switch sides.

Variation
- To increase the intensity of the rotation, turn further to look behind the body.

Coaching Cues
- Find a rhythm with your breath and the twist—inhale and twist, exhale to relax into the stretch, inhale to return to start, and exhale to finish the movement.
- With each repetition, feel the body surrendering to the stretch. Allow this to happen organically, without straining or jerking movements.

Side Stretch

Primary Muscles Worked
- Spinal lateral flexors
- Extensors

Instructions
1. Brace the left hand on the right thigh (or hold the side of the chair for support).
2. Inhale and raise the right arm.
3. Exhale and reach the right arm to the left, stretching sideways. Keep both buttocks on the seat.
4. Hold the side stretch for a count of three.
5. Return to the start position.
6. Repeat three to five times, then switch sides.

Variation
- Side stretching can be performed with the torso only. Hold on to the bottom of the seat and stretch to the side.

Coaching Cues

- Keep both feet firmly planted on the floor.
- Avoid overreaching.

Towel Squeeze

Primary Muscles Worked

- Hip adductors
- Pelvic floor

Instructions

1. Place a rolled towel (or a small pillow or Pilates ball) between the legs.
2. Align the knees over the feet and inhale.
3. Exhale and squeeze the towel while imagining stopping the flow of urine. (Do not practice this exercise while urinating.) Hold for a count of three, then release the squeeze.
4. Complete a total of 10 repetitions.

Variation

- Imagine squeezing a towel or ball without the tactile use of a prop.

Coaching Cues

- When inhaling, imagine the breath descending into the pelvis; when exhaling, imagine the breath floating away from the pelvis.

Deep Abdominal Work

Primary Muscles Worked

- Transversus abdominis

Instructions

1. Sit with good posture and with a hand over the belly.
2. Cough a few times.
3. Feel the belly forcefully move toward the spine. This is a contraction of the deep abdominal muscles that provide core strength and spinal support. Coughing or forcefully exhaling (e.g., as if blowing out a candle) helps to access these muscles.
4. Try to replicate the muscle contraction without coughing—just exhale and pull the navel to the spine.
5. Hold for a count of three, then relax.
6. Repeat 10 times.

Coaching Cues

- It will take time to learn to contract these muscles on demand.
- Think of pressing the navel to the spine like a plunger.

Heel Raises With Arm Press

Primary Muscles Worked

- Shoulder flexor
- Plantar flexor

Instructions

1. Inhale
2. Exhale and raise the right heel while pressing the left arm forward. Hold for a count of three. Switch sides.
3. Complete 10 repetitions (5 per leg).

Variation

- Progress the movement to lift the heel off the floor in a slow-motion march.

Coaching Cues

- Press the arms forward with resistance, as if moving through water.
- Lift the heel as if it were stuck to the floor.

Training Clients With Obesity and Postural Instability

John Bauer

Loaded locomotion is about traveling from one place to another while experiencing some sort of external resistance (i.e., holding a weight or pushing a sled). Such a training approach is beneficial for people with excess weight from a functional perspective because it is useful in everyday life to have the strength, endurance, stability, and postural control to be able to carry or move heavy things from one place to another. Also, these exercises stimulate most, if not all, of the major muscle groups necessary for activities of daily living, resulting in higher body functionality and quality of life among individuals with an unhealthy weight. More importantly, these exercises do not require high levels of skill, and thus, persons with obesity can experience the benefits right away, even if they have poor functional capacity and physical limitations. Loaded locomotion as a part of a workout can improve posture, grip strength, core strength, full-body strength, aerobic capacity, and caloric expenditure. Tables 13.84 to 13.86 offer sample postural instability programming.

Table 13.84 Postural Instability Sample Program

Training parameters		Notes
Frequency	Twice per week	There may be additional workouts in the week, but these two refer to those including loaded locomotion
Intensity	OMNI-RES of 6-8 out of 10	Moderate to vigorous intensity, with borderline discomfort and some heavy breathing
Time	60 min	—
Equipment type	—	Dumbbells or kettlebells, a sled that can be pushed and pulled, a cable machine, or bands

Note: OMNI-RES = OMNI resistance exercise scale of perceived exertion.

Table 13.85   Training Session 1: Carries With Upper-Body Push or Pull

WARM-UP PHASE	
General	5-10 min
Exercises	Walking, jogging, cycling, elliptical machine, stair stepper, or basic calisthenics
Dynamic	5-10 min
Exercises	Circular joint rotations, including movement of the wrists, shoulders, trunk, hips, knees, and ankles

CONDITIONING PHASE				
Exercise	**Sets**	**Reps or time**	**Load or intensity**	**Rest**
Loaded marching	1-4	20-30 s	OMNI-RES of 6-8	60-90 s
Farmer's carry	1-4	20-30 s	OMNI-RES of 6-8	60-90 s
Standing cable row	1-4	10-15	OMNI-RES of 6-8	60-90 s
Suitcase carry	1-2 each arm	20-30 s	OMNI-RES of 6-8	60-90 s
Standing cable press	1-4	10-15	OMNI-RES of 6-8	60-90 s

COOL-DOWN PHASE	
Time	5-10 min
Sets	1-2 sets of 30 s for each stretch
Stretches	Pecs, lats, hip flexors, glutes, hamstrings, and thoracic spine

Note: OMNI-RES = OMNI resistance exercise scale of perceived exertion, on a scale of 0 to 10.

Table 13.86   Training Session 2: Sled Push and Pull, Hinging, and Overhead Press

WARM-UP PHASE	
General	5-10 min
Exercises	Walking, jogging, cycling, elliptical machine, stair stepper, or basic calisthenics
Dynamic	5-10 min
Exercises	Circular joint rotations including movement of the wrists, shoulders, trunk, hips, knees, and ankles

CONDITIONING PHASE				
Exercise	**Sets**	**Reps or time**	**Load or intensity**	**Rest**
Overhead loaded marching	1-4	20-30 s	OMNI-RES of 6-8	60-90 s
Sled push	1-4	20-30 s	OMNI-RES of 6-8	60-90 s
Dumbbell RDL	1-4	10-15	OMNI-RES of 6-8	60-90 s
Sled pull	1-4	20-30 s	OMNI-RES of 6-8	60-90 s
Standing dumbbell overhead press	1-4	10-15	OMNI-RES of 6-8	60-90 s

(continued)

Table 13.86   Training Session 2: Sled Push and Pull, Hinging, and Overhead Press *(continued)*

COOL-DOWN PHASE	
Time	5-10 min
Sets	1-2 sets of 30 s for each stretch
Stretches	Pecs, lats, hip flexors, glutes, hamstrings, and thoracic spine

Note: RDL = Romanian deadlift; OMNI-RES = OMNI resistance exercise scale of perceived exertion, on a scale of 1 to 10.

Step Aerobics Workout for Clients With Obesity

Lauren Korzan, MA

Step aerobics has become increasingly popular in the fitness industry and weight loss programs since the 1990s (Olson et al. 1991). In recent years, group dance fitness programs have retained their appeal on a global scale for those engaged in physical exercise (Newsome et al. 2024). A step aerobics program is a combination of low-impact aerobic dance moves and step aerobics, aiming to improve cardiorespiratory fitness and body composition (Scharff-Olson et al. 1996). The choreography is repeated several times to music and uses different movements in an appropriate sequence (American College of Sports Medicine 2023). The present program is appropriate for most clients with excess body weight or obesity, provided that the necessary training considerations, safety concerns, and appropriate communication strategies are taken into account. Research shows that aerobic bench step exercises provide sufficient cardiorespiratory demand to increase aerobic fitness, improve physical fitness and functional capacity, and promote weight loss in sedentary women who are middle-aged or older and have overweight or obesity (Arslan 2011; Hallage et al. 2010; Olson et al. 1991; Sáez de Villarreal et al. 2023). The present workout offers an inclusive, group-based step aerobics class designed for clients with excess weight, intending to promote exercise engagement in a group fitness setting.

Class format: Step aerobics
Total time: 45 minutes
Equipment: Steps and risers
Goal: To improve participants' cardiovascular fitness through easy-to-follow step patterns set to upbeat music.
Music: Select music that is upbeat (118 to 128 beats per minute) with positive or motivational lyrics or with no lyrics. Use 32-count phrased music that syncs with the movement patterns.

Considerations and Safety Concerns

Provide modifications to allow participants to progress or regress in the movements as needed. Progressions include adding arm movements at chest level or above the head and adding propulsion to movements. Regressions include performing movements on the floor instead of the step and reducing the ROM (e.g., tap the step instead of lifting the knee, or keep the arms by the sides instead of performing bigger arm movements). Avoid using the terms *beginner* and *advanced* when showing different modifications to the step patterns. Instead, let participants choose the option that works best for them that day. In addition, note the following safety tips:

- Before class begins, make sure the room temperature is between 68 °F and 72 °F (20 °C and 22 °C) to prevent participants from becoming overheated.
- Check the pads on the bottom of the steps and risers to ensure they are free of dust and dirt, which will help prevent them from slipping.
- To prevent injury, instruct participants to place the whole foot on the step and make sure the heel does not hang off the back or the toes off the front.
- Include breaks between step patterns for participants to drink water and monitor their exercise intensity. For deconditioned participants, have them work at a moderate intensity, which can be easily monitored by rating of perceived exertion (RPE) or the talk test. On a 1-10 RPE scale, they should work between levels 3 and 5. If using the talk test, participants should be able to talk, but not sing, while exercising. As participants' aerobic fitness improves, they can progress to more vigorous intensities.
- Beginners should start with a 4 in. (10 cm) step (the height of the step platform) and can add 2 in. (5 cm) step risers as they become more conditioned and comfortable using the step. New or beginner participants can begin by performing the movements on the floor if they do not yet feel comfortable using the step.

Promote Inclusivity

It is important that everyone feels welcome and included in the class. This can be accomplished by arriving early and greeting each person as they enter the room. Also consider doing the following:

- Introduce yourself to new participants and learn their names.
- Let participants know that you are available to answer questions after class.
- Encourage social interaction before and after class. Making social connections in a group fitness class can help participants make exercise an enjoyable lifestyle habit as opposed to an unpleasant obligation.

Communication Strategies

Use positive messages that focus not on weight but on the benefits of exercise, such as having more energy and improved sleep. Also consider the following strategies:

- Encourage participants on their health journey. An example of this would be saying, "I noticed that you added arm movements to the step patterns this week. That's a great way to challenge yourself. Way to go!"
- When possible, face the participants during class instead of teaching with your back to them. This allows eye contact with participants, which can be encouraging and create a friendlier interaction with them.

Class Components

Here is the basic framework for structuring a full workout.

Warm-Up (10 Minutes)

Begin the warm-up with easy movements on the floor that start to increase the heart rate, followed by basic movements on the step that allow participants to rehearse the upcoming step patterns.

Conditioning (25 Minutes)

The conditioning phase of the workout will be performed on the step. The step patterns progress from basic to more complex and use repetition to help participants learn the movements. Once participants learn the three step patterns, have them perform all three patterns in a row as a finale. Each step pattern is 32 counts and self-reversing (performed with the right foot leading and then the left foot leading).

Cool-Down and Stretch (10 Minutes)

Begin the cool-down with easy movements on the floor, followed by the following standing static stretches for the lower body. Perform each stretch on the right and left sides. Hold stretches for 20 to 30 seconds and repeat as needed. If time allows, stretches for the upper body can also be included.

- *Hamstrings:* Place one heel on the step and hinge forward from the hips.
- *Calves:* Stand on top of the step and drop one heel off the back of the step.
- *Quadriceps:* Standing on the floor, go into a lunge position and tuck the back hip forward while keeping the front knee over the ankle.

Table 13.87 includes a sample step aerobics workout.

Table 13.87 Step Aerobics Sample Workout

Phase	Modality	Method	Reps*	Time
Warm-up	Dynamic movements	Increase heart rate while rehearsing step patterns	—	10 min
		Step touches on the floor	16	
		Hamstring curls on the floor	16	
		Basic step right	8	
		Basic step left	8	
		Knee ups	8	
		Hamstring curls	8	
		Repeat above movements	—	
		Toe taps on the step	16	
		Heel taps on the step	16	

Phase	Modality	Method	Reps*	Time
Condi-tioning	Step patterns, progressing from basic to complex	Learn three step patterns, then perform all three patterns in a row as a finale	32 counts per pattern; lead with right foot, then switch to lead with left foot	25 min
	Pattern A	Basic step	2	
		V-step	2 (8)	
		Knee up	2 (8)	
		3-count repeater knee	(8)	
	Pattern B	March on top of the step	4 (4)	
		March on the floor	4 (4)	
		L-step	2 (16)	
		Rocking horse	(8)	
	Pattern C	Rear lift, facing the front of the room	2 (8)	
		Turn step	2 (8)	
		Over the top	2 (8)	
		3-count repeater side leg lift	(8)	
Cool-down and stretch	Easy movements on the floor	Lower body If time allows, stretches for the upper body	—	10 min
		Step touch on the floor	16	
		Toe taps on the step	16	
		Heel taps on the step	16	
	Standing static stretches	Hamstrings	—	
		Calves	—	
		Quadriceps	—	

*The counts for each part of the pattern are in parentheses.

Yoga Workout for Clients With Obesity

Vula Bolou

An adapted Iyengar yoga program for people with excess weight aims to increase body awareness and coordination and build muscular strength and mobility while lowering stress levels, resulting in overall health enhancement (Iyengar 2001). The workouts can be applied under the supervision of a senior Iyengar yoga teacher within various exercise settings (i.e., gym, studio, or home) and formats (i.e., personal training or small group training) (Iyengar 2007).

In general, yoga practice has been documented as a feasible, effective, and injury-free mind–body fitness modality inducing beneficial psychophysiological alterations in adults with overweight or obesity (Batrakoulis 2022). Yoga incorporates a meditative component for identifying dysfunctional perception and cognition to reduce any pain while discovering inner peace and salvation. Such adaptations are critical for people with the physical limitations, poor body functionality, and impaired mental health commonly observed among individuals with overweight or obesity (Batrakoulis 2023).

Beginner

Begin with a 30-minute workout following the basic structure provided in table 13.88 and then progress to tables 13.89 and 13.90 as clients become more proficient.

Table 13.88   Beginner Yoga Workout (Duration: 30 min)

Pose	Mode	Time
Easy pose or simple sitting on chair	Right and left crossing of legs	1 min each side
Easy pose with upward bound hands pose	Crossing of fingers, both hands	30 s each
Easy pose with twist	Right and left	30 s each side
Bound-angle pose	—	1 min
Wide-angle seated forward bend	—	1 min
Half downward facing dog	Hands on the back of a chair or on top of a table	1 min × 2
Supported standing forward bend	Forehead on forearms on the back of a chair or on top of a table	1 min × 2
Mountain pose	—	1 min
Mountain pose with upward-bound hands pose	Crossing of fingers, both hands	30 s each
Extended triangle pose	Right and left	30 s each side
Warrior pose II	Right and left	30 s each side
Extended side angle pose	Right and left	30 s each side
Wide-legged standing forward bend I	—	1 min
Wind-relieving pose	On the floor, or on a bench if unable to lie down	1 min
Four feet pose	On the floor, or on a bench if unable to lie down	30 s × 2
Relaxation pose	Blanket for the head and a bolster under the knees	3 min

Intermediate

Progress is made by the different use of props: less in some cases so the effort is increased and more in others, where new asanas are introduced or greater mobility is required. Also, by staying in the asana longer, the practitioner improves their stamina.

Table 13.89 Intermediate Yoga Workout (Duration: 45 min)

Pose	Mode	Time
Easy pose	Legs crossed or simple sitting on a chair	1 min each side
Easy pose with upward bound hands pose	Crossing of fingers, both hands	30 s each
Easy pose twist	Right and left	30 s each side
Hero pose	—	1 min
Hero pose with upward bound hands pose	Crossing of fingers, both hands	30 s each
Hero pose twist	Right and left	30 s each side
Half downward facing dog pose	Hands on the seat of a chair	1 min × 2
Half upward facing dog pose	Hands on the seat of a chair	1 min × 2
Supported standing forward bend	Forehead on forearms on the seat of a chair or a bolster on the seat of a chair	1 min
Mountain pose	—	1 min
Mountain pose with upward bound hands pose	Crossing of fingers, both hands	30 s each
Extended triangle pose	Right and left	30 s each side
Half moon pose	Elbow or hand on a chair, right and left	30 s each side
Extended side angle pose	Right and left	30 s each side
Revolved triangle pose	Hand on the seat of a chair or yoga brick, right and left	30 s each side
Wide-legged standing forward bend I	—	1 min
Inverted staff pose with chair	—	1 min
Seated chair twist	Right and left	30 s each side
Four feet pose	On the floor, or a bench if unable to lie down	30 s × 2
Supported bridge pose	On brick or blocks	3 min
Inverted relaxation pose	Hips on a bolster against a wall	3 min
Relaxation pose	Blanket for the head and a bolster under the knees	4 min

Advanced

Progress is made by gradually longer stays in the inversions, which will invariably contribute to the reduction of stress hormones.

Table 13.90   Advanced Yoga Workout (Duration: 60 min)

Pose	Mode	Time
Easy pose	Legs crossed or simple sitting on chair	1 min each side
Easy pose with upward bound hands pose	Crossing of fingers, both hands	30 s each
Easy pose twist	Right and left	30 s each side
Supported standing forward bend	Forehead on forearms on the seat of a chair or a bolster on the seat of a chair	1 min × 2
Standing forward bend	—	1 min
Downward facing dog pose	—	1 min × 2
Mountain pose	—	1 min
Mountain pose with upward bound hands pose	Crossing of fingers, both hands	30 s each
Mountain pose with cow face arms	—	30 s each side
Extended triangle pose	Right and left	30 s each side
Half moon pose	Elbow on a chair, right and left	30 s each side
Extended side angle pose	Right and left	30 s each side
Standing forward bend	—	1 min
Warrior pose I	Right and left	30 s each side
Warrior pose III	Right and left	20 s each side
Wide-legged standing forward bend I	—	2 min
Half handstand	Feet on a wall or ledge	20 s × 2
Inverted staff pose with chair	—	2 min
Supported shoulder stand	—	3 min
Supported plow pose	—	1 min
Revolved abdomen pose	Right and left	30 s each side × 2
Full boat pose	—	30 s
Half boat pose	—	30 s
Supported bridge pose	On a brick or blocks	4 min
Inverted relaxation pose	Hips on a bolster against a wall	4 min
Relaxation pose	Blanket for the head and a bolster under the knees	5 min

Training Preadolescents With Obesity

Brett Klika, BS

The prevalence of obesity in children and adolescents is increasing at an alarming rate on a global scale (Zhang et al. 2024). It is recommended that exercise programs for preadolescents with overweight or obesity be designed with the specific intention of enhancing both health- and skill-related fitness components (American College of Sports Medicine 2021). A well-designed youth fitness program should include activities focusing on different movement patterns and motor skills. In addition, age-appropriate muscle-strengthening drills and creative activities should be included. Finally, play-oriented fitness games and activities can be implemented to improve movement skills and elevate cardiorespiratory fitness among preadolescents with excess body weight or adiposity (Faigenbaum et al. 2011). The implementation of such an exercise strategy has been observed to facilitate the engagement and efficacy of training among previously inactive youth populations. The concept of fun is a significant motivator for engaging children and adolescents in regular physical activity through inclusive and recreational movement-based programs (Dishman et al. 2005).

Balloon Volleyball

Target age group: 8- to 12-year-olds
Duration: 60 minutes
Level: Beginner

Equipment Needed
- One balloon for every three children
- Cones or markers to establish space

Instant Activity (5 Minutes)
This is an activity the children can do as they arrive to the training center to get them engaged immediately.

Instructions
1. Children are arranged randomly throughout a small space.
2. The coach hits one or more balloons into the air and instructs the participants to keep the balloons in the air and avoid letting them contact the floor.

Warm-Up (10 Minutes)
Creative Discovery (3-4 Minutes)
Creative discovery allows children to move in different and novel ways. The movement prompts should be familiar for beginners, progressing to more abstract and creative prompts as they advance.

Movement Words (1 Minute)

Begin by calling out a movement-based word, and have the children do that movement for about 10 seconds.

1. Reach
2. March
3. Jump
4. Skip
5. Shuffle
6. Jog

Movement Sentences (2-3 Minutes)

Once children can respond to individual movement words, put two or three of these words together and have the children transition from one movement to another, repeating for 10 seconds.

1. Reach, march, jump (repeat for 10 s)
2. Skip, shuffle, jog (repeat for 10 s)
3. Jog, jump, reach (repeat for 10 s)
4. Shuffle, march, jog (repeat for 10 s)

General Guided Discovery

Provide just enough instruction for the children to understand how to perform the movement and what the added variable looks like.

Movement Variables (5 Minutes)

Start by having the children perform a fundamental movement skill for 5 seconds. After that, add a movement variable to that movement.

1. Run (5 s), loud feet (5 s), soft feet (5 s), run (5 s)
2. Jump (5 s), fast (5 s), slow (5 s), jump (5 s)
3. Squat (5 s), while moving (5 s), one leg (5 s each leg), squat (5 s)
4. Lateral shuffle (5 s), feet close together (5 s), feet far apart (5 s), lateral shuffle (5 s)

Specific Guided Discovery for Skip (2 Minutes)

This simple activity familiarizes the children with the anatomy, coaching cues, and other prompts that will be used when instructing them how to perform the movement.

Simon Says:

- Weight on your heels
- Weight on your toes
- Weight on the ball of your foot
- Step hop in place, right knee up
- Step hop in place, left knee up
- Step hop in place, right knee up, right arm up
- Step hop in place, left knee up, left arm up
- Step hop in place, right knee up, left arm up
- Step hop in place, left knee up, right arm up

Movement Skill of the Day: Skipping (10 Minutes)

These activities, drills, and games aid in developing and practicing the specific movement skills of the day.

Moon Marches

1. Create a grid 20 to 30 yd (18-27 m) across.
2. Have the children line up shoulder to shoulder, with space between them.
3. Instruct them to skip across the grid.
4. As they skip, prompt them with *high gravity*, in which they skip low to the ground, and *low gravity*, where they focus on a high knee drive, bringing their body up off the ground.
5. Repeat.

Gear Runs (Use Skipping)

1. Instruct the children to line up at one end of the given space.
2. Explain how the movement has different speeds, or "gears."
3. Tell them they are a sports car with four gears.
4. First gear is slow (walk), second gear is half speed (jog), third gear is three-quarter speed (run), and fourth gear is full speed (sprint).
5. With the children starting at one end of the given space, call out progressive gear shifts as they move across.
6. Provide feedback if they are moving at the incorrect relative speed.

Fundamental Movement Skill Application (10 Minutes)

These drills and activities help develop a wide variety of movement skills involved with sports and other physical activities.

Partner Mirror Drill (20 Seconds for Each Partner; Each Partner Takes 2 Turns)

1. Have each child partner with another child or the instructor.
2. Choose one partner as the leader.
3. Instruct the partners to face each other, about 6 ft (2 m) apart.
4. The leader begins to perform movements in any direction.
5. The mirroring partner attempts to mirror the direction changes as quickly as possible.
6. Continue for an allotted time (20-30 s).
7. Encourage children to use a variety of movements.

Partner Tracking Tag (20 Seconds for Each Partner; Each Partner Takes 2 Turns)

1. Have each child partner with another child or the instructor.
2. One partner stands behind the other.
3. The partner in front stares straight ahead.
4. The partner behind lifts either hand on different sides of the body at different levels in their partner's periphery.
5. The first partner must turn their head to seek, then track the hands being raised behind them and attempt to tag their partner's hand with their own hand on the same side of their body.
6. Repeat for an allotted amount of time (20-30 s), then have the children switch partners.

Conditioning Circuit (10 Minutes)

These fundamental movement skill circuits develop strength and coordination.

Each station: 30 seconds

Transition: 10 seconds

Repetitions: 3-4 times through the circuit

Station 1: Alternating Lunges

Station 2: Single-Leg Balance Reach

Balancing on one leg, children are instructed to reach forward as far as possible without losing balance and placing the other foot on the ground.

Station 3: Push-Up

Station 4: Prone Extensions (Superman)

Perceptual Motor and Fundamental Movement Skill Game (10 Minutes)

These activities gamify the practice and development of movement skill in addition to improving aerobic fitness and strength.

Story Stop and Go

1. Have the children line up at one end of a 20 to 30 yd (18-27 m) grid, facing the other end.
2. Similar to the game of red light, green light, the children move and stop based on verbal cues.
3. In this version of the game, the instructor tells a story. Children are instructed to go or stop based on either certain words or the beginning letters in words. For example, if the word *red* is used in the story, that may mean *go*. If the word *blue* is used, it may mean *stop*. Alternatively, any word that starts with *R* could signify *go*, and any word starting with *B* could signify *stop*.
4. Similar to the game of red light, green light, any improper movement results in a return to the start.

Cool-Down and Self-Regulation (5 Minutes)

While standard stretching and flexibility exercises are effective for a cool-down, developing deep breathing and other self-regulation strategies can aid in returning parasympathetic tone as well.

Cone Breathing

1. Have the children lie on their backs, placing a cone on their navel.
2. Instruct the children to breathe in to fill their belly with air.
3. They will see the cone rise and fall if performed correctly.

Note: Time intervals include transitions and instruction.

CHAPTER 14

Case Study Scenarios

After completing this chapter, you will be able to

- interpret theory into practice through real-world cases, focusing on the needs and priorities of clients with overweight or obesity and considering their impaired psychophysiological profile;
- summarize the scientific knowledge and practice-oriented information obtained throughout the textbook and manage specific considerations for individuals with excess weight; and
- relate success stories that have emerged from the field to describe how to overcome common exercise barriers associated with obesity.

Obesity is a complex, multifactorial condition that requires a personalized, holistic approach to treatment and management. This chapter offers a large variety of case studies as a valuable resource for exercise professionals to better understand and communicate with clients who have obesity. By tailoring the exercise approach, communication style, and treatment plan to a client's unique psychophysiological preferences, exercise professionals can create a more personalized and effective obesity care experience in a real-world fitness setting. Exploring the case studies presented in this chapter and integrating science-based and practice-oriented information into obesity management can lead to improved client outcomes; stronger relationships between exercise professionals and clients; and more holistic, client-centered care.

The chapter presents practical solutions for eight real-world examples and four weight-management stories from the field of obesity management. The benefits of applying these solutions include the following:

- Improved client engagement and adherence to a treatment plan
- Increased client satisfaction and trust in the exercise professional
- Better alignment between the client's needs and the exercise professional's approach
- Optimization of communication and shared decision-making
- An understanding of actual cases involving clients with excess body weight or adiposity

REAL-WORLD EXAMPLES

Coaching Clients After Bariatric Surgery

Tracy L. Markley

Thirty-one years ago, a 39-year-old woman weighing 354 lb (161 kg) had bariatric surgery. It was 1992. She came to me for training a couple of years after her surgery. She described her eating portion size by sharing with me that she could eat three bites of a slice of pizza, and she was full; also, if she ate a 2.5 oz (70.9 g) Tootsie Roll candy, it filled her up. She also stated that it took her about 20 minutes to eat each of those items. After training with me for about 6 months, she began to have surgeries to remove excess skin. I was highly concerned for her when she told me she was going to have surgery once a week until she was all done with removing extra skin from her body. I am not a doctor, but I knew that a person being put under anesthesia once a week, with the physical trauma, fatigue, and healing that comes with and follows each surgery, was dangerous. Her body would not be recovered from the previous surgery when she proceeded to the next surgery, and it would take a dangerous toll on her. She said that she and her doctor shared the same religion, so she trusted that the doctor knew what she was doing. After the first three surgeries, my client almost died. She then stretched her surgeries out.

The Coaching Concept

The key points of my coaching strategy were as follows:

- Always be sure that the bariatric surgeon clears the patient or client for any exercise program.
- All patients undergoing bariatric surgery are recommended to avoid exercises that put strain on the abdomen for at least 6 to 12 weeks after their surgery. They should avoid lifting weights and engaging in abdominal exercises for at least 6 to 12 weeks. The surgery site and incisions need to heal. Following these guidelines will also help the client to avoid abdominal hernias near incisions and other complications.
- Low-impact exercise, such as walking, in the first several weeks as the body is healing from surgery is recommended if the surgeon has cleared the client to do so. Studies suggest getting between 10 and 30 minutes of such exercise a day. The client must only do what works for them and what their surgeon told them for their care. Each client is different.
- Very light weights may be used in exercise programs if the surgeon approves the individual to do so. Otherwise, patients are not advised to perform strenuous lifting or exercises.
- It is essential to develop good communication with the client to help the client listen to and understand their own body.
- The client needs to avoid overexertion, which can lead to injury and complications.
- Each client is different. When the client is cleared by the surgeon to proceed with further, and possibly more challenging, exercises, these exercises need to be planned around any injury, weakness, or other limitations the client may have developed due to obesity. These often include knee, foot, hip, and back weakness or injuries.

- In the first weeks after bariatric surgery, water exercises may be very helpful for gaining strength around the joints without causing undue stress on them. If the client can ride an exercise bike without causing discomfort or injury elsewhere in their body, a bike can be a comfortable option, especially for clients with foot issues that limit their ability to walk for cardiovascular exercise.

- Some studies also recommend delaying any balance exercises for 6 to 12 weeks or until receiving clearance from the surgeon. I find that having a bar on the wall to assist with exercises is essential.

- When clients are cleared by their surgeon for abdominal exercises, proceed with individual care and exercises. The core holds the torso upright and in proper posture. A strong core and posture are essential for gaining the proper alignment for the arms and legs to become stronger and to train to avoid injuries. However, exercises should be tailored to each client's needs. For example, abdominal crunches on the floor may be difficult or unattainable for some because clients may not be able to get to the floor. It is also important to understand that crunches do not fully strengthen the core.

- If a client is having a hard time standing up, having a chair in front of the balance bar can help them gain the inner core strength needed for standing and walking, but in a gentle way. When a surgeon clears a client to connect to engaging their abdominal muscles after the proper healing time has taken place, standing on balance pads, discs, and balance balls near a bar can also be extremely helpful and important for gaining strength in the core muscles of the spine and back, which are part of the balancing system.

- Teach the client how and when to engage their abdominals in movements and certain exercises. Know that the surgeon will not want the client to engage their core in the first 6 to 12 weeks (the time will vary per client). Be cautious.

- Hydration is extremely important for clients. Dehydration is one of the leading reasons patients are readmitted to the hospital following bariatric surgery. Dehydration can also add to fatigue. The following practices can help clients avoid dehydration:

  1. Sip water throughout the day.
  2. Do not drink water with meals.
  3. Do not drink carbonated beverages; bubbles in carbonated drinks can stretch the stomach and cause discomfort and bloating.
  4. Avoid caffeine. It is a diuretic and will make staying properly hydrated more challenging.

- Always understand that as a professional, when you have any questions, you should refer clients back to their physical therapist or surgeon when needed.

The Feedback

My client and I have stayed in touch, and each time we discuss her weight and the bypass surgery, she explains that the reason she gained and kept the weight on for all those years prior to her bariatric surgery was because she was sexually abused by her father when she was younger. Here is what she shared with me this week (31 years later) about her history of abuse and her bariatric surgery experience:

I hardly eat anything now. My father sexually abused me for a few years. Most people who are very obese have abuse of some kind. I have the aches and pains of aging now. I can't do much. I watch TV. I am glad I had it done. I had lots of extra skin removed too—30 surgeries over the years.

Based on my years of experience with clients and weight loss, this client's statement indicating that sexual abuse commonly leads to weight gain and obesity is true. I know this client has had years of psychological therapy to help her cope with the past abuse. A couple of years after we met, her son overdosed and passed away. She was devastated. This brought her more heartache and challenges. After she began her surgeries to remove excess skin, she never came back to train with me. She physically could not do it. She is the kindest and most caring individual. It is a shame that she endured such hard experiences in her life. She did everything she could to make her life better for herself. She was determined and worked hard. I am proud of her. She took care of herself and continued to have help with psychological therapy. She is 70 years old as I write this, and she has not regained the original weight she lost from the bypass surgery. Each client who has had bariatric surgery will be different, but at 5 ft 10 in. (178 cm) tall, this particular client weighs 180 lb (82 kg) today, 31 years later.

Coaching Clients With Obesity Through the DISC Model of Behavior

Michael R. Mantell, PhD

The DISC model of behavior is a theoretical personality test widely used to describe human behavior, based on four personality traits (e.g., dominance, influence, steadiness, and conscientiousness). Psychologist Dr. William Moulton Marston developed the test in the 1920s, and when used properly, this assessment can help coaches relate to clients in effective, helpful, and inspirational ways. Each personality style, with its own distinct characteristics, can be easily seen and identified within moments by a receptive coach. The DISC model is widely used in the fields of psychology, business, and personal development to improve communication, teamwork, and leadership skills (Owen et al. 2017).

Dominance Personality Trait

Let's start with the dominance (D) type of client. Such a person places emphasis on achieving goals and seeing the big picture. They are confident, sometimes blunt, outspoken, and demanding, as the following scenario illustrates.

Coach: "Good morning, Dennis. It's so great meeting you. I'm looking forward to getting to know you and helping you achieve your goals relating to your health. You have a good weekend?"

Client: "Uh, yeah, so what's the bottom line here? What are some tips you have? What are some useful suggestions that I can begin applying to help me lose some weight and win the contest I'm having with my neighbor? I mean, what's the point of this coaching if winning isn't my target?"

Coach: "Well, I see that you want to get right to the point, so I'll present some options and some solutions for you. After all, you're in charge of you, right? So, let's focus on some facts for you to help you get the results you want."

Key Points

- Notice the coach's emphasis on getting to the point and focusing on results.
- Notice the questions beginning with *what*.
- Notice the brevity.
- Notice the "ready, aim, fire" approach the client is inferring. This client is a classic dominant D.

Influence Personality Trait

Now, let's turn to the influence (I) type of client. Listen for the people-focused, "let's have some fun," charming manner of this type of client.

Coach (with a big smile): "Good morning, Iris. I enjoyed speaking with you over the phone—and you are so right about how much easier it is to be less formal. So, you said you had a fun weekend with family and friends after we spoke? You seem to be bubbling with joy! Sounds like you had a blast. Let's have some fun working on your goals of improving your health and attaining the target weight you say you'd enjoy living with. I want to tell you about another client who had similar goals and what we did. One thing we did is something I bet you'll really get a kick out of and find helpful. I'll go over the details with you, but I suspect you'll catch it all, so we can work together on this. We're a team, and I want to hear your opinions."

Key Points

- Notice the coach's more informal, enthusiastic, emotion-over-facts approach.
- Notice the focus on letting the client talk about herself, more than just talking to the client.
- Notice the friendly teamwork manner. That's what will generally work best with an influencer.

Steadiness Personality Trait

Time to check in with the steadiness (S) type of client. This is the client who will appreciate a slow, steady, calm, patient, and gentle manner from the coach, and this is also the client who will appreciate direct communication.

Coach: "Good morning, Steve. It was very helpful speaking with you about your goals, and I appreciate you clarifying how you'd like to proceed—slow and steady, one step at a time, will always win for you. I value your being involved in the planning of our coaching approach from the beginning."

Client: "Thanks, coach . . . we seem to be connecting, and I feel comfortable sharing some of my previous attempts at improving my health that obviously didn't work."

Coach: "It's good to know that, and I feel that getting to know you is so important to our working together. Can you share some thoughts on what got in the way of achieving the goals you had in the past?"

Client: "Well, to be honest, I didn't have real goals in the past, just some general plans. But it's clear that I do need some help with that. I'm not someone who sticks to plans too easily."

Coach: "Would you feel comfortable discussing some specific goals you have in mind, so we can create a clear, step-by-step action plan together?"

Key Points

- The client benefits from a reserved, people-oriented style, with the client taking more of a directing role. This approach works best when the coach asks more indirect questions than direct questions.
- If the coach comes across as very bottom-line, the coach might appear aggressive to a steady type of client.

Conscientiousness Personality Trait

And now for the conscientiousness (C) type of individual. You'll see the careful, logical, organized, "do it right" style come through with this client.

Client: "Hi coach. I've been doing a great deal of reading on well-researched ways to gain health and lose weight. As you can tell, for me, it's all about the details and avoiding any slipshod methods."
Coach: "Yes, we share a similar, 'do it the right way' attitude, with a focus on 'how.' Please know that I welcome your direct questions, and I prefer to get right to the task at hand, without wasting your time with small talk."
Client: "Perfect! Just give me the pros and cons of your suggested approach and we can go from there."
Coach: "Excellent. So let's begin by telling you about this very objective approach developed at Harvard Medical School. I'd like to share some data with you and hear what you think."

Key Points

- Note the avoidance of discussing personal issues; the patient, slow approach of using facts and not emotions; and the detail-driven focus.
- You'll notice analytical thinking and a more reserved and systematic mindset in this type of client.
- These clients are motivated by opportunities to gain knowledge and want to show the coach their own expertise.

Coaching Clients With Obesity-Related Metabolic Health Impairments

Maurice Williams, MS

Your client is a 50-year-old married mother of three who works as a full-time accountant assistant. Her body mass index (BMI) is 35 kg/m², her waist circumference is 37 in. (94 cm), and her waist-to-hip ratio is 0.9. She has been overweight most of her life and currently has elevated blood pressure, insulin resistance, and an impaired blood lipid profile. She weighs herself daily, sometimes multiple times per day. She has no prior history of exercise or regular physical activity and does not like exercising. She also feels a lot of psychological stress because of a lack of free time, and sometimes she feels depressed.

Behavior Change Strategies

Metabolic syndrome is a complex condition combining several disorders, such as abdominal obesity, raised blood pressure, prediabetes or type 2 diabetes, and dyslipidemia (Klaric et al. 2021). Regular exercise is a proven intervention to reduce the effects of metabolic syndrome (Myers et al. 2019). As a fitness professional, it is important to understand that changing a client's behavior is a process. Behavior change can be uncomfortable and goes against what is normal (Sutton 2022). The five-stages-of-change model (e.g., precontemplation, contemplation, preparation, action, and maintenance) is effective for assisting clients with an unhealthy weight and with metabolic syndrome. As a fitness professional, it is your responsibility to determine your client's initial stage. A few helpful questions to ask them include the following:

- What is their past exercise history?
- What has kept them from consistent exercise?
- What worked well when they were regularly exercising?

SMART Goals

Setting realistic fitness goals is another aspect of behavior change. This is where SMART goals are appropriate; as a fitness professional, you must help your clients set specific, measurable, attainable, realistic, and timely goals (Sutton 2022). For example, one of the disorders of metabolic syndrome is obesity, so a SMART goal for obesity could be the following: the client will lose 1 to 2 lb (0.5-1 kg) each week by exercising 5 days per week for 30 minutes each day, getting 7 to 9 hours of sleep each night, and reducing their stress levels by practicing meditation three times per week for 10 minutes. Also, healthy eating patterns are critical for cardiometabolic improvements related to weight loss in patients with metabolic syndrome. Thus, exercise professionals should refer their clients to a registered dietitian to address nutritional behavior in order to avoid providing services that are outside the scope of practice of a fitness professional.

Effective Communication

Effective communication strategies require active listening and affirmations. Therefore, verbal and nonverbal communication tools are valuable for exercise professionals when serving clients with major metabolic health impairments (Sutton 2022). An exercise professional should listen to what their clients say and do not say. When exercise professionals actively listen to their clients, it shows they care and respect each client's perspective (Sutton 2022). Open questions should be used, aiming to create enough space for an honest and productive conversation and to promote professionalism, empathy, and encouragement. Such a client-centered communication approach would be appreciated by every client.

Health and Fitness Assessments

To establish a baseline, the exercise professional needs to perform assessments with clients. The first assessment is to ensure the client has had a recent physical. If they have not had one in the past year, they must have one before they begin formal exercise. For a client who has metabolic syndrome, medical clearance is mandatory. A thorough fitness assessment includes subjective (general and medical history) and objective (body composition, cardiorespiratory fitness, and postural assessment) information.

Common assessments include a physical activity readiness questionnaire, resting heart rate and waist and hip circumference measurements, the Rockport walk test, and posture assessments (such as the overhead squat assessment) (Sutton 2022). Each assessment provides a general overview of the client and aids in the design of the exercise program. The Rockport walk test helps determine appropriate cardiorespiratory exercise, and the overhead squat assessment provides important information related to the client's flexibility and mobility limitations, their core strength and endurance, and what muscles need strengthening to reduce the chance of injury (Sever et al. 2023).

Exercise Programming

Exercise programming for a client with abdominal obesity and metabolic syndrome should be simple yet effective. It should include every aspect of physical activity and all the things aforementioned. For example, flexibility, aerobic, and resistance training are important components of a comprehensive training program for this client. In addition, rest is important. Table 14.1 is a sample 30-day exercise program for a medically cleared, beginner client with metabolic syndrome.

Table 14.1   Sample Exercise Program for Metabolic Health

Exercise type	Aerobic (walking) and resistance (circuit-based) training
Frequency	Aerobic: 3 d/wk Resistance: 3 d/wk
Intensity	Aerobic: 50%-65% of HRR Resistance: 50%-70% of 1-RM
Time	Aerobic: up to 30 min Resistance: 15-30 min
Flexibility training	Static stretching: 1 set of 30 s holds on areas of the body that are overactive, based on the overhead squat assessment
Resistance training	1-3 sets of 12-20 reps at a slow tempo with 0-90 s of rest between sets; total body circuit training, using as many compound exercises as possible, is recommended
Special considerations	Include balance and core training, monitor heart rate by having the client wear a heart rate monitor or using the talk test, make sure there is a proper warm-up and cool-down, and reassess the client every 4-6 wk to regress or progress programming

Note: 1-RM = 1-repetition maximum; HRR = heart rate reserve

Coaching Pregnant Clients With Obesity

Farel B. Hruska

This case involves a 36-year-old white woman in her 11th week of pregnancy. The client is 5 ft 5 in. (165 cm) tall and weighs 295 lb (134 kg). She has a history of being sedentary and in a cycle of unhealthy eating based on generational learnings. This is her third pregnancy and will be her third child.

The client's exercise experience is minimal and includes walking occasionally; her preferred exercise is gentle-impact walking. She desires an exercise community and social support for exercise. She has a history of undiagnosed knee pain, assumed to be due to carrying extra weight, and a limited range of motion in all joints. Her hip mobility is especially limited, with pain at the pubic symphysis. She also has low-back pain, and her prepregnancy lordosis is exaggerated with the additional anterior weight load caused by pregnancy.

The client's postural issues include painful kyphosis with increased weight and larger breasts. She is concerned because each postural issue is exacerbated with the growth of the baby. Her exercise frequency is unknown, because most sessions feel uncomfortable.

The Workout Concept

The guidelines in table 14.2 explain the general concept for constructing a workout for the client. Medical clearance is recommended, and gradual progression from the baseline levels should be implemented in a fully supervised exercise setting (ACOG 2015; Mottola et al. 2019).

Table 14.2   Exercise Guidelines for Pregnant Clients

PRENATAL ASSESSMENT	
Mobility and balance	Single-leg balance: 3 s stable on each leg to assess ankle weakness and hypermobility
	Squat assessment: shallow squat with balance aid available (there will be an exaggerated Q angle in first trimester)
	Gait length, with stability assessed at baseline and then throughout the pregnancy
Movement patterns: • Make a balance aid available to the client, and ensure pain-free range of motion • Address muscular imbalances in positions of stability	Prone, quadruped, seated, and standing, with a balance aid available if needed
	Kyphosis: emphasis on strengthening the mid-lower trapezius and rhomboids and muscular release of pectorals and upper trapezius
	Lordosis: emphasis on strengthening 3-dimensional, cylindrical core musculature in all 3 planes of motion and muscular release of the iliopsoas and erector spinae
Frequency	Two times per week, progressed to three times per week in the second and third trimesters
Sessions	Mobility and stability in a full-body workout program
POSTNATAL ASSESSMENT	
Movement patterns are important to consider when designing a program that leads to mental and physical preparation for motherhood once the baby is home	Balance challenges holding and caring for the baby (putting the child on the hip while performing other duties, such as talking on the phone or carrying other items)
	Asymmetric load when putting the baby in a crib or car seat, putting the car seat in the car, etc. (as the baby grows, so does the resistance; the movements intensify as the baby develops)

Structure

A main aspect of the structure needed for this client is a psychologically safe space created before any programming. The lines of communication around fears, insecurities, feeling uncomfortable, and so on need to be open throughout the program. There may be some days when the planned programming is not accessible for the client that day for mental, emotional, or physical reasons. Flexibility is needed in the location (privacy helps with self-confidence), intensity, and selection of exercises (Kuhrt et al. 2015).

Phase 1: Warm-Up

Instructions
Start slowly, progressing only when physical and mental safety is felt.
- March in place (2-3 min)
- Wide-stance frontal and sagittal pelvic rocks
- Shallow forward and reverse lunges with overhead reach
- Wide-stance rotational swings, light on the feet with the toes and knees aligned

Phase 2: Conditioning

Instructions
Plan a full-body session with foundational movement patterns, such as squat, hip hinge, lunge, push, pull, carry, and rotation (see table 14.3 for a sample). Start slowly, progressing only when the client feels physically and mentally safe. All muscle-strengthening exercises should be performed with either dumbbells or resistance bands.

Table 14.3   Sample Conditioning Session for Pregnant Clients

Exercise	Muscles engaged	Equipment	Instructions	Sets	Reps
Sumo squat with biceps curl	Quadriceps, gluteus maximus, biceps	Resistance band anchored on feet	Start with no resistance, and progress slowly with weight and repetitions that feel manageable Keep knees and elbows soft at extension	3	8
Forward lunge with rear fly	Quadriceps, hamstrings, posterior deltoids, mid-lower trapezius, and rhomboids	Resistance band anchored anteriorly	Start with no resistance, and progress slowly with weight and repetitions that feel manageable	2	8
Side lunge with chest press	Quadriceps, gluteus medius, gluteus maximus, anterior deltoids, and pectorals	Resistance band anchored around the upper back or external anchor	Start with no resistance, and progress slowly with weight and repetitions that feel manageable	3	8

Exercise	Muscles engaged	Equipment	Instructions	Sets	Reps
Hay bailer and squat with rotation	Quadriceps, hamstrings, gluteus maximus, internal and external obliques	Resistance band anchored on outside foot or weight lowered to the same leg for resisted rotation	Start with no resistance, and progress slowly with weight and repetitions that feel manageable	2	8
Cat–cow	Rectus abdominis and erector spinae	—	Emphasis on spinal flexion in strengthening the three-dimensional core and core release in the extension (can also return to neutral spine if pain occurs in spinal extension)	—	—

Phase 3: Cool-Down

Instructions
Mimic warm-up movement patterns after a brief 5-minute walk.
- Wide-stance frontal and sagittal pelvic rocks
- Shallow forward and reverse lunges with overhead reach
- Wide-stance rotational swings, light on the feet with the toes and knees aligned
- Seated stretch
  - Figure-4 stretch with ankle on the opposite knee
  - Single-leg hamstring stretch
  - Cross-legged torso rotation
  - Three deep breaths with arms overhead each time

Exercise Programming

The top priorities should be (1) awareness of fatigue and imbalance challenges and (2) free communication of thoughts and feelings. Table 14.4 provides a sample of seven days of exercise programming and table 14.5 outlines recommended training parameters.

Table 14.4   Sample 7-Day Program for Pregnant Clients

	Day 1	Day 2	Day 3	Day 4	Day 5	Day 6	Day 7
Modality	1. Muscle strengthening 2. Flexibility	Rest	Cardiorespiratory fitness (walking)	1. Muscle strengthening 2. Flexibility	Rest	1. Muscle strengthening 2. Flexibility	Cardiorespiratory fitness (walking)
Time	1. 15-30 min 2. 10-15 min	—	15-30 min	1. 15-30 min 2. 10-15 min	—	1. 15-30 min 2. 10-15 min	15-30 min

Table 14.5 Training Parameters

Frequency	1-3 sessions per week, depending on the client's fitness level *Muscle strengthening* • 2 d/wk during the first trimester • Progress to 3 d/wk during the second and third trimesters if the client feels ready and the exercise routine is tolerated *Cardiorespiratory fitness and flexibility* • 2 d/wk • Progress to 3 d/wk during the second and third trimesters if the client feels ready
Intensity	Avoid muscle failure and discomfort throughout the session (RPE of 11-13 on the Borg 6-20 scale)
Time	30-45 min/session, including warm-up and cool-down
Type	Intersession concurrent training (i.e., session A: muscle-strengthening and flexibility; session B: cardiorespiratory fitness)

Note: RPE = rating of perceived exertion.

Coaching Tips

Overall coaching methods should center around clarity about the purpose of each movement and patience with the client's emotional and mental state. Mental and emotional considerations include the following:

- Feelings of losing sense of self
- Concern about exercising during pregnancy, because of fears that it could harm the baby
- Worry about feeling winded and fatigued before movement
- Feelings of defeat when balance is challenged and when a movement pattern is unattainable at first

Movement, no matter how low the intensity, is good and helpful. Coaching the client to be patient and kind to herself is key (Evenson et al. 2014).

Coaching Clients With Obesity Through SMART Goals

Stephanie Cooper, PhD

A new gym member requests an appointment with a certified fitness professional for one-on-one training. The fitness professional schedules an initial meeting with the client to discuss their health history, assess current fitness levels, and develop goals for training. During the initial meeting, the client indicates having had a hard time adhering to an exercise plan and healthy eating plan in the past. Being unsuccessful at adopting long-term health-promoting behaviors led the client to undergo bariatric surgery (sleeve gastrectomy) to promote substantial weight loss. It has been 1 year since the surgery, and the client has lost 110 lb (50 kg). The bariatric surgeon and primary care physician have provided medical clearance to exercise. The information in table 14.6 was measured or provided through answers on a questionnaire.

Table 14.6   Client Vital Statistics

Sex	Male
Age	42 y
Height	5 ft 11 in. (180 cm)
Weight	190 lb (86 kg)
Body mass index	26.6 kg/m^2
Resting heart rate	64 bpm
Age-predicted maximal heart rate	179 bpm
Resting blood pressure	128/80 mm Hg*

Note: bpm = beats per minute.

*The client takes medication to help control blood pressure.

The client discloses that their current physical activity engagement is best described as "irregular." They walk 1.5 to 2.0 mi (2.4-3.2 km) a few times per week at a moderate intensity (about 3.5 mph [5.6 kmph]), which usually takes 25 to 35 minutes; however, the client admits to skipping the walk when their work schedule is too busy. The reason the client is seeking professional help is to become more consistent with their walking schedule and begin a resistance training program in order to maintain weight loss, enhance muscular fitness, and promote overall health.

Before developing an exercise plan, the fitness professional and client create SMART goals together. They focus on the client's desire to improve consistency in walking habits and to achieve muscular hypertrophy through the new resistance training program. The two sets of goals can be found in tables 14.7 and 14.8.

Table 14.7   SMART Goals for Consistent Walking

GOAL 1: WALKING	
Specific	Walk at a moderate intensity for 30 min 5 times per week
Measurable	Achieve a heart rate of 110-132 bpm while walking (40%-59% of HRR)
Attainable	Increase weekly walking frequency from 1 or 2 times per week to 5 times per week through gradual progression across 3 mo
Relevant	The client enjoys walking for exercise, has a desire to be more consistent, and wants to promote overall health
Time-bound	In 3 mo, the client will consistently walk for 30 min 5 times per week at a moderate intensity

Note: bpm = beats per minute; HHR = heart rate reserve.

Table 14.8 SMART Goals for Consistent Resistance Training

GOAL 2: RESISTANCE TRAINING	
Specific	Engage in 3 d of full-body resistance training per week while focusing on muscular hypertrophy
Measurable	Complete 1-3 sets of 8-12 reps at 67%-80% of the 1-RM for 8 movements that focus on various muscle groups (i.e., total body) for each training day
Attainable	Begin with 1 set of 8-12 reps for each exercise and gradually progress to 3 sets of 8-12 reps per exercise across 3 mo
Relevant	The client wants to focus on muscular hypertrophy to enhance muscular fitness and promote overall health
Time-bound	In 3 mo, the client will regularly engage in muscular hypertrophy training 3 times per week

Note: 1-RM = 1-repetition maximum.

After the SMART goals are developed, the fitness professional creates a general training plan for the next 3 months. It involves training sessions that focus primarily on resistance training, includes moderate-intensity walking as a warm-up, and prescribes walking sessions to be completed independently either outside or at the gym. At the end of each month, the fitness professional and the client revisit the goals and discuss the progress being made toward each. During these conversations, the fitness professional helps the client identify challenges that have occurred in trying to achieve the goals and strategize ways in which those barriers can be overcome. For example, after 1 month, the client is still skipping a walk once a week, if not more often, due to a busy work schedule. The fitness professional suggests a few strategies to overcome this challenge:

- Block off time on a weekly planner for exercise and treat this time as if it is an important meeting that cannot be missed.
- If needed, divide the 30-minute walks into shorter bouts throughout the day (e.g., two 15-min walks).
- Identify any meetings that could be conducted as walking meetings.
- Allocate additional time before or after the training sessions to complete a prescribed walking bout.

At the end of 3 months, the client has met their goals. Now that they have been consistent in their walking and resistance training schedule, they want to focus their next set of SMART goals on improving cardiorespiratory fitness and muscular endurance. The fitness professional uses the new goals to guide the next phase of training.

Coaching Clients With Obesity Through Behavioral Versus Nonbehavioral Goals

Erin Nitschke, PhD

In the world of health and exercise, the battle against unhealthy weight is a prevalent concern for professionals and clients alike. Clients seeking help at the gym often present with a variety of goals, including weight-centered or body-centric goals, such as weight loss and body transformation. However, the path to achieving these goals can differ significantly based on whether the approach is behavioral or nonbehavioral (Brehm

2014). This case study explores the practical implications of behavioral (process-oriented) and nonbehavioral (outcome-oriented) goal setting in a gym environment and the communication skills required from health and exercise professionals to effectively guide and coach clients toward goal success.

Imagine a bustling urban gym named FitLife, where clients of all ages, fitness levels, abilities, and backgrounds come seeking guidance for their health and weight-related concerns. FitLife offers a comprehensive range of services, from personal training to group classes, and attracts clients with diverse goals. Let's examine two different client personas, John and Emily.

1. *John (nonbehavioral goal):* John, a 35-year-old software engineer, has been struggling with obesity for years. He has set a nonbehavioral goal to lose 50 lb in 6 months in order to attend his high school reunion feeling confident.

2. *Emily (behavioral goal):* Emily, a 28-year-old marketing executive, wants to improve her overall health, fitness, and energy. She has set a behavioral goal to attend at least three gym sessions per week consistently and meet with her health coach every 2 weeks.

Behavioral Goals and Strategies (Process)

Behavioral goals focus on specific actions and habits that lead to desired outcomes. In Emily's case, her goal is to attend gym sessions regularly as well as meet with her health coach, fostering a sustainable, long-term approach to fitness, wellness, and energy.

Goal-Setting

As Emily's personal trainer or health coach, it is essential to help her set SMART (specific, measurable, achievable or attainable, relevant, and time-bound) goals. This involves discussing her weekly gym attendance targets, identifying her nutritional intake and eating habits or style, and gradually increasing her workout intensity. Because Emily is also interested in improving her energy, it is essential to also encourage her to monitor her sleep and energy levels.

To assist Emily in identifying each component of the SMART goal she intends to pursue, ask open-ended questions to help her establish the necessary approach. "Pocket questions" such as the following are useful.

- What do you want to achieve? (Specificity)
- How will you know you've achieved the goal? (Measurability)
- What is a reasonable timeline to achieve this goal? (Achievability)
- What is important about this for you? (Personal meaning and relevance)
- What are possible obstacles you might face? How can you confront them? (Overcoming barriers and identifying high-risk situations)
- What external resources do you envision yourself needing to support your progress? (This might include tools, support groups, individuals, or online resources)

Self-Monitoring

Encourage Emily to keep a fitness journal to track her gym sessions, diet, and any challenges faced. Invite her to make note of her daily energy levels and how they fluctuate from morning to evening. This will help her stay accountable and identify areas for improvement. This type of tracking also helps the fitness professional identify patterns or trends in behavior.

Positive Reinforcement

Provide regular positive feedback, and celebrate small victories with Emily. Acknowledging her progress can boost Emily's motivation and adherence to her behavioral goals.

Education

Educate Emily about the importance of consistent exercise, nutrition, and sleep for achieving her overall health and fitness objectives. A well-informed client is more likely to stay committed.

Nonbehavioral Goals and Strategies (Outcomes)

Nonbehavioral goals and strategies, as demonstrated by John, emphasize the end result without a clear roadmap of actions. These goals are often unpredictable and do not offer a clear timetable or accountability actions. These goals generally lead to short-term motivation but lack a foundation for lasting and meaningful behavior change.

Outcome Focus

John's primary focus is losing 50 lb in 6 months. It is crucial for his trainer to understand his motivations but also to gently guide him toward breaking this outcome into manageable steps.

Short-Term Gratification

Nonbehavioral goals often lean on quick fixes and extreme diets. It is essential to educate John about the potential risks of these approaches and the importance of sustainable habits.

Emotional Support

Clients like John may face emotional challenges during their weight loss journey. Being empathetic and providing emotional support can help him stay motivated.

Communication Skills for Fitness Professionals

Effective communication is the cornerstone of helping clients with their weight management goals. Here are some key skills required:

1. *Active listening:* Listen attentively to both John and Emily to understand their unique needs, fears, and motivations. Active listening builds trust and helps tailor strategies accordingly.
2. *Empathy:* Empathize with clients' challenges and feelings. Understanding their emotions can help you provide appropriate support and motivation.
3. *Goal alignment:* Ensure clients' goals align with their values and lifestyle. Help them set realistic goals that fit into their daily routines.

4. *Educational communication:* Provide clients with evidence-based information about nutrition, exercise, and healthy habits. Use simple language to ensure comprehension.

5. *Motivational interviewing:* Use motivational interviewing techniques to evoke clients' intrinsic motivation for behavioral changes. Encourage them to express their own reasons for change (Miller and Rollnick 2013).

Challenges and Solutions

Clients' programs are as unique as the clients themselves. However, certain challenges typically surface during the fitness process. The following are some common types of challenges your clients might face and solutions you can apply to help them.

1. *Resistance to behavioral goals:* Some clients may resist setting behavioral goals due to a preference for quick fixes. In such cases, it is important to explain the long-term benefits of behavioral changes and provide evidence of their effectiveness.

2. *Unrealistic expectations:* Clients like John may have unrealistic expectations regarding weight loss. Gently guide them toward setting achievable goals, and educate them about a healthy rate of weight loss.

3. *Plateaus and setbacks:* Clients, especially those with nonbehavioral goals, may become discouraged when they hit plateaus or experience setbacks. Encourage resilience and provide strategies for overcoming obstacles.

Conclusion

In the dynamic world of exercise and weight management, understanding the distinction between behavioral and nonbehavioral goals is essential for fitness professionals. By adopting a behavioral approach, clients like Emily can build sustainable habits that lead to long-term success, while clients like John may require guidance to transform nonbehavioral goals into actionable steps. Effective communication skills are pivotal in helping clients navigate their unique weight management journeys, ultimately leading them to healthier, happier lives. In the gym setting, FitLife's fitness professionals strive to bridge the gap between clients' aspirations and their actions, transforming their goals into tangible results.

Coaching Clients With Obesity Through the Transtheoretical Model of Health Behavior Change #1

Mary Yoke, PhD

"I just hate to exercise," says Ms. Reluctant, a 48-year-old woman with a BMI of 39 kg/m^2 and a waist circumference of 45 in. (114 cm) who has come to you because her doctor insists that she become more physically active. Ms. Reluctant has hypertension, high cholesterol, knee osteoarthritis, and prediabetes. She sits almost continuously for 8 to 9 hours per day at work, then gets take-out food, goes home, and watches television. Ms. Reluctant is not happy with her weight and appearance; however, she lacks motivation to do anything about it. She reports that she does not know what to do at the gym and feels as if everyone stares at her.

Preparation-Stage Objectives

According to the transtheoretical model (TTM), Ms. Reluctant is in the preparation stage (DiClemente et al. 1998; Prochaska et al. 1994), and she has come to ask you to help her get going. The following objectives can be beneficial to her success.

1. *Find something active that she enjoys.* In order to increase the intention to change according to the reasoned action approach (RAA), the new behavior must be pleasurable, enjoyable, and fun (Fishbein et al. 2010).

2. *Make physical activity as convenient for her as possible.* The RAA states that ease of access is a critical determinant in increasing a person's intention and subsequent action. Help Ms. Reluctant devise a convenient home exercise program, which will help her avoid feeling stigmatized at the gym.

3. *Help her to perceive physical activity as normal.* Both the RAA and the TTM emphasize the importance of social norms. Walking with a friend or as part of a walking group normalizes physical activity. Alternatively, Ms. Reluctant could exercise along with a streaming or recorded class for people with weight challenges.

4. *Help her develop self-efficacy.* This is a key construct in both the TTM and the social cognitive theory (SCT) (Bandura 2023). Self-efficacy is the feeling a person has when they are confident that they can do a particular task. Choose exercises and goals that help Ms. Reluctant feel successful and self-empowered.

5. *Set appropriate, short-term, approachable SMART goals.* A short-term goal—1 week or less—is best for developing self-efficacy. An approachable goal is positive, enjoyable, and something to look forward to (example: "This week I will take a 30-minute walk on the beach at sunset on Friday with my friends"). A SMART goal is a goal that is specific, measurable, action-oriented, relevant, and timed. The example given here is a SMART goal.

6. *Emphasize the immediate (today!) benefits of physical activity.* These include decreased anxiety and depression; improved mood, energy, and productivity; improved cognitive functioning and self-esteem; and better sleep.

7. *Remember that too much, too soon, is a major cause of injury and dropout.* Research shows that exercise perception is not the same when a person is struggling with their weight. Imposing a walking speed that is just 10% higher than what overweight women would have self-selected has been shown to lead to a significant decline in pleasure (Ekkekakis et al. 2006).

Action Stage: Weeks 1-4

Depending on how long it takes Ms. Reluctant to become consistent, the action stage of her exercise program is estimated to take up to 4 weeks (see table 14.9 for an action-stage sample plan for weeks 1-4). The following objectives can be beneficial to her success.

1. *Encourage her to move throughout the day.* Set SMART goals to minimize Ms. Reluctant's sedentariness throughout the day.

2. *Have her engage in frequent movement-snack goals.* These smaller daily goals can include the following:

- Taking one flight of stairs every hour
- Walking the long way to the restroom
- Standing up and stretching every hour
- Marching in place for 1 to 2 min during TV commercials
- Walking around while talking on the phone

Table 14.9 TTM Action-Stage Sample Plan, Weeks 1-4

Monday	Tuesday	Wednesday	Thursday	Friday	Saturday	Sunday
Walk 10 min after lunch	Walk 10 min after lunch	Walk 10 min after lunch	Walk 5 min after breakfast, then 10 min after lunch	Walk 10 min after lunch	Take an aquatic exercise class or exercise to a streaming or recorded class at home	Walk 10 min after lunch

Note: Encourage Ms. Reluctant to walk with a friend, significant other, or walking group, ideally in a very convenient and enjoyable place. It is important for her to associate physical activity with pleasure.

Action Stage: Weeks 5-8

Once Ms. Reluctant is consistently physically active every day, progress the program as follows (table 14.10). Be careful not to plan too many sets, repetitions, and exercises. If Ms. Reluctant starts to drop off, reduce the frequency (e.g., provide a complete rest day) or reduce the duration. The goals are consistency and enjoyment.

Table 14.10 TTM Action-Stage Sample Plan, Weeks 5-8

Monday	Tuesday	Wednesday	Thursday	Friday	Saturday	Sunday
Walk 15 min after lunch 2 × 10 assisted squats Chair stretches: chest, erector spinae, seated hamstrings, standing calf, and hip flexors	Walk 15 min after lunch 2 × 30 s wall plank	Walk 15 min after lunch 2 × 10 s assisted squats Perform same stretches as on Monday	Walk 10 min after breakfast, then 10 min after lunch	Walk 15 min after lunch 2 × 30 s wall plank	Walk 10 min after breakfast Take an aquatic exercise or streaming or recorded class	Walk 15 min after lunch Perform the same stretches as on Monday

Action Stage: Weeks 9-12

After Ms. Reluctant has been adhering to the above program for 2 to 4 weeks, gradually begin to add additional exercises and increase the duration, as in table 14.11.

Table 14.11 TTM Action-Stage Sample Plan, Weeks 9-12

Monday	Tuesday	Wednesday	Thursday	Friday	Saturday	Sunday
Walk 20 min after lunch	Walk 20 min after lunch	Repeat Monday's plan	Walk 15 min after breakfast, then 15 min after lunch	Repeat Tuesday's plan	Walk 15 min after breakfast	Walk 15 min after lunch
3 × 10 body-weight squats	2 × 8-10 inclined standing push-ups				Take an aquatic exercise class	Repeat Monday's stretches
1 × 10 standing unilateral hamstring curls	1 × 10 seated, banded high rows					
1 × 10 supported standing stationary lunges	1 × 10 seated, banded, unilateral triceps press-downs					
1 × 10 supported standing calf raises	1 × 10 seated dumbbell biceps curls					
Chair stretches: chest, erector spinae, seated hamstrings, standing calf, and hip flexors	1 × 10 seated abdominal roll-backs					
	1 × 10 seated spinal extension press-backs					

Note: Weekly, even daily, goal setting is strongly encouraged. Have your client use reminders such as Post-It notes, screen-saver messages, or wearable apps.

Coaching Clients With Obesity Through the Transtheoretical Model of Health Behavior Change #2

Cherie O'Neill (Kroh), EdD

The client in this case study is Muhammed, a 35-year-old individual weighing approximately 350 lb (159 kg), with a BMI of 45 kg/m². Muhammed has expressed a desire to become more active and improve his overall health. Muhammed has said he would like to go to a local gym but has no experience with weight training. He is in the stage of preparation, because he has stated he is ready to get started.

Sample Program Objectives

The objective of the program is to design a 4-week, tailored workout plan that is sensitive to Muhammed's physical needs, promotes gradual behavior change, and considers his stage of change in the transtheoretical model. The workout plan will include low-impact cardiorespiratory fitness activities and muscle-strengthening exercises that accommodate Muhammed's body size and potential physical limitations, aiming to empower bodily movement. The following are some additional considerations to keep in mind throughout the 4-week period:

- Muhammed should be encouraged to listen to his body and provide feedback on the difficulty of the exercises.
- The weights suggested are starting points. If Muhammed finds the initial weights too easy or too challenging, adjustments should be made.
- Rest between sets should be 1 to 2 minutes, depending on Muhammed's recovery needs.

Week 1: Introduction to Exercise—Upper Body

The focus of the first week should be to achieve familiarization and establish a baseline with exercise movements concentrating on the upper body. Here are some basic guidelines:

- Warm up for at least 5 minutes, focused on the upper body.
- Consider using a heart rate monitor or the talk test.
- Choose weights that allow Muhammed to complete the sets comfortably, focusing on form.

See table 14.12 for a sample TTM program for week 1.

Table 14.12   Sample TTM Program: Week 1

Day of week	Modality	Type	Intensity (%HRR)	Time	Resistance training	Volume	Load
Monday	Aerobic exercise	Walking or cycling	40-50	10 min	—	—	—
	Resistance training	—	—	—	Seated dumbbell curl	2 sets of 8-10 reps	5-10 lb (2-5 kg)
	Resistance training	—	—	—	Seated dumbbell shoulder press	2 sets of 8-10 reps	5-10 lb (2-5 kg)
	Resistance training	—	—	—	Seated dumbbell fly	2 sets of 8-10 reps	5-10 lb (2-5 kg)
Wednesday	Aerobic exercise	Walking or cycling	40-50	10 min	—	—	—
	Resistance training	—	—	—	Seated triceps extension	2 sets of 8-10 reps	5-10 lb (2-5 kg)
	Resistance training	—	—	—	Seated lat pull-down (band)	2 sets of 8-10 reps	Resistance band
	Resistance training	—	—	—	Seated abdominal twist (band)	2 sets of 8-10 reps	Resistance band
Friday	Aerobic exercise	Walking or cycling	40-50	12 min	—	—	—
	Resistance training	—	—	—	Seated shoulder press	2 sets of 8-10 reps	5-10 lb (2-5 kg)
	Resistance training	—	—	—	Seated row (band)	2 sets of 8-10 reps	Resistance band
	Resistance training	—	—	—	Modified plank (knees)	2 sets of 15-20 s	—

Note: HRR = heart rate reserve; TTM = transtheoretical model.

Week 2: Introduction to Exercise—Lower Body

The focus of the second week should be to achieve familiarization and establish a baseline, with exercise movements concentrating on the lower body. Here are some basic guidelines:

- Warm up for at least 5 minutes, focused on the lower body.
- Consider using a heart rate monitor or the talk test.

- Ensure Muhammed maintains good posture during seated exercises.
- Adjust the resistance band as needed for comfort and effectiveness

See table 14.13 for a sample TTM program for week 2.

Table 14.13   Sample TTM Program: Week 2

Day of week	Modality	Type	Intensity (%HRR)	Time	Resistance training	Volume	Load
Monday	Aerobic exercise	Walking or cycling	45-55	12-15 min	—	—	—
	Resistance training	—	—	—	Seated leg press (band)	2 sets of 8-10 reps	Resistance band
	Resistance training	—	—	—	Lying hip bridge	2 sets of 8-10 reps	Body weight
	Resistance training	—	—	—	Calf raise	2 sets of 8-10 reps	Body weight
Wednesday	Aerobic exercise	Walking or cycling	45-55	12-15 min	—	—	—
	Resistance training	—	—	—	Standing leg curl (band)	2 sets of 8-10 reps	Resistance band
	Resistance training	—	—	—	Bird dog (low back)	2 sets of 8-10 reps	Resistance band
	Resistance training	—	—	—	Seated abduction (band)	2 sets of 8-10 reps	Resistance band
Friday	Aerobic exercise	Walking or cycling	45-55	15-17 min	—	—	—
	Resistance training	—	—	—	Seated leg extension (band)	2 sets of 8-10 reps	Resistance band
	Resistance training	—	—	—	Standing adduction (band)	2 sets of 8-10 reps	Resistance band
	Resistance training	—	—	—	Seated wall squat	2 sets of 8-10 reps	Body weight

Note: HRR = heart rate reserve; TTM = transtheoretical model.

Week 3: Introduction to Mixed Upper and Lower Body

The focus of the third week should be to establish a full-body routine, preparing Muhammed for continued fitness progression. Here are some basic guidelines:

- Warm up for at least 10 minutes, focused on full-body dynamic movements to prepare the muscles for exercise.
- Consider using a heart rate monitor or the talk test.
- Encourage Muhammed to maintain a controlled breathing pattern, especially during abdominal exercises.
- Adjust the resistance or weight as needed, based on Muhammed's feedback and comfort level.
- Emphasize the importance of rest and recovery, especially after workouts involving the lower back.
- Include a cool-down period with stretching to promote flexibility.

See table 14.14 for a sample TTM program for week 3.

Table 14.14   Sample TTM Program: Week 3

Day of week	Modality	Type	Intensity (%HRR)	Time	Resistance training	Volume	Load
Monday	Aerobic exercise	Walking or cycling	50-60	17-20 min	—	—	—
	Resistance training	—	—	—	Modified squat	2 sets of 10 reps	Body weight
	Resistance training	—	—	—	Standing oblique crunch	2 sets of 10 reps	Body weight
	Resistance training	—	—	—	Calf raise	2 sets of 10 reps	Body weight
Wednesday	Aerobic exercise	Walking or cycling	50-60	17-20 min	—	—	—
	Resistance training	—	—	—	Seated dumbbell row	2 sets of 10 reps	8-10
	Resistance training	—	—	—	Lying hip bridge	2 sets of 10 reps	Body weight
	Resistance training	—	—	—	Standing wall push-up	2 sets of 10 reps	Body weight
Friday	Aerobic exercise	Walking or cycling	50-60	17-20 min	—	—	—
	Resistance training	—	—	—	Seated shoulder press	2 sets of 10 reps	8-10
	Resistance training	—	—	—	Standing leg curl (band)	2 sets of 10 reps	Resistance band
	Resistance training	—	—	—	Modified plank (knees)	2 sets of 30 s	—

Note: HRR = heart rate reserve; TTM = transtheoretical model.

Week 4: Progressive Overload Continuation

The focus of the fourth week should be to solidify the exercise routine and prepare for future progression. Here are some basic guidelines:

- Continue to focus on form and controlled movements.
- Encourage Muhammed to communicate any discomfort or pain immediately.
- Adjust the resistance or weight as needed based on Muhammed's feedback and comfort level, ensuring Muhammed can complete the sets with good form but still feel challenged by the last 2 repetitions.
- Regular reassessment will help to tailor the program to Muhammed's evolving fitness level.
- Emphasize the importance of rest and recovery.
- Include a cool-down period with stretching to promote flexibility.

See table 14.15 for a sample TTM program for week 4.

Table 14.15   Sample TTM Program: Week 4

Day of week	Modality	Type	Intensity (%HRR)	Time	Resistance training	Volume	Load
Monday	Aerobic exercise	Walking or cycling	55-65	20-25 min	—	—	—
	Resistance training	—	—	—	Modified squat	2-3 sets of 10 reps	Body weight
	Resistance training	—	—	—	Modified side plank on knee	2-3 sets of 10 reps	Body weight
	Resistance training	—	—	—	Calf raise	2-3 sets of 10 reps	Body weight
Wednesday	Aerobic exercise	Walking or cycling	55-65	20-25 min	—	—	—
	Resistance training	—	—	—	Seated dumbbell row	2-3 sets of 10 reps	10-15 lb (5-7 kg)
	Resistance training	—	—	—	Lying hip bridge	2-3 sets of 10 reps	Body weight
	Resistance training	—	—	—	Standing wall push-up	2-3 sets of 10 reps	Body weight or add resistance band

(continued)

Table 14.15 Sample TTM Program: Week 4 *(continued)*

Day of week	Modality	Type	Intensity (%HRR)	Time	Resistance training	Volume	Load
Friday	Aerobic exercise	Walking or cycling	55-65	20-25 min	—	—	—
	Resistance training	—	—	—	Seated shoulder press	2-3 sets of 10 reps	10-15 lb (5-7 kg)
	Resistance training	—	—	—	Standing leg curl (band)	2-3 sets of 10 reps	Resistance band
	Resistance training	—	—	—	Modified plank (knees)	2-3 sets of 30 s	—

Note: HRR = heart rate reserve; TTM = transtheoretical model.

Sustaining Motivation During the Action Stage

The questions in this section are designed to facilitate a conversation that helps the individual reflect on their actions, reinforce their commitment, and plan for sustained change. These questions also serve to strengthen the therapeutic alliance and support and validate the individual's efforts.

Exploring the Change

- What motivated you to start making this change?
- Can you tell me about the steps you've taken so far?
- How does engaging in this new behavior make you feel compared to before?

Supporting Self-Efficacy

- What strengths do you draw upon to make these changes?
- How confident do you feel about continuing your new activities?
- What have you learned about yourself through this process?

Identifying Successes and Challenges

- What successes have you experienced since you began making changes?
- What challenges have you encountered, and how have you dealt with them?
- In what ways has your life improved since you started this action?

Enhancing Commitment

- What keeps you motivated to continue with your action plan?
- How important is it for you to maintain these changes, and why?
- What future goals do you have in mind now that you've started this journey?

Problem-Solving

- How do you plan to overcome any obstacles that might arise in the future?
- What strategies have worked best for you when facing difficulties?
- Who or what could support you in staying on track with your goals?

Reflecting on Outcomes

- How has this change affected your daily life?
- What differences have others noticed in you since you started this action?
- How do you see these changes affecting your future?

Planning for the Future

- What are the next steps you plan to take to maintain your progress?
- How do you envision your life a year from now if you continue with these actions?
- What might you need to keep yourself motivated and moving forward?

WEIGHT MANAGEMENT STORIES FROM THE FIELD

Story 1

Louise Valentine, MPH

A woman aged 44 years was seeking strength training, running, and nutrition coaching with a goal to lose weight, increase strength, and run an injury-free marathon and ultramarathon despite living with excess body weight. With a BMI of 33.7 kg/m², she had recently lost a significant amount of weight with a very low-calorie diet program and prepackaged processed foods. She was experiencing fatigue, bloating, and frustration with a weight loss plateau despite running more and eating less. Self-reported barriers to success included a high-stress, sedentary job; family demands; and an evening sweet tooth.

In the client's initial session, we agreed her running program would include running 4 days per week and strength training 3 times per week. Cardiovascular exercise included easy-paced aerobic short runs, long runs that progressed in distance every other week, and anaerobic speedwork to support her metabolic health. She was provided with two time-efficient strength plans to accommodate her busy lifestyle. The lower-body program included core, hip extension, posterior chain, stability, and running-specific injury-prevention exercises. Targeted strength exercises were included to address common women's health and runner concerns, such as pelvic floor pain, diastasis recti, runner's knee, sacroiliac joint dysfunction, back pain, and urinary incontinence. The upper-body plan was designed to maximize building lean muscle and strength—working with the physiology of a woman aged 35 years or older—by targeting a repetition range of no greater than 10. Because estrogen, progesterone, and testosterone decrease for most women beginning around age 35, the client's body responded best to lifting heavy weights that provided enough stimulus to effectively build muscle.

Follow-up sessions focused on adherence to her program with proper time for muscle recovery, mindset strategies to overcome self-doubt, and addressing emotional triggers to overeat. Realistic movement strategies to break up periods of prolonged sitting at her sedentary job were identified to support mitigating insulin resistance, weight gain, and negative health outcomes. She agreed to move at least once every hour and for at least 2 minutes after any snack or meal. We discussed realistic ways to move more and sit less, such as walking to refill her water, doing posture-corrective exercises at her desk, and walking up and down stairs when possible. Nutrition strategies were provided to fuel her best hormonal health, energy, and running performance, with a focus on replacing processed foods with whole foods she enjoyed. Other barriers identified and addressed included restoring damaged metabolism from a history of underfueling and mitigating common pathology for women aged 35 or over, including insulin resistance, premenstrual syndrome (PMS), mood swings, loss of lean muscle and bone, gut dysbiosis, and nutrient deficiencies. Finally, decreased use of caffeine was encouraged, to be replaced with energy-supporting suggestions for adequate protein intake, timing, and sport nutrition strategies.

As coaching progressed, the client found motivation in a local running community. Highly motivated to lose weight, she began to run more mileage than discussed. Via multiple sessions, we discussed the symptoms and consequences of overtraining, underfueling, and underrecovery, including low mood, damage to hormonal and metabolic health, compromised immunity, and increased injury risk. Upon discussion of fatigue and a persistent upper respiratory infection, it was a breakthrough in the coaching relationship when I told her, "If you drain your health, energy, and hormone tank with too much cardiovascular exercise and not enough fuel, not only will you not feel good on a day-to-day basis, you may never make it to race day due to injury, illness, or burnout."

With a newfound understanding, the client adhered to her program and was thrilled to run her first marathon and ultramarathon with optimal energy and strength and without injury, despite being a larger-bodied individual.

Upon completion of the client's races, we agreed to support more aggressive weight loss with reduced running volume, a strategic reduction in caloric intake, and an increased focus on building lean muscle to support her best metabolism. Weight lifting increased to 4 days per week, alternating between a new upper- and lower-body program. Because she enjoyed running, we agreed to include 3 shorter runs per week, to include a high-intensity interval training (HIIT) session and two easy-paced aerobic runs.

A month into the revised program, the client expressed she was again experiencing fatigue, low mood, exacerbated PMS, and lack of weight loss. After discussing barriers to program adherence, we agreed it was time to decrease running volume further, as it was triggering hunger and cravings and contributing to a cycle of overstress, overeating, and attempts to burn excess calories through longer-than-discussed training runs.

As with all client journeys, finding the sweet spot of an exercise mode one enjoys, paired with proper nutrition, mindset, stress reduction, and lifestyle movement habits, was essential to success. With an increased focus on the benefits of building lean muscle, the client found her weight-lifting sessions empowering. While she missed marathon training, an understanding of the benefits of treadmill incline walking, shorter HIIT runs, and one weekend run for joy led to a healthy balance of cardiovascular exercise to support sustained weight loss over time. A change in her employment supported an overall reduction in lifestyle stress but did not eliminate stress-induced overeating. However, with consistent coaching support, the client learned how to work with her female physiology to understand root causes of cravings, energy crashes, and weight loss plateaus. She completed coaching feeling stronger, pleased with body composition changes, and confident that she had effective tools to support continued weight loss.

Key Points

- Excessive cardiovascular exercise and calorie restriction are counterproductive to successful weight loss. Warning signs of excessive exercise include low mood, fatigue, and frequent illness.
- Strength training is essential to build lean muscle and support hormonal and metabolic health. Consider injury prevention and sex-specific exercises.
- If you identify disordered eating or undereating, refer the client to a nutrition professional if it is not in your scope of practice to support them.
- Consider clients holistically, reviewing barriers to success in lifestyle habits, family support, sedentary behavior, and stress management.
- A collaborative approach will guide clients to best results and sustainable success. Discuss program modifications that best fit the client's preferences and lifestyle.

Story 2

Brian Richey, BS

"Why should I work with you as a trainer when you are so fat?" This sharp and stinging comment was said to me during an initial assessment I had with a client. You could see that she meant it. If I couldn't take care of myself and keep myself in shape, why should she trust me to keep her in shape? As a fitness professional and as an international lecturer on topics of anatomy, kinesiology, and medical and corrective exercise, this is a question that I wrestled with myself. But I will say, hearing it come out of someone's mouth was a slap in the face.

Growing up in Kailua, Hawaii, I was always the biggest kid in the class, both by weight and height. Fortunately, or unfortunately, my personality and temperament led me to be the one who was bullied rather than being the bully. I was picked on and teased every day in school, even by the teachers. It was a very different time and not uncommon to be ridiculed for weight, even by those who should know better. Sticks and stones may break my bones, but words will do far more damage.

By the time I was 12, I was well over 200 lb (91 kg), partially because of a failed experiment of my mother's psychologist at the time, whose advice was to give me a daily food allowance and have me shop for and prepare my own meals. I was given 5 dollars a day. It wasn't much, and with no education about proper nutrition, my food choices weren't stellar. In fact, they were probably the worst choices I could make. I would eat one meal a day. I discovered I could buy 2 lb (1 kg) of 80% ground beef, a loaf of bread, and a can of chili for around 4 dollars. I could get a Super Big Gulp of soda with the change. And all that food became my daily meal. Like I said, not a stellar choice. After the failed experiment for most of a year, my weight shot up and never looked back.

By the time I graduated from high school, I weighed in at over 420 lb (191 kg) at a height of 6 ft (183 cm). The only scale that could weigh me was at the airport shipping dock—a tad embarrassing, to say the least. It was in my freshman year of college that I turned things around. Granted, up until this point, I had been on every fad diet on the market. Nothing worked. What did work was a combination of eating a little less, not eating late at night, and walking 5 miles (8 km) a day. Combined with the fact that I was young and had the benefit of teenage hormones helping me, I lost over 200 lb (91 kg) over the next couple of years, and for the most part, I kept it off by living on a highly restrictive diet and exercising like crazy 6 to 7 days a week.

I fell in love with fitness and devoted my life to it. I would do 60 to 90 minutes of cardio a day and then weight training for an additional hour 6 days a week. Being young, my body was able to do that. My diet was very restrictive—basically, a bodybuilder contest diet, except I did it year-round. My metabolism was never the same again.

I began gaining weight easily. My body had gotten used to existing on so few calories that any time I ate more than it was used to, I gained weight. Then I freaked out and starved myself, and the downward spiral went lower and lower. My weight ping-ponged between 217 lb (98 kg) and 270 lb (122) for 15 years. It would crawl upward and then I would strip it back down by eating even less. By the time I was in my late 40s, I couldn't lose any more weight. I was exercising for 2 or more hours a day, weights and cardio, but any time I ate more than 1,200 kcals a day, I gained weight.

It was highly embarrassed coming to fitness conferences, teaching classes, and being the worst-looking person in the room. I was definitely the "before" picture, while all my students were the "after."

I sought help from over 20 endocrinologists. What I heard time and time again was "Your blood work is perfect. I guess you have a slow metabolism. What do you want me to do about it?" I did find a couple of physicians who worked with me to try to get my metabolism revved back up. I tried all available prescription medications on the market. None of them worked. I worked with many nutritionists, all of whom told me I needed to eat more, not less. One of these times, I gained 40 lb (18 kg) in a month eating exactly what I was told to—2,100 kcals/d. The nutritionist said that was impossible. I said, "Welcome to my world."

Today I am 190 lb (86 kg) and around 10% to 12% body fat. What eventually worked for me? A physician and good friend of mine recommend I investigate bariatric surgery. He wasn't sure it would work, but it was the last-ditch try. Without going into too much detail, during the surgery, my surgeon found some things in my stomach that he was able to correct, which may have contributed to my inability to lose weight after a gastric bypass. With a combination of getting my body to work correctly on top of the surgery itself, I lost the weight. Before surgery, I was 298 lb (135 kg), and within 6 months after surgery, I was 185 lb (84 kg). My eating habits have changed, of course. I eat a lot less than I used to. I exercise in moderation and live a very active lifestyle. This choice was not an easy one to make, and the experience was the hardest thing I have ever done. It is still a challenge. It's no wonder why so many people drop out of the program before the surgery. Those who say it is a shortcut have no idea what they are talking about. But it was worth it. I now look in the mirror and see the person I always thought I should be, could be. And that feels pretty good.

Story 3

Daniel Green, BA

Several years ago, I completed a behavior-change project, powered by one of the world's leading fitness certification organizations, that involved adhering to the Physical Activity Guidelines for Americans and Dietary Guidelines for Americans for a full year and documenting the changes in my health, fitness, and overall wellness. Part of the catalyst for that project was the quest for new ways to motivate and inspire health and exercise professionals—and their clients—by sharing the value of true lifestyle change. The other consideration was my own health. I was at a point where I knew I had to do something dramatic to get myself moving and eating more healthfully. I had counted calories and steps. I had lifted weights and installed a suspension trainer under my deck. I had done everything I could think of, yet my chronic headaches were worsening and I was slowly and steadily gaining weight. So, I offered myself up as a test subject and chronicled my journey along the way.

I've been working in the health and fitness industry since 1998. In that time, I've written dozens of articles meant to help health and exercise professionals motivate their clients to get and stay active and eat more healthfully. The truth is, I'd squandered a tremendous opportunity. For each article, I interviewed sought-after experts at length. My writing relies on my ability to take the complex science they describe and reframe it so that it becomes usable for health and exercise professionals who are tasked with inspiring their clients each and every day. Unfortunately, I never took that next step and inspired myself. For over two decades, I'd been reading and writing about the best workouts for beginners, how to motivate clients who are stuck on fitness plateaus, how to stay active when traveling, and the best advice for training older adults (as well as youths, pregnant women, people with obesity, and even firefighters), all while spending long days at my desk, eating trail mix and drinking Diet Mt. Dew.

As my doctor said when I told him about my plans, I had timed the beginning of my lifestyle-change journey perfectly, as I was prediabetic and had obesity and stage 1 hypertension. He said that while I wasn't truly sick yet, I was on the brink of having a lot of issues. The aforementioned headaches were one of the bigger obstacles to regular participation in physical activity, as I would often start a workout regimen, be consistent for a few weeks, then fall off track when the headaches kicked it. So, that was goal number one: to better manage the headaches and find types of physical activity that didn't cause pain. Goal number two was weight loss, and I was well aware that the two issues were undoubtedly linked. I worked with a functional movement specialist and personal trainer to develop a program, which initially consisted of foam rolling and other forms of myofascial release, a full-body flexibility routine, and a lot of mobility exercises, planks, and bodyweight exercises. The objective was to develop proper movement patterns before adding external loads.

Over the course of the next few months, we slowly added external resistance in the form of free weights and weight machines, as well as introducing the suspension trainer and heavy ropes. We advanced the complexity of the mobility exercises and added the rowing machine to a cardio routine that had largely consisted of walking. Soon, steady-state exercise on the elliptical trainer transformed into high-intensity interval training as my fitness levels progressed.

Importantly, both the frequency and severity of my headaches improved, which meant I was able to become more consistent than I had ever been when it came to exercise. Another clear sign of progress was that whenever I went hiking—my preferred form of cardio—I noticed that I felt considerably better during and after the hike and required less recovery time.

In addition to monitoring how I was feeling over the course of the year-long project, I had undergone an extensive amount of baseline testing with both my doctor and my functional movement specialist and personal trainer. Every measurable element of my health improved over the course of the year. Table 14.16 shows what I call the final faceoff between my old self and my new self, taken 365 days apart.

Table 14.16   The Results of 1 Year of Lifestyle Change

Test or measurement	Day 1	Day 365
Weight	244.5 lb (110.9 kg)	210.0 lb (95.3 kg)
BMI	37.2 kg/m^2—grade II obesity	31.9 kg/m^2—grade I obesity
Blood pressure	124/82 mm Hg—stage 1 hypertension	118/76 mm Hg—normal
Total cholesterol	205 mg/dL—elevated	185 mg/dL—normal
LDL cholesterol	128.2 mg/dL—normal	128.6 mg/dL—normal
HDL cholesterol	33 mg/dL—low	33 mg/dL—low
Triglycerides	219 mg/dL—elevated	117 mg/dL—normal
Hemoglobin A$_{1C}$	5.8%—prediabetes	5.4%—normal
Fasting blood glucose	96 mg/dL—normal	98 mg/dL—normal
Body fat, % (skinfolds)	26.9%—obese	22.2%—average
CIRCUMFERENCES		
Hips Waist Abdomen Biceps Chest Thigh	42.5 in. (108.0 cm) 46.0 in. (116.8 cm) 45.7 in. (116.1 cm) 17.5 in. (44.5 cm) 48.0 in. (121.9 cm) 24.6 in. (62.5 cm)	40.9 in. (103.9 cm) 40.4 in. (102.5 cm) 42.1 in. (106.9 cm) 15.4 in. (39.1 cm) 45.3 in. (115.1 cm) 23.2 in. (58.9 cm)
Waist-to-hip ratio (target is <0.95)	1.08—at risk	0.99—at risk
PERFORMANCE ASSESSMENTS		
Push-up test Curl-up test Bodyweight squat test 1-mi walk test	21 reps—very good 28 reps—poor 58 reps—excellent 17:03—poor	31—excellent 43—above average 80—excellent 14:31—low average

Note: BMI = body mass index; HDL = high-density lipoprotein; LDL = low-density lipoprotein.

I'd like to share some lessons learned that exercise professionals can share with their clients to empower them to change their lives in the same way that structured and methodical exercise did for me.

- Before getting started, take the time to examine your current habits.
- Find partners who will hold you accountable.
- Small changes add up quickly, so be mindful each time you eat a meal or perform a workout.
- Have daily and weekly goals.
- Treat a vacation as a break from stress, not as a break from the things that keep you happy, healthy, and centered.
- Find activities you enjoy.
- Try not to focus on your failures.
- Focus on progress, not perfection.

A consistent physical activity program that featured progressive exercise and was aligned with my goals and values was an essential element of this life-changing journey. By combining better nutrition, a holistic approach to wellness that featured mindfulness and checking in with how I was feeling before and after meals and workouts, and an understanding that true change takes time and commitment, the exercise program changed the course of my life. Free from the daily pain I had been suffering, I was able to enjoy my life in ways I had never been able to before. And shouldn't that be the ultimate goal?

Story 4

Jonathan Ross

I'm going to get something to eat," I said to my father. "I'll see you when I get back." But I didn't see him when I got back. I never saw him again. When I was 24 years old, my father died of a heart attack. He was 56 years old and weighed 424 lb (192 kg). Those were the last words we spoke. He was at the hospital, and they were running tests on him. We had already been there for many hours. I left to get something to eat, and when I came back, he was gone. Not gone from the hospital, but gone from existence. Not long after this, I chose a career in fitness, inspired directly by a desire to lead the countless people living lives like my father was—if you can call it living—toward a different everyday experience and a different outcome.

Jay

Many years later, I met Jay. He knew he needed help and hired me to provide it. He was in his mid-30s, with a demanding job featuring work shifts in three different time blocks. He had 1-year-old and 10-year-old sons, and he was getting married in the coming year. He also weighed 360 lb (163 kg), and he knew his health was headed in the wrong direction. At the same time, he was lost as to how to navigate the fixed parts of his life while successfully changing his lifestyle.

During our first session, Jay knew he needed to get healthier and lose weight, because there is no healthy version of 360 lb (163 kg). However, he did not—on a meaningful personal level—know why he needed to lose weight. This is very common. By this point in my career, I had learned to be what I have humorously begun to refer to as usefully annoying. I kept asking Jay, "Why is this important to you?" After many rounds of unsatisfying, superficial answers, followed by my repeating of the question, we finally hit the jackpot.

Jay mentioned that he and his 10-year-old son enjoy amusement parks—specifically, riding roller coasters together. He began telling me a story about how, the previous summer, they were in line to ride a roller coaster, and as they were almost to the point of getting on the ride, the operator had to prevent Jay from riding due to safety restrictions related to his excess weight. The moment he began telling this story, I noticed the change to the tone of his voice, which grew lower, softer, and more serious. I noticed the look in his eyes as they got shinier and focused on some far-off spot recalling the memory of that day. I imagined what that must have felt like—to stand there and be told you cannot ride due to legitimate, yet no less crushing, safety concerns. I imagined how devastating it must have felt—the embarrassment of this happening in front of so many strangers and the confusion Jay's son must have felt, because he was unlikely to understand the nuances of why they were prevented from riding. And I was also excited. I was excited because I knew, in that moment, we had discovered the essential motivational fuel to keep Jay going. No one wants to lose weight just to get healthier. They want to enjoy the things they love to do with the people they care about. In Jay's case, this was riding roller coasters with his son. The reason for seeking weight loss is unique to each person. Discover it and you find an almost limitless source of motivation. What Jay did with this realization was moving, as we will soon see.

Time

I have learned that when beginning training sessions with a fitness professional, a client will often give best-case-scenario answers when asked, "How much time do you have to exercise?" Jay was no different. He gave me an hour each workday. His plan was to work out on the way to, or on the way home from, work, as determined by his schedule on any given day. But I knew better. None of us have very many best-case-scenario days, especially when you are raising children while working a demanding, full-time job. Jay gave me 60 minutes. I used only 30. To give him a useful mixture of the two main essential types of exercises, I had him perform a full-body resistance training circuit and aerobic interval training for 15 minutes each. No matter where he was in the circuit, at the 15-min mark, I had him stop and immediately switch to 15 minutes of the aerobic work. Around 3 weeks into his workouts, after missing only one planned workout due to some unavoidable circumstances, Jay told me that the 30-minute workout was a wise choice (even though he had initially challenged me on whether it was long enough at the beginning). He shared that there were numerous days where, given how much the day had taken out of him, had he been facing a 60-minute workout, he would likely have skipped it. At 30 minutes, the commitment of time felt small enough that Jay would still do his workout, even when conditions in his day were not ideal.

Endless Motivation

Finally—and it is essential to point out that this idea did not come from me—Jay figured out how to motivate himself. With his awareness that his real goal was to have cherished experiences with his son, he took a picture of his family and a picture of a roller coaster, taped them to a small piece of cardboard, laminated it, brought it to every workout, and placed it on the display of whichever cardio machine he was using. And he just stared at it while exercising. I could not have thought of this for him, and even if I had, it would have been less powerful for having come from me.

Takeaways

- Help clients find the emotional relevance of exercise and physical activity. This provides the motivation from within.
- Have clients do whatever they can for however long they can at first. Consistency is key. The body a person lives in is the product of their consistent behaviors.

Chapter Quiz and Case Study Answers

Chapter 1

Chapter Quiz Answers

1. c
2. d
3. a
4. d
5. a
6. b
7. a
8. a
9. b
10. b

Case Study Answers

1. b
2. a
3. Identify two limitations of using BMI as the only measure of weight status when working with this participant.
   - BMI does not consider an individual's gender, ethnicity, body shape, or body composition.
   - Using only the BMI ignores adverse bias and stigma associated with this measure.
4. Describe two behavioral factors that affect obesity and are within the scope of the exercise professional to discuss with the participant.
   - Low levels of physical activity
   - Prolonged bouts of sedentary behavior

5. How can you take a person-centered approach to developing the exercise prescription and working with this participant?
   - Do not assume weight loss is the participant's goal.
   - Avoid weight bias and stigmatizing language.

Chapter 2

Chapter Quiz Answers

1. b
2. d
3. a
4. b
5. b
6. a
7. d
8. d
9. b
10. b

Case Study Answers

1. d
2. b
3. b
4. What barriers to Martina's becoming more physically active can you identify from the information provided?

   Suggested answer: Highly sedentary job; need for child care if she were to attend classes outside of school or work hours; finding time to exercise; although her employer provides a benefit related to physical activity, the location is close to work but not necessarily close to her home.

5. What are some of the challenges Martina may face when trying to change her dietary intake?

    Suggested answer: Lack of a grocery store near her home, changing caloric intake while also managing her high blood pressure and type 2 diabetes, and creating a meal plan that meets her needs in addition to those of her children.

Chapter 3

Chapter Quiz Answers

1. a
2. c
3. b
4. b
5. b
6. a
7. c
8. b
9. b
10. d

Case Study Answers

1. d
2. c
3. b
4. b
5. d

Chapter 4

Chapter Quiz Answers

1. b
2. c
3. c
4. a
5. c
6. b
7. d
8. a
9. d
10. b

Case Study Answers

1. Given Penny's sense of urgency to improve both her own and Roy's physical activity behaviors and weight loss goals, you deduce that she is using key tenets of the health belief model (HBM), such as perceived threats. Based on the HBM, explain both the perceived threats and the outcome expectations that Penny may have regarding her partner's health status.

    Suggested answer: Examples of perceived threats may include that Roy's health conditions (prediabetes and hypertension) pose a large threat to his quality of life and that Roy's diagnoses and his doctor's advice should be taken seriously to improve his health. Outcome expectations, either positive or negative, may include that if Roy starts exercising, it might be easier for him to manage his weight, and if he doesn't start exercising, he may be at higher risk for a cardiac event.

2. a

3. You are strategizing about your communication approach with Roy, knowing that Penny is bringing him in to meet with you. Using the strategies of motivational interviewing, what are three examples of questions you might ask him?

    Suggested answers:

    1. You've already taken the hardest step by coming in here today. What physical activity have you tried in the past?
    2. I can see that you have great social support and encouragement from your wife, Penny. Tell me about the conversations the two of you have had to lead up to our time together today.
    3. Thanks for sharing that with me. It sounds like you're hesitant to start any type of resistance training or lifting program, since it's been about 15 years since you've been in a gym. Can you tell me a little bit more about that?

4. What lifestyle behaviors could potentially be affecting Roy's blood test, blood pressure, and BMI results? How would you facilitate self-awareness and self-regulation of Roy's lifestyle behaviors?

    Suggested answers: Lifestyle factors that could be affecting Roy's clinical results include nutrition, eating, and hydration patterns; physical inactivity; poor sleep; stress; and the amount of social support present at home and work. Self-monitoring—either using technology or a paper record—may help Roy to develop self-awareness.

5. Two evidence-based ways to improve self-efficacy include verbal persuasion and vicarious experiences. If you were to use these strategies to improve Roy's self-efficacy, what would that look like? Provide at least three examples of tactics that may be useful.

Suggested answers:

1. *Vicarious experience example:* You could tell Roy about a current client of yours who shares the same life stage as Roy and has seen improvements in physical function and other health markers since starting to exercise two days per week.

2. *Verbal persuasion example:* You could explain the reasoning behind the first month of exercise programming in terms that align with Roy's personal goals and what matters to him. For instance, if you've learned that Roy and Penny have grandchildren on the way, you can discuss the importance of his being able to lift, carry, and play with his future grandchildren.

3. *Vicarious experience example:* You could ask Roy to recall a friend or family member who has started a physical activity program and has seen mental or physical health benefits after consistently sticking with it.

Chapter 5

Chapter Quiz Answers

1. d
2. b
3. a
4. c
5. d
6. a
7. c
8. a
9. d
10. d

Case Study Answers

1. According to the ACSM preparticipation guidelines, should Andre get medical clearance before starting an exercise program?

2. Which cardiovascular disease risk factors does Andre have?

ACSM Preparticipation Screening Responses	
Currently participates in regular exercise?	No
Known cardiovascular, metabolic, or renal disease?	No
Signs or symptoms suggestive of cardiovascular, metabolic, or renal disease?	Yes
Desired exercise program intensity?	No
Is medical clearance recommended for Andre?	Yes
CVD Risk Factor Analysis Using ACSM Criteria	
Age	Yes
Blood glucose level	Yes
Blood pressure	Yes
Body mass index and waist circumference	Yes
Cigarette smoking	No
Family history	No
Lipids	No
Physical inactivity	Yes

Note: ACSM = American College of Sports Medicine; CVD = cardiovascular disease.

Chapter 6

Chapter Quiz Answers

1. d
2. b
3. c
4. d
5. d
6. e
7. a
8. b
9. d
10. c

Case Study Answers

1. What health-related assessments would you perform on Mrs. Penelope?
   - 6-minute walk test for cardiorespiratory fitness
   - timed up and go test for functional motor control
   - testing of all vital signs, including height, weight, skinfold measurements, arm circumference, and waist-to-hip ratio
   - YMCA bench press test
   - 60-second sit-to-stand test

2. Which field test would best accommodate Mrs. Penelope to measure her cardiorespiratory fitness? Explain why you chose this test.

   Suggested answer: The 6-minute walk test would best measure her cardiorespiratory fitness. She stated that she tires easily walking up stairs but can walk some distance on flat ground, so this test will give a good indication of her abilities.

3. Does this client have any contraindications that would preclude you from conducting certain fitness tests on her? If so, what tests should be avoided, and why might they be unsafe for this individual? If not, indicate why you would be comfortable with conducting any of the fitness assessments.

   Suggested answer: At this time, the client does not have any contraindications that would preclude performing any of the assessments. I would be sure to monitor her blood pressure prior to and following the assessments, given that it is slightly elevated,

but I feel that Mrs. Penelope will tolerate the assessments fine.

4. How would you assess Mrs. Penelope's muscular endurance? Which test, or tests, would you use and why?

   Suggested answer:
   - I would use the YMCA bench press for upper-extremity strength. It can be easily administered and would provide better results than a push-up test.
   - I would use the 60-second squat test for her lower-extremity strength. This test is simple to administer, and Mrs. Penelope has expressed that her legs tire with stair climbing, so this test would provide some information that could assist with program planning.

5. Would you prescribe cardiorespiratory exercise, resistance training, or both? Provide a rationale for your answer.

   Suggested answer: I would prescribe both cardiorespiratory exercise and resistance training, because both parameters are critical for optimal health and function. However, I would focus on the cardiorespiratory exercise a bit more, initially, and begin resistance training with light hand weights, kettlebells, and circuit-type training to give Mrs. Penelope the confidence to increase resistance training. She feels that she has a strong upper body, so I want to encourage her in an area in which she is confident.

Chapter 7

Chapter Quiz Answers

1. b
2. a
3. b
4. b
5. a
6. c
7. c
8. b
9. b
10. b

Case Study Answers

1. b
2. d

3. Name three ways Meg can build Beth's comfort level with her and the facility.

   Suggested answer: Find a quiet space away from the mirrors, set up a space where Beth can move freely between pieces of equipment, and use welcoming and inclusive language.

4. Based on what you know of Beth's experience with exercise and her limitations, what is one warm-up drill you would recommend that Meg avoid?

   Suggested answer: Meg should have Beth avoid bodyweight exercises on all fours until she has a better understanding of Beth's wrist limitations.

5. Based on what you know of Beth's experience with exercise and her likes and dislikes, what is one warm-up drill you would recommend that Meg include?

   Suggested answer: Beth enjoys treadmills and stationary bikes, so Meg could incorporate some movement on those pieces of equipment.

Chapter 8

Chapter Quiz Answers

1. b
2. a
3. d
4. b
5. a
6. c
7. a
8. d
9. c
10. b

Case Study Answers

1. What mode of resistance training should John perform for his muscular fitness program to meet his goals from both a physiological and psychological perspective?

   Suggested answer: Foundational movement patterns using body weight, dumbbells, and a diverse range of elastic bands may be a feasible and effective muscle-strengthening concept for John. Additionally, partner-assisted manual resistance using isometric holds can also be used as an adjunct strategy, offering a safe and engaging exercise experience. This approach can be easily implemented in a personal training studio or John's home, where stationary weight training machines and barbells may not be available.

2. How would you program the muscle-strengthening routine in terms of the number of exercises, volume, intensity, and rest intervals?

   Suggested answer: A progressive circuit resistance training program can be used, incorporating 4 to 12 exercises for all major muscle groups, performed in a circuit fashion with 8 to 20 repetitions (30-60 s) for each exercise, with rest intervals lasting anywhere from 10 to 30 s. Two to three rounds of the circuit should be performed, with 2 to 3 minutes of rest between rounds. All prescribed exercises should respect John's physical limitations and musculoskeletal health profile, ensuring a pain-free muscle-strengthening experience.

3. What type of physiological responses might John expect when performing this exercise routine?

   Suggested answer: John will probably experience an increase in heart rate, ventilation, systolic blood pressure, and sweat rate (due to an elevation in body temperature) as well as an increase in blood flow and oxygen delivery to the working muscles. These responses will fluctuate in accordance with the working sets and rest intervals yet will likely remain elevated in comparison to resting conditions.

4. When will John begin to see results from his new workout routine, and what physiological adaptations can he expect with regard to his health and fitness profile?

   Suggested answer: The physiological effects of the circuit-based muscle-strengthening program may be seen as early as 4 weeks for cardiometabolic indices, with the majority of alterations occurring closer to 8 or 12 weeks. These changes may include a reduction in resting heart rate, blood pressure, blood lipids, and fasting glucose levels, as well as a reduction in body mass (particularly when combined with healthy eating habits) and improved body composition (i.e., an increase in lean body mass and a reduction in body fat mass). Additionally, there should be an increase in muscular strength and muscular endurance. The aforementioned adaptations will likely lead to notable enhancements in functional capacity and overall health.

5. Besides biological benefits, what other psychological and mental benefits might John experience from his new resistance training routine?

Suggested answer: As the resistance training routine is performed and improvements are observed, John may experience an increase in self-confidence, self-esteem, and self-efficacy. Furthermore, he may report positive affect, an improved mood state, increased energy arousal, and feelings of happiness. It is possible that such psychological and mental alterations may enhance John's quality of life over the long term.

Chapter 9

Chapter Quiz Answers

1. b
2. d
3. b
4. a
5. b
6. a
7. c
8. c
9. d
10. a

Case Study Answers

1. If you were Sharon's personal trainer, explain how you would guide her after discovering her story during her initial assessment.

Suggested answer: Sharon has a history of unfortunate events that have led her to a very lonely state of living. There are many changes that need to occur, but after discovering her low motivation, adherence will be key before focusing on other changes. The prime goal, initially, is for Sharon to develop a habit and keep her appointments. Performing exercises that feel good for her body, along with deep breathing, can help promote adherence. Once her initial exercise goal is met, then adding additional changes will be easier.

2. Explain your role, or scope of practice, with regard to helping Sharon live a healthier life.

Suggested answer: Many of Sharon's deeper psychoemotional issues would be best worked through with a therapist. However, a trainer can guide her to resources, classes, and breathing exercises that can help her overall well-being and boost her confidence.

3. Explain how Sharon's lifestyle choices of television and junk food contribute to her negative health cycle, regardless of her thyroid situation.

Suggested answer: Many processed foods negatively affect the metabolism while also increasing inflammation. Television and junk food go hand in hand, and both are addictive and demotivating. They can keep people like Sharon in a vicious loop; to cope with trauma, she escapes with junk food and movies, but what she consumes is detrimental to her health and well-being.

4. Given Sharon's history, explain how mind–body exercise could benefit her.

Suggested answer: Sharon is unbalanced in various aspects of her physical, mental, and emotional well-being. Mind–body exercise would be beneficial and maybe even like a one-stop shop for Sharon, aiding with her stress, physical health, and confidence. Physically, Sharon would be able to participate in low-impact exercise that focuses on deep breathing, and this would reduce her stress and help her sleep. The positive hormones released during an activity such as yoga might also help to give Sharon a better outlook on herself and on life.

5. If you were guiding Sharon, how would you convince her of the benefits of mind–body exercise to encourage her to try it? Share three examples.

Suggested answers:

• Since Sharon has an autoimmune disorder, her autonomic nervous system is already compromised. Mind–body exercise would not only help her physically move, but she would also be caring for her nervous system, which would help her body regulate imbalances.

- Mind–body exercise can improve both mental and physical health. When the body feels better, people often choose healthier foods, which would help Sharon produce more energy and feel better in general.
- Deep breathing and mind–body exercises can help Sharon organically process her past trauma and let go of any pain or suffering from inside.

Chapter 10

Chapter Quiz Answers

1. a
2. c
3. a
4. c
5. b
6. c
7. b
8. a
9. d
10. c

Case Study Answers: Cardiorespiratory Fitness

1. What mode of exercise should Aubrey perform for her HIIT program, and how should she set up her initial intervals?

   Suggested answer: Aubrey should perform her HIIT workouts on her stationary cycle to avoid overstressing her foot injury. While she could perform workouts on her commuter bike, it may be easier to track with the stationary cycle initially. She should set up her intervals using a 1:2 work-to-rest ratio lasting 3 minutes. The intensity should be monitored using the rating of perceived exertion, making sure the high-intensity bout is either hard or somewhat hard and the low-intensity bout is light.

2. How would you program the hybrid-type interval training in terms of the number of exercises, sequence, and rest intervals?

   Suggested answer: The hybrid-type interval training should involve full-body exercises performed in a circuit format, where 8 to 10 exercises are performed for 20 to 40 seconds each, with rest intervals lasting anywhere from 20 to 40 seconds. At least two rounds of the circuit should be performed.

3. What type of physiological responses might Aubrey expect when performing these exercise routines?

   Suggested answer: For both routines, Aubrey should expect to experience increases in heart rate, ventilation, systolic blood pressure, perspiration (due to increased body temperature), blood flow to working muscles, and oxygen delivery to the muscles. These responses will undulate with the high- and low-intensity intervals but will remain elevated compared to resting conditions.

4. When will Aubrey begin to see results from her new routine, and what physiological adaptations can she expect?

   Suggested answer: The physiological benefits of the program might be observed after as few as 4 weeks for metabolic markers, with the majority of changes occurring closer to 8 weeks. These changes may include a reduction in resting heart rate and blood pressure, a decrease in body weight (particularly when combined with dietary improvements), and enhanced body composition (i.e., an increase in lean body mass and a reduction in body fat mass). Additionally, there should be an increase in maximal oxygen consumption and an improvement in tolerance to aerobic exercise and activity.

5. Besides physical benefits, what other psychological and mental benefits might Aubrey gain from her new routine?

   Suggested answer: She may report feelings of improved self-efficacy, affect, and enjoyment or pleasure as she begins to observe improvements in her performance of the exercise routine. However, it should be noted that these feelings are not universally experienced by all individuals who perform these types of routines.

Case Study Answers: Dance Fitness

1. For someone like Nicole, what are three reasons dance fitness may be beneficial for her health and exercise adherence?

   Suggested answer:
   - Nicole already enjoys dancing, and clients are more likely to adhere to exercise that they enjoy the most.
   - Since dancing is fun for Nicole, she can obtain the traditional physical

benefits from dancing and enhance her emotional well-being by meeting new friends.

- Dance fitness moves the body in all planes of motion to stimulate muscles that Nicole does not regularly use.

2. As an exercise professional, what would you say to Nicole for encouragement to attend dance fitness sessions, even if her attendance is irregular?

   Suggested answer: People lead busy lives in this modern time, and clients have to be realistic with what they can fit into their schedule. Working in the medical field is stressful, with long hours. Nicole should attend dancing as much as she can around her lifestyle. Encourage Nicole by telling her that dancing is not only an effective form of exercise for physical well-being but a great form of stress release that can also stimulate the creative side of life.

3. Nicole's past experiences of attending fitness classes have left her sore and unable to walk much for days. As an exercise professional, what recommendations do you have for her to ease into dance fitness so she does not experience the same results?

   Suggested answer: Shorter, online dance videos are an effective way for her to build endurance and tolerance of multidimensional movement before going from a sedentary lifestyle to hour-long dance classes. Encourage her to attend moderate classes before more advanced programming and to take breaks when needed.

4. Based on the theory you learned above, why is dance fitness so much more appealing for many people than traditional exercise?

   Suggested answer: Dance fitness is more appealing to many people because it seems closer to our human design of being upright, moving, and free. Coupled with music, many people encounter states of flow and have a positive association linked to this movement.

5. Besides physical benefits, what other emotional or mental benefits can Nicole gain from dance fitness?

   Suggested answer: Dancing can be an escape from her stressful day job as a way to enjoy an hour of fun along with boosting her mood. Since she started dancing, Nicole

has slept better, and sleep affects mental health. Social support is a component of emotional and mental well-being, so if Nicole also develops a social life with fellow dancers, this community support may make her feel better.

Chapter 11

Chapter Quiz Answers

1. d
2. b
3. a
4. c
5. c
6. d
7. b
8. a
9. c
10. d

Case Study Answers

1. Do you think someone like Aditya is within your scope of practice?

   Suggested answer: There are aspects that are within and outside of a fitness professional's scope of practice. Aditya's constant pain issues for everyday movements may require physical therapy or a doctor's analysis of his joints. Within the fitness professional's scope of practice would be a focus on a variety of corrective exercises to build joint mobility and stability as well as bodyweight exercises that mimic everyday movements. The goal is to make sessions enjoyable and not associated with pain. Working on behavioral changes and stretches to release low-back pain also might be beneficial for Aditya.

2. Within your scope of practice, how would you structure Aditya's fitness program?

   Suggested answer: Aditya needs fitness training to enhance his well-being. Everyday movements with constant hip flexion have triggered hip pain, so Aditya needs corrective exercise for the major joints in his body. Warming up with walking and then progressing to corrective exercises, followed by everyday movements, is a good structure for the bulk of the program. Cooling down with walking, deep breathing, and several major stretches will benefit his program.

3. Knowing that Aditya's hip pain flares up with the specific exercises mentioned, what cool-down exercises would you incorporate into his program?

   Suggested answer: Because Aditya needs conditioning, walking would be an effective exercise to cool down the body while increasing his conditioning. Thoracic mobility exercises may also help, because he sits for long periods of time.

4. What stretches would you incorporate into Aditya's cool-down program?

   Suggested answer: A supported hip hinge, high lunge with pectoral and calf stretch, and elevated forward fold could help alleviate Aditya's low-back pain and focus on postural improvement.

5. What SMR techniques would you incorporate, knowing that Aditya should not sit on the foam roller?

   Suggested answer: Aditya should not perform traditional foam rolling until he is better conditioned. He can use a massage ball, or even his thumb or palm area, to gently apply pressure to the top of the quadriceps and lateral hip. In addition, gently rubbing out the pectoral muscles may reduce tension caused in these areas from poor posture.

Chapter 12

Chapter Quiz Answers

1. a
2. d
3. b
4. b
5. d
6. b
7. a
8. b
9. c
10. c

Case Study Answers

1. What mode of training should Mary perform to meet her cardiorespiratory, muscular, and neuromotor and functional needs, priorities, and goals, from both a physiological and psychological perspective?

Suggested answer: Mary should perform cardiorespiratory, resistance, flexibility, and neuromotor exercises (balance and agility exercises) as recommended. Considering her older age, hip arthritis, body weight, and low functional capacity, she should select exercises that are low impact, such as low-intensity walking, cycling, swimming, or training on an elliptical machine. Strength training could involve bodyweight movements, comfortable stationary machines, elastic bands, or dumbbells with lighter weights. If a particular exercise exacerbates her pain, she should modify it with the help of her trainer to target the same muscle groups. Most importantly, Mary should choose exercises that she enjoys. She could also join group fitness classes or a walking group, which would provide her with valuable emotional and social support to stay motivated.

2. How would you program the aerobic and muscle-strengthening routine in terms of the number of exercises, volume, intensity, rest intervals, and type of equipment?

   Suggested answer:
   - Mary can begin aerobic exercise by starting with 2 or 3 days per week and gradually increasing to 5 days. She should choose activities that involve major muscle groups, such as walking, cycling, or swimming. She should start with 30 to 60 minutes of exercise per week and progress to 150 minutes; for weight loss, she should aim for 250 to 300 minutes per week, beginning at a low intensity and working toward moderate intensity, using the talk test to gauge effort. She should progress by increasing exercise time by 5 to 10 minutes per week over 6-8 weeks before adjusting frequency, intensity, or type.
   - Mary can start resistance training 2 days per week with a full-body workout consisting of 8 to 10 exercises targeting major muscle groups. She should begin at a lighter intensity, gradually increasing to moderate or vigorous intensity using the rating of perceived exertion scale. She should start with 1 set of 12 to 15 repetitions and progress to 2 or 3 sets of 8 to 12 repetitions. She

should use bodyweight movements, stationary machines, elastic bands, or dumbbells for exercises and increase the weight when she is able to complete 2 or 3 sets of 12 to 15 repetitions.

- All progressions should be very gradual. Stretching and neuromotor exercises should also be included to improve balance and agility, which is especially important considering Mary's age.

3. What type of physiological responses might Mary expect when performing a comprehensive exercise routine?

Suggested answer: Mary can expect several physiological changes when following a comprehensive exercise routine. These changes may include increased muscular strength and endurance, power, bone density, muscle mass, balance, and cardiorespiratory fitness as well as reductions in body weight and in both visceral and subcutaneous body fat. These improvements may enhance her ability to perform daily tasks, such as climbing stairs, rising from a chair, and walking with reduced fatigue. Additionally, she may experience fewer falls, reduced joint swelling, and less pain. Exercise could also help lower Mary's cardiovascular disease risk factors, such as cholesterol and blood pressure, and improve her overall heart health.

4. What should be a priority for Mary with respect to her health and fitness profile, especially regarding her behavior outside the gym? Suggest client-centered program design strategies.

Suggested answer: Mary should prioritize all four components of fitness. This does not have to be only through structured exercises; it could be physical activities outside the gym, such as taking the stairs instead of the elevator, dancing, gardening, walking or hiking, playing pickleball or tennis, or doing household chores. It is important that she does not ignore strength training, because weight loss is usually accompanied by muscle and bone loss, which can lead to a decline in physical function.

5. Besides biological benefits, what psychological and mental benefits might Mary experience from a personalized exercise routine?

Suggested answer: Mary may experience psychological and mental benefits from a personalized exercise routine, including reduced stress; improved mood, self-esteem, self-efficacy, self-confidence, and cognitive function; and better sleep. Regular exercise can also help reduce anxiety and depression, promoting Mary's overall mental well-being and quality of life.

Glossary

active isolated stretching—A method of muscle lengthening and fascial release that is a type of athletic stretching technique intended to provide effective, dynamic, facilitated stretching of major muscle groups.

activities of daily living (ADLs)—Skills needed to live independently.

acute responses—Immediate physiological changes that occur during or immediately after a resistance training session, such as increases in heart rate, hormonal changes, and muscle fiber activation.

acute stress—The stress experienced daily from minor situations.

adaptations—Physical changes that occur with training. Typically, adaptations are classified as neurological, muscular, or metabolic changes that occur with a training stimulus.

adherence—Maintenance of or commitment to a training program.

adipokines—Cytokines secreted by adipose tissue; they play roles in metabolism and inflammation and can be altered as a result of obesity.

adipose tissue—Loose connective tissue composed mostly of adipocytes; also known as body fat.

adiposity distribution—Distribution of white adipose tissue in the human body, including subcutaneous fat, visceral fat, yellow bone marrow, intermuscular fat, and breast tissue fat.

aerobic—Referring to the use of oxygen for energy regeneration during an activity.

affect—An instinctive mood response that does not require considerable thought and is associated with pleasure or displeasure and tension or calmness.

air displacement plethysmography—A body composition analysis technique for measuring body composition that uses air displacement to determine body volume; typically measured using a device known as a Bod Pod.

anaerobic—Referring to energy regeneration without the use of oxygen during an activity.

android obesity—Obesity characterized by the distribution of adipose tissue mainly around the trunk and upper body; also called *apple-shaped obesity*.

anthropometrics—The practice of taking measurements of the human body and providing categorized data.

anti-obesity medications (AOMs)—Medications prescribed to aid in weight loss by affecting appetite, metabolism, or nutrient absorption.

arrhythmogenic—Producing or tending to produce cardiac arrhythmia.

asymmetric—Not symmetrical; lacking symmetry; misproportioned.

autonomic nervous system—A component of the peripheral nervous system that regulates involuntary physiologic processes including heart rate, blood pressure, respiration, digestion, and sexual arousal.

ballistic stretching—A type of stretching that uses the momentum of a moving body or a limb in an attempt to force a joint beyond its normal range of motion.

bariatric surgery—A surgical procedure used to manage obesity and obesity-related conditions.

barriers to behavior change—Impediments to one's ability to make forward progress with health-related goals, including actual barriers (e.g., lack of access, bodily ability, or transportation) or perceived barriers (e.g., lack of time or competence).

barriers to entry—Specific conditions that make it less likely for someone to buy or take part in something.

basal metabolic rate (BMR)—The rate at which the body expends energy to maintain basic physiological functions at rest; also referred to as resting energy expenditure (REE).

beats per minute—The pace of music, measured by the number of beats occurring in 60 seconds.

behavioral modification—The use of behavior change techniques to alter eating and activity habits in order to achieve weight loss.

beiging—The process by which white adipose tissue takes on characteristics similar to brown adipose tissue, including increased metabolic activity and heat production.

bioelectrical impedance analysis (BIA)—A body composition analysis technique that uses an electrical current and resistance encountered by the electrical current to estimate body composition.

blood glucose—The main type of sugar in the blood and a main source of energy for the body's cells.

blood pressure—The pressure exerted by the blood on the arteries, measured in millimeters of mercury (mm Hg).

body composition—The body's amount of fat mass relative to fat-free mass.

body mass index—An index of weight relative to height, calculated by dividing body weight in kilograms by height in meters squared.

body temperature—A vital sign that measures how well the body produces and releases heat, typically 37 °C at rest and increasing to up to 40 °C during exercise.

bodyweight exercise—A type of exercise in which individuals use their own body weight as resistance, rather than equipment.

bradykinesia—Slowness of movement and speed (or progressive hesitations or halts) as movements are continued.

branding—The creation of a particular feeling about a company, individual, or service in the mind of the target market.

cardiac output (*Q*)—Volume of blood pumped per minute.

cardiorespiratory fitness (CRF)—Ability to perform large-muscle, dynamic, moderate- to vigorous-intensity exercise for prolonged periods.

cardiovascular preparedness—State in which the heart and circulatory system are primed for increased activity through gradual increases of intensity with warm-up exercise.

catecholamines—Hormones, such as adrenaline and noradrenaline, released during stress and exercise, which help to increase heart rate, blood pressure, and energy supply.

central nervous system—The part of the nervous system consisting of the brain and spinal cord; plays a key role in initiating muscle contraction during resistance training.

chronic disease—Conditions that last 1 year or longer and require ongoing medical attention, limit activities of daily living, or both.

chronic responses—Long-term physiological adaptations resulting from consistent resistance training over a period of time, including increases in muscle size and strength and improvements in metabolic function.

chronic stress—A prolonged, often overwhelming feeling of stress that can negatively affect a person's daily life.

client-centered—Characterized by placing clients at the center of professional–client relationship to best support clients in setting and meeting their exercise goals.

clinical exercise physiologist—Degreed exercise professional who specializes in managing long-term, noncommunicable health conditions using a scientific, rehabilitative, individualized exercise prescription.

combined training (CT)—A combination of resistance training and continuous endurance training in a single training session.

comorbidity—The state of having more than one disease or medical condition at the same time.

continuous endurance training (CET)—Performance of a single type of rhythmic exercise for a prolonged period at a low to moderate intensity.

cool-down—The act or an instance of allowing physiological activity to return to normal gradually after strenuous exercise by engaging in less strenuous exercise.

core activation—The engagement and strengthening of the muscles in the torso, including the abdominals, obliques, and lower back, to stabilize the spine and support movements during exercise.

cortisol—A glucocorticoid hormone produced and released by the adrenal glands.

cytokines—Signaling proteins that regulate the inflammatory response within the body, enabling the immune system to mount an effective defense against pathogens and other substances that can cause illness.

dance—Moving one's body rhythmically to music, usually as a form of artistic or emotional expression; one of the most primitive forms of human communication and expression and considered to be one of the most synchronized activities performed by the body.

dance fitness—A full-body workout routine incorporating dance movements.

dance therapy or movement therapy—The psychotherapeutic use of movement to promote emotional, social, cognitive, and physical integration of the individual for the purpose of improving health and well-being.

Davis's law—Describes how soft tissue is modeled according to imposed demands.

decisional balance—A fundamental construct of the transtheoretical, or stages of change, model which involves weighing the pros and cons of engaging in a health behavior and the outcome of changing the behavior.

dietary restriction—A reduction in calorie intake through intentional dietary planning.

dual-energy x-ray absorptiometry (DEXA)—A body composition analysis technique that uses a low-dose x-ray to measure body composition, including estimates of fat mass, lean mass, and bone mineral density.

dynamic warm-up—A series of active movements that prepare the body for exercise by increasing heart rate, blood flow, and flexibility.

dynamometer—A device that measures static force.

efferent motor pathways—Nerve pathways that carry signals from the central nervous system to the muscles to initiate movement.

emotional intelligence—The ability to process emotional information and use it in reasoning and other cognitive activities; typically described as having four components: (1) self-awareness, (2) self-regulation, (3) situational awareness, and (4) situational regulation.

entrepreneurial myth (e-myth)—The mistaken belief that if one knows the skills for doing a job (e.g., personal training), they have the skills to run a business that provides that service.

endogenous opiates—Naturally occurring opiates in the body, such as endorphins, that can enhance mood and provide pain relief.

energy balance—The state achieved when energy intake equals energy expenditure, resulting in stable body weight.

energy expenditure—The total amount of energy used to maintain essential body functions (respiration, circulation, and digestion) and as a result of physical activity.

energy intake—The amount of energy attained from food consumption.

excess postexercise oxygen consumption (EPOC)—The increased rate of oxygen intake following strenuous activity, contributing to higher energy expenditure during recovery.

exercise—A type of physical activity that is planned, structured, and repetitive and has an objective of improving or maintaining physical fitness.

exercise physiologist—Degreed exercise professional who develops physical activity and exercise programs to help people improve components of their physical fitness, including cardiovascular fitness, muscular strength, muscular endurance, and flexibility.

extrafusal muscle fibers—Muscle fibers outside the muscle spindle; most muscle tissue is composed of extrafusal fibers.

exercise preparticipation health screening—A brief process designed to identify people who may be at risk for exercise-related acute myocardial infarction or sudden cardiac death.

exercise professional—An individual who is trained in designing and implementing exercise programs to promote physical activity engagement and meet the physical activity needs and goals of a client; these professionals may be certified by educational organizations.

exerkines—A group of signaling molecules released during physical exercise that can affect various tissues and cellular pathways, including metabolic regulation, anti-inflammatory effects, muscle adaptation and growth, cognitive health, and cardiovascular health.

extrinsic motivation—A type of motivation that involves engaging in a behavior or activity for a reward or recognition from others.

flow state—A mental state that occurs when someone is completely immersed in a task or activity.

gait—The manner of walking or moving on foot.

glycated hemoglobin (HbA$_{1c}$)—The average blood glucose level over a 3-month period.

glycogen stores—Reserves of glucose stored in the muscles and liver and used as energy during physical activity.

Golgi tendon organs—Sensory receptors located within a tendon that provide the brain with information about muscle tension to prevent muscle damage.

gravity—The force that attracts a body toward the center of the earth or toward any other physical body having mass.

gynoid obesity—Obesity characterized by fat accumulation in the hips and thighs; also called *pear-shaped obesity*.

health—The absence of any disease or impairment, or a state of balance that allows an individual to adequately cope with the demands of life.

heart rate—The number of times the heart beats within a specific period, typically 1 minute.

high-intensity interval training (HIIT)—A type of physical training that uses repeated, high-intensity bouts of exercise interspersed with low-intensity bouts of recovery.

homeostasis—A state of balance among all the body systems needed for survival and correct body function.

hybrid training—training that uses any intermittent, multicomponent exercise mode engaging both the cardiovascular and musculoskeletal systems throughout a single session.

hypertension—A condition in which the pressure of blood in the blood vessels is too high (140/90 mm Hg or higher); also known as high blood pressure.

insulin sensitivity—The efficiency with which cells respond to insulin, affecting how well the body can use glucose for energy.

interdisciplinary—Relating to more than one branch of knowledge.

intrafusal muscle fibers—Muscle fibers inside the spindle.

intrinsic motivation—A type of motivation that involves engaging in a behavior or activity for inherent satisfaction, such as personal accomplishment or enjoyment.

isometric exercise—Contractions of a specific muscle or group of muscles without noticeably changing the muscle's length.

kyphosis—Excessive forward curvature of the spine.

lactic acid—A chemical the body produces when the cells break down carbohydrates for energy.

lean body mass—An aspect of body composition defined as the difference between total body weight and body fat weight; it includes the mass of all organs except body fat, including the bones, muscles, blood, and skin.

left ventricular hypertrophy—An increase in the size of the left ventricle of the heart, often as a chronic adaptation to increased workload from training.

limited range of motion—Occurs when a joint does not move fully and easily in its normal manner, due to a number of factors, including a mechanical problem within the joint, tissue swelling around the joint, muscle spasticity, pain, and disease.

linear periodization—A programming method that gradually increases intensity relative to a person's 1-repetition maximum (1-RM) while simultaneously reducing volume.

lipids—Fatty compounds that perform a variety of functions in the body, facilitating the movement and storage of energy, absorption of vitamins, and synthesis of hormones.

loaded locomotion—A task-specific, multiplanar activity that integrates the whole body and involves moving or resisting an external load.

lordosis—Excessive inward curvature of the spine.

low-impact exercises—Exercises that place minimal stress on the joints.

manual resistance—A type of external resistance applied manually; it requires a partner or a trainer to provide and control the resistance throughout the entire range of movement.

medical clearance—Approval from a health care professional to engage in exercise.

medical history—Information regarding the health and well-being of a client, usually obtained through an interview or a form.

Mind–body fitness—Physical exercise executed with an inwardly-directed focus.

mitochondrial function—The performance of mitochondria, the energy-producing organelles in cells; it is crucial for energy metabolism.

moderate-intensity continuous training (MICT)—Performance of aerobic activity at a moderate intensity in order to improve aerobic fitness.

motivation—Personal reasons for doing something, such as exercising.

motivational interviewing—A communication approach that helps individuals define their current and ideal selves and isolate behaviors that influence movement toward the ideal self.

motor cortex—Area of the brain responsible for planning, controlling, and executing voluntary movements, including those involved in resistance training.

motor skills—Movements and actions that require the coordinated use of large and small muscle groups to complete whole-body movements (gross skills) and precise movements (fine skills), respectively.

motor units—The basic functional units of muscle contraction, consisting of a motor neuron and the muscle fibers it innervates.

multijoint—Referring to coordinated movements or exercises that focus on movements of two or more muscle groups and joints.

multimorbid conditions—The co-occurrence of at least two chronic conditions in the same individual.

multiplanar—Refers to movement of a joint in more than one plane of motion (sagittal, frontal, or transverse).

muscle activation—The stimulation and engagement of specific muscles during exercise to generate force and movement.

muscle hypertrophy—Muscle enlargement that occurs when muscle protein synthesis exceeds muscle protein breakdown, resulting in a positive net protein balance in cumulative periods.

muscle spindles—Sensory receptors within muscles that sense changes in muscle length, playing a crucial role in maintaining muscle tone and coordination.

myofibrillar hypertrophy—Increase in muscle size due to the growth of muscle fibers, primarily through resistance training.

myofilaments—Protein structures within muscle fibers that are involved in muscle contraction and are susceptible to damage during resistance training.

myokines—Inflammatory cytokines that are produced by muscle fibers in response to damage and play a role in muscle repair and adaptation.

neuromotor exercise—Exercise that incorporates various motor skills, such as balance, agility, gait, coordination, and proprioception.

neuromuscular activation—The recruitment and stimulation of nerves and muscles during exercise to perform a specific movement or task.

neuropathy—A nerve condition that can lead to pain, numbness, weakness, or tingling in one or more parts of the body.

neuroplasticity—The ability of the nervous system to change its activity in response to intrinsic or extrinsic stimuli by reorganizing its structure, functions, or connections after an injury, such as a stroke or traumatic brain injury.

neurotropic—Having an affinity for or localizing selectively in nerve tissue.

neurotransmitter—A signaling molecule secreted by a neuron to affect another cell across a synapse.

niche market—A specific demographic that is being targeted.

nonalcoholic fatty liver disease (NAFLD)—A condition characterized by excessive fat buildup in the liver not due to alcohol consumption; often associated with obesity and metabolic syndrome.

obesity—Abnormal or excessive accumulation of body fat, marked by a body mass index classification of 30 kg/m² or greater.

1-repetition maximum (1-RM)—The maximum force that a specific muscle or muscle group produces at one time and one time only.

operant conditioning—A learning theory suggesting that individuals' behaviors are shaped by the consequences that follow them.

osteoporosis—A bone disease that develops when bone mineral density and bone mass decrease or when the structure and strength of bone changes.

overweight—Body weight higher than what is considered healthy for a person's height, marked by a body mass index classification of 25.0 to 29.9 kg/m².

palpitation—A skipped, extra, or irregular heartbeat.

parasympathetic nervous system—A network of nerves that relaxes the body after periods of stress or danger and also helps in the performance of life-sustaining processes, such as digestion, during times when a person feels safe and relaxed.

person-first language—Language that names the individual before their disease or disability to prioritize the individual, not the medical condition.

perceived value—The value of a product or service in the mind of the target market (i.e., what they believe it is worth).

phenotypic variables—Observable traits or characteristics of an individual, such as body weight, that can affect energy expenditure.

physical activity—Any bodily movement produced by skeletal muscles that results in energy expenditure.

Physical Activity Readiness Questionnaire for Everyone (PAR-Q+)—A self-guided questionnaire that determines a person's readiness to exercise based on general health questions.

physical fitness—A set of attributes that are either health- or skill-related and can be measured.

Pilates—A system of exercises using special equipment and designed to improve physical strength, flexibility, and posture while enhancing mental awareness.

posttraumatic stress disorder (PTSD)—A mental health condition triggered by either experiencing or witnessing a terrifying event.

prevalence—The proportion of a population that has a specific characteristic in a given time period.

principles—Concepts based on scientific evidence in the research.

prone—A position in which the front or ventral surface of the body is facing downward.

proprioception—The sense of the relative position of one's own body parts and the strength of effort being used in movement; often affected by excess body weight.

proprioceptive neuromuscular facilitation (PNF)—A technique that involves both stretching and contracting (activation) of the muscle group being targeted to achieve maximum static flexibility.

psychophysiological—Refers to the relationship between the mind and body.

quadruped—A position where both hands and knees are on the ground.

rate pressure product—The product of the systolic blood pressure and the heart rate, often used during exercise to represent the oxygen demands of the heart muscle; also known as the double product (DP).

rating of perceived exertion (RPE)—A subjective, self-reported measurement of exercise intensity.

range of motion (ROM)—The extent to which a body part can be moved round a given joint.

rapport—A connection built on mutual understanding and trust that helps exercise professionals best meet clients' needs.

reflective listening—A component of the motivational interviewing approach; it combines eye contact, body language, and phrases like "I hear you saying…" and "I recall you mentioned that…" to show the coach is truly listening and to help the client feel understood.

registered dietitian—A food and nutrition expert who obtained a graduate degree from an accredited dietetics program, completed a supervised practice requirement, passed a national exam, and completes continuous professional development.

repetition—A single execution of a particular movement or exercise.

risk factor—Any attribute, characteristic, or exposure that increases an individual's likelihood of developing a disease or injury.

rhythm—A regular, repeated pattern of movement or sound.

safety—The condition of not causing injury or harm to clients by delivering programs that meet their needs and ability levels.

satiety—The feeling of fullness and the suppression of hunger after eating, influenced by various physiological signals.

self-efficacy—An individual's belief in their capacity to execute behaviors necessary to reach specific goals.

self-myofascial release—A self-massage technique using a device such as a foam roll or roller massager.

skinfold measurement—A method of estimating body fat percentage that involves using calipers to measure the thickness of subcutaneous fat at several sites on the body.

sleep–wake cycle—A recurring 24-hour cycle of sleeping and waking that is part of the body's internal clock running in the background to carry out essential functions and processes; also known as the circadian rhythm.

SMART goal framework—A well-recognized goal-setting strategy for promoting health behavior change; the acronym stands for specific, measurable, attainable, realistic, and timely or time-bound.

social–ecological model—A comprehensive perspective on health that encompasses various factors affecting an individual's well-being and conceptualizing several layers that can affect health behaviors, starting with intrapersonal factors and zooming out to societal or policy factors.

sphygmomanometer—A device consisting of a blood pressure cuff and a manometer to measure blood pressure.

spirit—The force within a person that is believed to give the body life, energy, and power.

static stretching—A series of movements that involve holding stretches for a certain period to gradually increase muscle flexibility.

steady state—The maintenance of a relatively constant physiological state during exercise, analogous to homeostasis at rest.

strength and conditioning coach—An exercise professional who uses individualized exercise prescriptions to improve the performance of competitive athletes or athletic teams.

stroke volume (SV)—The volume of blood the heart pumps per beat.

steroid hormones—Hormones, including testosterone and cortisol, that are synthesized from cholesterol and are involved in the body's stress response and muscle building.

strategy—A plan of action based on a scientific principle.

SWOT analysis—A strategic planning tool that systematically evaluates strengths, weaknesses, opportunities, and threats and can aid in professional development for certified exercise professionals.

sympathetic nervous system—A network of nerves that helps the body activate the fight-or-flight response; its activity increases when an individual experiences stress, is in danger, or is physically active.

tai chi—A Chinese martial art and system of calisthenics consisting of sequences of very slow, controlled movements.

talk test—Assessment of ventilatory demands during exercise, based on an individual's ability to engage in conversation or counting.

technique—An exercise or movement selected to address a specific program strategy.

tempo—The speed or pace of a given composition; also known as beats per minute.

tidal volume—Amount of air moved in and out of the lungs per breath.

timed up and go (TUG) test—A test to determine functional mobility; individuals are at risk of falls if it takes them over 10 seconds to complete it.

transtheoretical model—A structured, multidimensional model that helps individuals progress through various stages when adopting and sustaining health-promoting behaviors; also referred to as the stages of change.

trauma—A deeply distressing experience resulting from exposure to an incident or series of events that is emotionally disturbing or life-threatening and has lasting adverse effects on functioning and mental, physical, social, emotional, or spiritual well-being.

uncoupling protein 1 (UCP1)—A protein found in the mitochondria of brown fat that is involved in generating heat by uncoupling respiration from adenosine triphosphate (ATP) synthesis.

undulating periodization—A nonlinear programming method in which volume and intensity increase and decrease, either weekly or daily, within the training period.

unique selling proposition (USP)—The difference between an individual's or business's product or service and that of their competition; the thing that makes a product or service different.

$\dot{V}O_2$**max**—The maximum rate of oxygen consumption measured during incremental exercise; a higher $\dot{V}O_2$max indicates better cardiovascular fitness.

waist-to-hip ratio (WHR)—A measurement that assesses the relationship between a person's waist and hip circumferences, indicating fat distribution and identifying the type of obesity.

warm-up—An essential preparatory phase that precedes the main exercise session to gradually increase body temperature, heart rate, blood flow, and muscle flexibility.

weight-related biases—Negative attitudes, beliefs, judgments, or stereotypes based on a person's body weight; can be thought of as an act of discrimination based on body weight and may impact a person with excess adiposity from seeking medical and health-related care.

wellness—Striving for health while also integrating one's perceptions of physical and mental health with the environment.

yoga—A group of physical, mental, and spiritual practices or disciplines that originated in ancient India and aim to control and still the mind.

Index

About the Editor

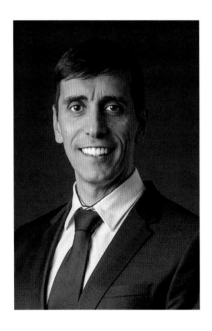

Alexios Batrakoulis, PhD, CSCS,*D, ACSM-EP, FACSM, has been involved in the health and fitness industry since 1995. He currently works as a personal trainer, exercise physiologist, fitness educator, speaker, author, subject matter expert, and adjunct professor and is based in Greece. He holds a bachelor's degree in physical education and sport science, a master's degree in exercise and health, a doctorate in clinical exercise physiology, and numerous certifications through the American Council on Exercise (ACE), American College of Sports Medicine (ACSM), National Academy of Sports Medicine (NASM), and National Strength and Conditioning Association (NSCA). His primary research interest is the study of hybrid-type, multicomponent interval training in obesity. He has authored over 100 international peer-reviewed publications on exercise, including research articles, textbook chapters, and translated books.

He has won multiple awards for his fitness expertise: He received global recognition as a 2017 IDEA Personal Trainer of the Year finalist, the 2018 IDEA Personal Trainer of the Year, the 2019 IDEA China Fitness Innovator, the 2020 NSCA Personal Trainer of the Year, a 2020 MedFit Professional of the Year finalist, the 2021 PFP Trainer of the Year, a 2021 ACSM Certified Professional of the Year finalist, and the 2022 ACSM Certified Professional of the Year.

He has been a member of EuropeActive's Professional Standards Committee, leading the technical experts group that developed educational standards for the occupational role of Weight Management Exercise Specialist. He has served on several committees for ACSM and NSCA, is an ACSM fellow, and is a member of the NSCA board of directors. Lastly, he is the founder of the International Obesity Exercise Training Institute (IOETI), teaching internationally approved continuing education courses in 45 countries across five continents and empowering over 3,000 fitness professionals since 2017.

Contributors

Anoop Balachandran, PhD

Rodiel Kirby Baloy, DPT

Amy Bantham, PhD

John Bauer

Alison C. Berg, PhD

Vula Bolou

Lee Boyce

Ryan Carver, BS

Christine M. Conti, MEd

Stephanie Cooper, PhD

Landon Deru, PhD

Grace DeSimone, BA

Daniel Green, BA

Farel B. Hruska

John M. Jakicic, PhD

Brett Klika, BS

Lauren Korzan, MA

Sara Kovacs, PhD

Elizabeth Kovar, MA

Meir Magal, PhD

Michael R. Mantell, PhD

Tracy L. Markley

Jonathan Mike, PhD

Erin Nitschke, PhD

Tony Nuñez, PhD

Mark A. Nutting

Cherie O'Neill (Kroh), EdD

Michael Piercy, MS

Rachele Pojednic, PhD

Rachelle Acitelli Reed, PhD

Susie Reiner, PhD

Brian Richey, BS

Deborah Riebe, PhD

Keli Roberts

Renee Rogers, PhD

Jonathan Ross

Melody Schoenfeld, MS

Lauren Shroyer, MS

Summer Sides

Michael Stack, BS

Leslie A. Stenger, EdD

Kathleen S. Thomas, PhD

Louise Valentine, MPH

Christie L. Ward-Ritacco, PhD

Kia Williams, MS

Maurice Williams, MS

Mary Yoke, PhD

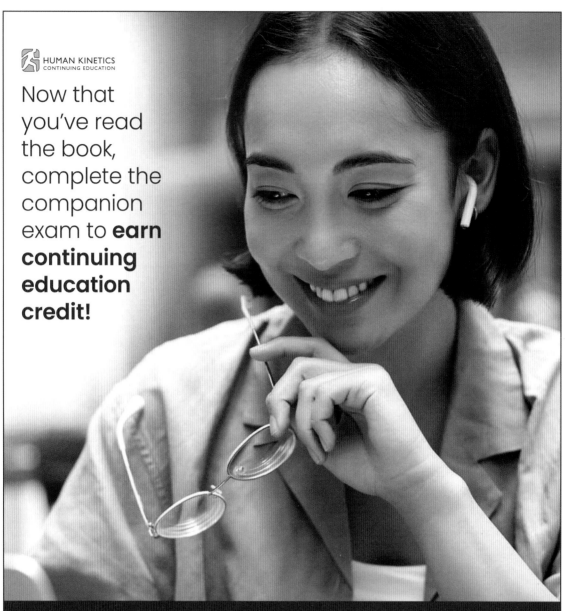
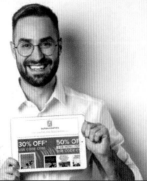